Fundamentals of Evolutionary Biology

Evolution is a stochastic process, and given the amount of data generated in biological sciences today, there is a pressing need for people with a quantitative background to understand and contribute toward the understanding of evolution, leading to better interaction between stakeholders. This book equips engineers and physical scientists to make biologically relevant quantitative representations of evolutionary processes. The concepts of evolution are introduced via semi-quantitative treatment with graphical illustrations and explain how evolution experiments are conducted in a laboratory.

Features:

- Discusses background, concepts of evolutionary biology, and experimental evolution.
- Helps readers develop a geometric view of evolutionary processes.
- Covers both biological and mathematical foundations in equal measure.
- Illustrates coding exercises supported by pertinent MATLAB codes for the provided problems.
- Includes homework problems and a solutions manual.

This book is aimed at senior undergraduate and graduate students in engineering and physical sciences.

Fundamentals of Evolutionary Biology

An Introductory Guide for Physical Scientists, Engineers, and Biologists

Supreet Saini

CRC Press
Taylor & Francis Group
Boca Raton London New York

CRC Press is an imprint of the
Taylor & Francis Group, an **informa** business

Designed cover image: © Supreet Saini

First edition published 2026
by CRC Press
2385 NW Executive Center Drive, Suite 320, Boca Raton FL 33431

and by CRC Press
4 Park Square, Milton Park, Abingdon, Oxon, OX14 4RN

CRC Press is an imprint of Taylor & Francis Group, LLC

ISBN: 978-1-032-98436-0 (hbk)
ISBN: 978-1-041-06083-3 (pbk)
ISBN: 978-1-003-63366-2 (ebk)

DOI: 10.1201/9781003633662

Typeset in Times
by SPi Technologies India Pvt Ltd (Straive)

Contents

About the Author

Supreet Saini is a Professor of Chemical Engineering and Fellow of DBT/Wellcome Trust (India Alliance) at the Indian Institute of Technology Bombay, Mumbai, India. He studied Chemical Engineering at undergraduate level at Indian Institute of Technology Delhi, India. He obtained his Ph.D. from the University of Illinois, Urbana-Champaign, US. His Ph.D. thesis focused on using systems biology approaches to understand *Salmonella* pathogenesis. His research group works, using experiments with yeast and bacteria and theory, to answer open questions in evolutionary biology.

Preface

At its core, evolution is a stochastic, yet logical process. It is based on and follows principles that, once understood, reveal a coherent and elegant framework that governs the living world. The mechanisms of evolution – natural selection, genetic drift, mutation, and gene flow – operate through well-defined rules, making the study of evolution as rigorous as any other scientific discipline. This book is structured to help the reader appreciate the logical underpinnings of evolutionary biology.

To truly grasp evolutionary principles, a graphical intuition is extremely valuable. Evolutionary processes unfold over time and space, and visualizing these changes is key to developing a deep understanding. Throughout this book, graphical representations accompany biological details, reinforcing both conceptual and empirical insights. This interplay between visualization and biological complexity helps clarify concepts but also builds intuition.

The structure of this book reflects the way evolutionary biology, in my opinion, is best understood. It begins by describing what is natural selection and how it was discovered. Science is also stories, and one about the discovery of theory of natural selection by Charles Darwin, Alfred Wallace, and Patrick Matthew is particularly fascinating (Chapter 1).

While a deep understanding of biological detail is not necessary to grasp evolutionary biology – after all, many foundational ideas in the field were developed before the structure of DNA was even known – modern molecular insights have greatly enriched our perspective. To appreciate these advances, it is essential to learn the Central Dogma of molecular biology. Understanding how genetic information flows from DNA to RNA to protein allows us to connect molecular mechanisms to broader evolutionary processes. We discuss this in Chapter 2. This is all the biology that one needs for this book, and hence, after reading this chapter, readers with a background in physical science and engineering will find this book completely accessible.

Evolutionary biology, when studied in the context of prokaryotes versus eukaryotes, presents two very different perspectives. The tools, analytical approaches, and experimental techniques used to study microbial evolution differ vastly from those applied to sexually reproducing organisms. Because of this, early on in our exploration of evolutionary biology, we must decide whether we are examining evolution through the lens of prokaryotic organisms or eukaryotes. This distinction shapes how we interpret evolutionary processes and patterns. We make this call in Chapter 3.

In the next section of the book, the core, we lay out the fundamental concepts of evolutionary biology (Chapters 4–11), which form the unifying principles of the field. Biological details can be intricate – even overwhelming at times – but the underlying concepts remain standard and essential. By focusing first on these core ideas, we establish a solid foundation upon which all further details can be built. These foundational chapters will be accessible to biologists with no formal training in mathematics. The ideas discussed here are concepts and are discussed from a geometric perspective. We discuss these concepts through very simple examples, and try and develop an intuition for the subject.

Once the conceptual groundwork is in place, the book moves into experimental detail (Chapters 12–16). This progression ensures that experimental evidence is interpreted within a robust theoretical framework rather than as an isolated collection of observations. By maintaining this approach, the reader is encouraged to think critically about data and its implications within the broader context of evolutionary theory.

To enhance engagement and deepen comprehension, this book includes sections titled 'Before Moving Ahead'. These are designed as interludes, inviting the reader to pause and consider specific problems or issues before proceeding. These exercises are meant to sharpen biological intuition, fostering an active learning experience. I strongly encourage readers to take these sections seriously, as they provide valuable moments for reflection and insight.

Additionally, the exercises in this book often take an open-ended approach, inviting readers to explore evolutionary concepts beyond the confines of rigid answers. Some problems may require the use of computational tools and coding, but these should not be seen as barriers. Instead, I encourage readers to embrace these aspects as opportunities to engage with the subject in a hands-on and interactive manner. Evolutionary biology is a field rich with quantitative and computational applications, and gaining experience with these tools will only enhance one's understanding of the subject.

This book is meant to serve as an entry point into the vast and fascinating world of evolutionary biology. While it provides a structured path through key concepts and experimental approaches, it is important to recognize that we are only scratching the surface.

I hope that readers approach this book with curiosity, patience, and a willingness to engage deeply with the material. Evolution is not just a subject to be studied; it is a lens through which we can understand the very nature of life itself.

Acknowledgments

My journey into studying evolution started when, in 2014, I started attending Population Genetics and Evolution Schools at International Centre for Theoretical Sciences (ICTS), Bengaluru. These schools have been organized by Dr. Deepa Agashe (National Centre for Biological Sciences, NCBS) and Dr. Kavita Jain (Jawaharlal Nehru Centre for Advanced Scientific Research, JNCASR), who graciously accommodated me in every iteration of the schoolsince then. For that, I am very thankful to Deepa, Kavita, and ICTS.

Back at IIT Bombay, much of what I learned in evolution was a collaborative effort with a colleague, Dr. P. Jayadeva Bhat. From 2015 to 2020, we both learned from and taught each other evolution. We floundered around, chased dark alleys, but were patient with each other and learning the subject. For his time, enthusiasm, and patience, I am thankful to Jayadeva Bhat.

Thanks to Sarvesh Baheti, an undergraduate student at IIT Jodhpur and an intern in my lab for the past two years, for making the landscape figures used in this book. Thanks to Neetika Ahlawat, a post-doctoral researcher in my group, for taking the pictures of flasks and plates that are used in the book.

Thanks to Pavithra Venkataraman, a former Ph.D. student in my group, for discussions regarding many trivial and non-trivial issues about structuring the book.

I am grateful to all present and past members of my group – for learning the subject with me. Finally, I am grateful to my peers in this field, whose work, and efforts to uncover evolution have greatly inspired me.

1 The Theory of Evolution by Natural Selection

1.1 INTRODUCTION

Making sense of all life on Earth is a challenging task! There are tens of millions of species on the planet. How we make sense of all this biodiversity? Is there a unifying principle with which life forms evolve and diversify? What is this principle and how does it operate?

The 20th-century geneticist and evolutionary biologist Theodosius Dobzhansky remarked, *nothing in biology makes sense except in the light of evolution*. Why did Dobzhansky say this, and why is this statement quoted by scientists so often?

Dobzhansky is trying to say that evolution is the common framework and principle which can explain the diversity of life forms. Evolution via natural selection is the one common principle which guides all biological change and the resulting organization of life forms. Hence, *nothing in biology makes sense except in the light of evolution*.

Questions regarding evolution of life have intrigued people since the time of Greek philosophers. It was commonly thought that species are unchanging, fixed entities. How life arose on the planet was something philosophers wondered about for a long time before Darwin. However, mere ponderings about how life evolved were unlikely to make serious progress toward answering the question. The formal development of the idea of organic evolution needed Darwin.

The development of a framework in which we can best understand the process of organismal evolution started in earnest with Darwin's publication of the *Origin of Species* in 1859. The idea of species being mutable had been proposed prior to Darwin too, but the idea was never laid out in such careful detail and with inexhaustible evidence from natural and artificial settings.

The publication of the *Origin* also laid out issues and shortcomings in the theory. In this chapter, we briefly discuss the ideas of evolution prevailing prior to Darwin's publication, and then move to Charles Darwin's proposal of the theory of natural selection as a means of evolution, and then develop the scientific ramifications of this proposal.

We started this chapter by saying that there are millions of species. Remember that we do not even know about most of the species that exist on the planet. So, how do we study life forms when we do not even know them fully? One answer to that is that instead of studying each species separately, we rely on classification of living species into groups which make sense. The grouping should reflect some property or hierarchy of living beings which reflects an order that exists in life forms. What is this order? This is a question which has occupied biologists for a long time.

DOI: 10.1201/9781003633662-1

Organisms could be classified based on their morphology, cellularity (single/multicellular), biochemistry, habitat, etc. However, which classifications are going to provide us with information that is critical to understanding how life arose and evolved? What are the criteria we must use which reflect an underlying common biological theme of life, and explain continuity of life from its most primitive forms to today? These are not trivial questions!

While attempts to classify living beings started centuries ago, Carl Linnaeus (1625–1705) is credited with developing a first comprehensive classification system. In one sense, the naturalists of Linneaus' time were working on problems which needed modern late 20th-century tools. After hundreds of years of classification of organisms based on a multitude of features (morphology, where they live, what they eat, etc.), it was in the late 20th century that classification was fundamentally and forever changed by sequencing technology.

Using very primitive and tireless techniques, Carl Woese at the University of Illinois, Urbana-Champaign, US, figured out that the tree of life contained three major groups (archaea, bacteria, and eukaryotes), and not two (bacteria and eukaryotes), as previously thought. This was a major departure from what we thought was an apt arrangement of life on Earth. The key idea is that sequencing technology (however primitive) was needed before classification of life into three domains could be proposed.

The first person to refute the concept of species as a fixative entity was Jean Baptiste de Lamarck. Lamarck first introduced the idea of species as evolving entities in 1802, in which he claimed life arose 'directly' (or spontaneously) from non-living matter. Over extremely long time (Lamarck proposed, 'thousands to millions of centuries'), these forms, when acted upon the surrounding environment, moved toward greater complexity and generated the life forms that we today see around us today. In his 1809 book, *Philosophie zoologique*, Lamarck formalized his argument through proposal of two laws,

First, in every animal that has not reached the end of its development, the more frequent and sustained use of any organ will strengthen this organ little by little, develop it, enlarge it, and give to it a power proportionate to the duration of its use, while the constant disuse of such an organ will weaken it, deteriorate it, progressively diminish its faculties, and finally cause it to disappear.

Second, Lamarck proposed that, depending on the environment an individual is exposed to, individuals gain or lose an organ or a part. This gain or loss is conserved through generations in the new individuals descending from them.

While Lamarck's idea did not stand the test of time, he was successful in generating an intellectual atmosphere where future ideas on evolution could arise and be debated. It is in this context that we will begin our study of evolution by discussing the story of how the theory of evolution by natural selection came into being, and the events that led to the publication of the *Origin of Species by Natural Selection* (*Origin*) by Charles Darwin in 1859.

1.2 ALFRED RUSSELL WALLACE AND HENRY BATES

Alfred Wallace and Henry Bates, in the years between 1848 and 1852, traveled to South America. Together, they collected samples of living entities and fossil remains of organisms they encountered, to be sent to collectors and museums in Europe. While Bates remained there for a long time, Wallace took a ship back to Europe in 1852.

The scientific question that the two were interested in was the following:

where do species come from?

Unfortunately, as Wallace's ship was returning to England, it caught fire. The fire destroyed all samples, specimens, and notes that Wallace was bringing back after four years of arduous work. He was himself injured in the accident, but eventually found support in a lifeboat. After being rescued from the sea by a ship passing by, Wallace finally made it back to Europe and took a vow to never go to sea again.

1.3 CHARLES DARWIN AND THE VOYAGE OF THE *BEAGLE*

Wallace and Bates did not know at the time that the question they had been pondering over had also been thought about by another naturalist in the UK – Charles Darwin. Darwin was born in 1809, and when he was 22, got an opportunity to travel around the world on the ship *HMS Beagle*. His mandate on the ship was to be the ship's Captain's (FitzRoy) dining mate, and to be the amateur naturalist on board. The *Beagle*'s mandate under FitzRoy was measurement of the coordinates of several landmasses on the American continent.

Darwin was seasick most of the journey. In fact, in a letter to his sister on 4 August 1836, he wrote, *I loathe, I abhor the sea, & all ships that sail on it.* But what happened on the ship was to change the history of human intellectual journey forever.

1.3.1 On the East Coast of South America

Beagle, during its journey, spent a considerable time on the East Coast of South America. During this time, while the ship made measurements of the latitudinal and longitudinal coordinates, Darwin would often venture inland to study and collect samples.

One of the first things that struck Darwin was that, at any given place, the fossils of the organisms present there bore a striking resemblance to the extant (currently existing) organisms in that region. From this, Darwin concluded that spread of living organisms was not random. In fact, organisms present in a geographical location were co-incident in structure with the nature and form of the fossils in that region.

What did this mean? Since divine creation was the then accepted explanation of how living beings came into existence, did God create a certain type of organisms and place them at a particular place on the planet?

Why should that be so?

1.3.2 On the Southern Tip of South America

As the *Beagle* waited for summer to cross over from the Atlantic to the Pacific, Darwin came in contact with tribes that had remained completely cut-off from the 'civilized' world that he came from. The 19th-century prevailing view was that humankind was the pinnacle of creation. However, looking at these tribes, Darwin questioned this assertion, and doubted the hierarchical view of life that holds prevalence in the minds of 19th-century elite.

1.3.3 Galapagos Islands

A few miles off the coast of Ecuador, in the northwest of South America, are 18 islands, collectively called the Galapagos Islands. In 1835, the *Beagle* stopped at these islands for five weeks to map their coordinates. The islands are barren, dry – and when Darwin first saw them, he commented that if hell had any gardens, this is what they would look like. The time at Galapagos proved to be a great time in leading Darwin to the idea that evolution proceeds via the process of natural selection.

While on the islands, Darwin collected samples of several organisms, among them finches. As the ship sailed away from the islands toward Tahiti, as Darwin studied the finches he had collected, he noticed a curious feature. He observed that each island's finches were unique, when compared to finches present on other islands. For example, islands with seeds as food source were occupied by finches with short, stout, and strong beaks. Whereas, islands where the primary food source was a flower's nectar, finches with long, slender beaks flourished, as it allowed them access to the food source deep in the flower.

It seemed as if the finches occupying a particular island were best suited to survive and reproduce in that island's particular environment. To Darwin, this was astonishing!

How did this change come about?

The main food at the Galapagos for the *Beagle*'s crew was tortoise meat. While at the islands, to Darwin's surprise, locals from the area could tell – just by looking at the design pattern on a tortoise's back – which island a particular tortoise had come from. It was curious to Darwin that tortoise from different islands had their unique, characteristic taste.

Why should this be so?

Note the three questions above. Imagine Darwin as he grapples with these questions. What must have been going through his mind? How does he answer them? Everything that he is noticing around him tells him that species are continuously changing, and specialize in the respective environments where they reside. How did such an arrangement of life come to be?

Before Moving Ahead,

➔ What do you think explains the three questions Darwin was posed with?

*(Throughout this book, we will frequently encounter this section called '***Before moving ahead***'. You should try and attempt to think about the questions posed in these sections. Often, they reflect open-ended inquiries. Sometimes, they may not have a right or wrong answer. But thinking hard about these questions will sharpen your biological intuition.)*

The experience with finches and tortoise, told Darwin, that there is some degree of specialization happening in organisms, and organisms best suited to survive in a particular environment thrive, while the others – less well suited – are eliminated by competition.

Darwin and the *Beagle* made way around the world (Australia to South Africa, a detour to South America, and finally back to England), and eventually returned to England in 1836. Darwin was a meticulous record keeper, and throughout his explorations, had been sending back samples and specimens of creatures from around the world. As a result, by the time he returned to England, Darwin was already a celebrated naturalist, not only in England but also in all of Europe.

Upon his return, Darwin published a record of his travels in a book titled, *The Journey of the Beagle*. Evolution or the idea of natural selection, is conspicuously absent from this book. However, soon after his return, Darwin started sketching a solution to what was considered the 'mystery of mysteries' – where do species come from?

Note that this is the same question that Bates and Wallace were working on, almost a decade later. Darwin started working on this question much earlier, but kept his thoughts to himself, in his private notes.

In 1842, Darwin wrote a short note (~30 pages) on how he thought organisms change with time, and how natural selection acts, leading to evolution. Darwin was notoriously sick for much of his adult life. While writing the 1842 note, he told his wife Emma that, should he not survive his illness, she should make sure that the note is made public. Within a few years, Darwin was able to expand the note to 200 pages. However, he did not publish his views on natural selection and mutability of living species till 1859 in the *Origin*. However, in this time, he did share his views on the subject with Charles Lyell (a geologist, whose texts had shaped Darwin's early views on evolution) and Joseph Hooker (a botanist, who helped Darwin with his research during the 1840s).

1.4 WALLACE GOES BACK TO SEA

After being rescued by a passing ship in the Atlantic, Wallace vowed to never go to sea. However, soon after his return, Wallace went to the *Malay* Archipelago, to collect samples for private benefactors and museums. During his travels between the different islands, Wallace studied patterns of variations in populations spread over different islands and reached similar conclusions as Darwin.

While Darwin arrived at the thought of natural selection from his observations on finches, Wallace did the same using his observations on butterflies. In addition, while there, Wallace noticed that there seems to be a line cutting through the islands, to the southeast of which, marsupials reside on islands and to the northwest of which apes reside (this line is now called 'Wallace Line').

Why did God draw up an imaginary line and place these animals at specific geographies?

Wallace began to theorize and wrote a research monograph on the subject. In 1858, Wallace wrote a summary of how evolution via natural selection works and sent it to Darwin for his comments. In the letter, Wallace writes,

> *The life of wild animals is a struggle for existence··· and to provide for an infant offspring.*
>
> *Perhaps all of variations must have some definite effect, however slight in the habits and capacities of the individuals··· a variety having slightly increased powers··· must inevitably in time acquire a superiority in numbers.*

Darwin, in the meantime, had been working on putting together his magnus opus, in which he aimed to propose the theory of evolution by natural selection. Darwin envisioned the book to be several thousand pages long, in which he would lay down all arguments and evidence in support of natural selection. However, before *Origin of Species* was complete, Darwin received a letter from Wallace. The similarity of the idea that the two men had can be gauged by a comparison between the above text from Wallace's letter and *Origin*'s chapter 5,

> *Chapter 5: The struggle for existence as bearing on natural selection*;
>
> *All nature is at war. The struggle very often falls on the egg and the seed, or on the seedling··· any variation, however infinitely slight, if it did promote during any part of life even in the slightest degree, the welfare of the being, such variation would tend to be preserved or selected.*

The words of Darwin and Wallace are remarkably close to each other's. Darwin shared Wallace's letter with Lyell and Hooker. The two men knew that Darwin was the first to have arrived at the idea of natural selection, and hence, proposed a compromise regarding who was to get credit for the discovery and proposal of the theory of natural selection.

The meeting of the Linnean Society was to be held in the summer of 1858, and Lyell and Hooker jointly wrote to the Society President, communicating independent papers by Darwin and Wallace on the idea of natural selection (see Note I). The two papers were accepted and read during the Society's meeting. Neither Darwin nor Wallace, however, attended the meeting. While Wallace was away in Asia, Darwin was mourning the death of a child.

Remarkably, in summarizing the 1858 meeting of the Linnean Society, the president noted that nothing of great importance was reported in that particular year's meeting!

Wallace's letter precipitated the publication of *Origin*. In 1859, Darwin published *The Origin of Species by Natural Selection*. Despite Darwin anticipating that the *Origin* was going to be several thousand pages, it ended up being around only 500 pages. He calls the book an 'abstract'. While approaching the publisher John Murray, Darwin expressed his hope that his book would not cost the publisher money. All 1,250 copies of the *Origin* were sold on the day it appeared for sale.

1.5 BATESIAN MIMICRY

The scientific response to the *Origin of Species* was surprisingly accepting. There were no major challenges regarding the fact that evolution takes place, and that species are indeed mutable.

Upon reading the *Origin*, Henry Bates (Wallace's companion in South America) reported an observation. Bates had found that predators of butterflies, just by looking at the wing pattern and color, could tell which butterflies were poisonous and hence, not to be eaten. As a result, they focused their predatory efforts on catching non-poisonous butterflies.

In such a scenario, variations in the wing color and pattern among the non-poisonous butterflies, which made them appear like the poisonous butterflies, were helpful – since these variations meant that the butterfly would not be predated upon. Hence, the number of non-poisonous butterflies carrying wing patterns and colors similar to their poisonous counterparts grew. This was direct demonstration of natural selection in action, and is popularly called Batesian mimicry.

1.6 PATRICK MATHEW – SOLVER OF THE *ORIGIN OF SPECIES* PROBLEM

The March 1860 edition of the magazine *Gardner's Chronicle and Agricultural Gazette* carried a review of the *Origin*. Darwin had long subscribed to the magazine, being interested in breeding experiments with plants and animals. This review was read by a Scotsman, Patrick Mathew.

Mathew had inherited land, on which he aspired to grow the best timber so that Britain could maintain its naval supremacy, critical in Mathew's mind to maintain her global dominance. Toward this, in 1832, he published a book titled *On Naval Timber and Arboriculture*. Upon reading the March 1860 review of the *Origin of Species*, Mathew wrote a letter to the editor of *Gardner's Chronicle and Agricultural Gazette* in which he made a remarkable claim that the theory of natural selection was first proposed by him in his 1832 book.

Darwin, upon reading Mathew's letter, read Mathew's book and responded to Mathew's letter by acknowledging that Mathew indeed had arrived at the theory of natural selection prior to Darwin. In the letter, Darwin mentions that should there be subsequent editions of the *Origin*, he will acknowledge Mathew's contribution. Hence, in the third edition of the *Origin* onward, Darwin credits Mathew with having proposed the theory of natural selection prior to Darwin.

Mathew cut a frustrated figure at not having received public credit for the proposal of the theory of natural selection. History has also not been kind to Mathew, and his name has largely been ignored from the list of people who contributed toward the proposal of the theory of natural selection. See Note II for the correspondence between Mathew and Darwin, via the *Gardner's Chronicle*.

1.7 ELEMENTS OF THE THEORY OF NATURAL SELECTION

Darwin and Wallace's arrival at the idea of natural selection was influenced by an 1798 essay by the economist Thomas Malthus. In his publication on growth of human population, Malthus argues that human population grows exponentially (Figure 1.1). On the other hand, the agricultural produce increases linearly, as more and more land is brought under cultivation. In such a scenario, there will eventually be a time when demand for food outgrows the supply. This mismatch will then trigger off a competition for resources among the members of the population. In this competition, only those most suited to obtain food will survive, while the others will perish. These ideas crystallized, in Darwin's and Wallace's minds, the essential elements of the theory of natural selection.

We have come a long way since Darwin's time. And through this book, aim to understand evolution in its contemporary context. Thus, before moving ahead, we will familiarize ourselves with two terms.

a. *Phenotype*. A phenotype of an individual is a physical manifestation of certain part of his/her physiology. For example, height is a phenotype. So is eye color, or length of finger. Size of a bacterium is also a phenotype and so is the number of fingers on my hand.
b. *Genotype*. The phenotype is dictated by the underlying DNA sequence of an individual. This sequence is referred to as the genotype of the individual. All traits listed above have a genetic component (i.e., a particular gene sequence confers a particular eye color).

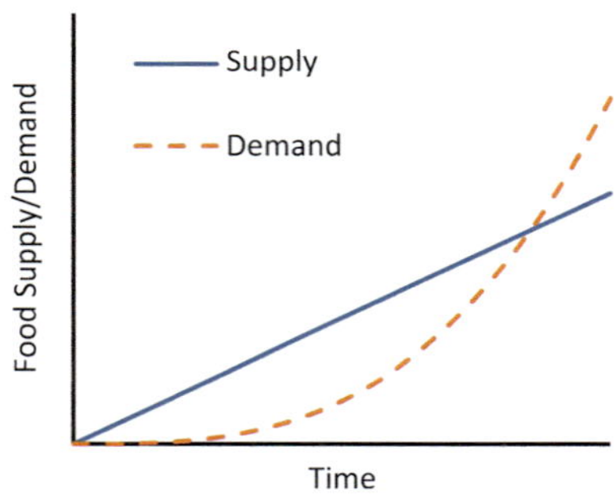

FIGURE 1.1 Malthus was concerned with the growth of human populations. According to him, as more and more land is brought under agriculture, food production (supply) increases linearly with time (blue, solid line). However, population growth is exponential (demand), shown as red dashed curve. Because exponential curve increases faster than a linear curve, there will come a point when the demand for food exceeds the supply (where the two curves meet). Beyond this point, the food supply is insufficient for the population size. As a result, competition sets in for food, where only those that are fit will get food. This idea of competition and fitness influenced both Darwin and Wallace, leading to their proposals of the theory of natural selection being responsible for evolutionary change.

1.8 THREE COMPONENTS OF NATURAL SELECTION

The idea of the theory of natural selection rests on satisfying the following three criteria. If these criteria are satisfied, evolution via natural selection follows quite logically. In this section, we will discuss these three criteria of the theory of natural selection.

1. Variation exists between members of a population with respect to a certain trait (phenotype). A trait is any manifestation of an organism's being (height, for instance).
2. The variation leads to differential reproductive success of members of the population, and
3. The variation is heritable (i.e., variation [or at least a part of it] has a genotypic basis).

Let us consider natural selection in action via the above three steps using an example from 19th-century United Kingdom.

(1) *Variation* – a population contains individuals which exhibit variations in a trait.

A population of moths exists where individuals have either light- or dark-colored wings. This satisfies the first condition for evolution by natural selection – i.e., variation exists in the population. The trait or phenotype of interest here is the color of the moth's wings.

(2) *Differential Reproductive Success* – trait value is linked with reproductive success.

Since prior to Industrial Revolution, there was little or no pollution in the English countryside, the colors of tree trunks were light. As a result, the light-colored moths camouflaged with the tree background. The camouflage hid the light-colored moths from predators. The dark-colored moths, on the other hand, stood out and were easily predated upon. Early predation led to lesser number of offsprings by the dark-colored moths, as compared to the lighter-colored moths. Thus, the trait in question is linked with differential reproductive success (light-colored moths have more offsprings than dark-colored moths). This satisfies the second criteria of the requirement for natural selection to be in action.

(3) *The trait under question is heritable* – the trait is genetically determined.

The color of a moth's wings is a genetic trait. That is, a dark-colored moth gives birth to an offspring with dark-colored wings. Similarly, a light-colored moth gives birth to a light-colored offspring.

Thus, our example satisfied all three criteria listed above. Let us now see how natural selection will act in this scenario. If we start with an equal number of light- and dark-colored moths, gradually the light-colored moths will become much greater in number as compared to the dark-colored moths.

Interestingly, as Industrial Revolution spread, the pollution from industries settled as soot on tree trunks, thus darkening them. As the tree trunks darkened, it was the dark-colored moths which were camouflaged better. On the other hand, light-colored moths now stood out against the dark tree trunk background. As a result, the light-colored moths were more easily predated upon, and hence, as time progressed, their numbers decreased in the population, while those of the dark-colored moths increased.

This is natural selection in action!

1.9 FITNESS

In evolutionary biology parlance, we will say that prior to Industrial Revolution, the light moths were more fit (or fitter) than the dark-colored moths. After Industrial Revolution, the light-colored moths were less fit than the dark-colored moths. The term *fitness* is of exceptional importance in study of evolution (and as we will see, very difficult to define in an ecological context), and we will keep revisiting it throughout this book.

We can think about fitness in the following way. Every individual, through his or her children, passes on their genes to the next generation. The more offsprings a certain individual has, the greater the representation of his/her genes in the next generation. Thus, for sexually reproducing organisms, fitness can be simply quantified as the number of offsprings an individual has. If I, as an individual, have no children, then I have a fitness of zero.

Having said that, I can still influence evolution – for instance, by providing for well-being of offsprings in my family, geographical area, sect, religion, society, etc. In this context, fitness can be viewed in a number of alternate ways. These ideas, where fitness lies outside of an individual, are commonly referred to as 'group' or 'kin' selection.

For now, we can simply define fitness of an individual as the following,

$$\text{Fitness, } f = \text{Number of offsprings} \tag{1.1}$$

For the most part, in this book, we will discuss evolution in microbial systems. We will discuss why we do this in the next chapter. There is a fundamental difference between populations of complex species (such as moths) and bacteria, and how fitness is differently understood in these two populations.

Unlike complex, sexually reproducing species, bacteria reproduce asexually. One bacterium divides, giving rise to two daughter cells. That is, reproduction is uniparental. For such an organism, we have to think of fitness alternatively. Fitness for bacteria is thus inversely proportional to the time it takes to divide. We can, thus, quantify this idea with the following simple equation,

$$\text{Fitness, } f = \frac{1}{\text{time of division}} \tag{1.2}$$

In my laboratory, I have strains of the common bacterium *Escherichia coli*, which can divide in 30 minutes, when grown in lab conditions. I have also isolated *Escherichia coli* strains from a nearby lake. The strain from the lake takes 50 minutes to divide in lab conditions. Hence, as far as the lab environment is concerned, the lab strain of *Escherichia coli* is 'fitter' than the lake strain.

On the other hand, in the lake environment (where nutrients are scarce), the lake strain divides in 3 hours, whereas the lab strain divides in 5 hours. Thus, in the lake environment, the lake strains are 'fitter' as compared to the lab strain.

Organisms are well adapted to the environments where they have had the time to evolve and adapt.

This brings us to another key point about fitness. Fitness is not a function of the organism alone. It is a combined function of the organism and the environment. For example, in the pre-Industrial Revolution environment, the fitness of dark-colored moths was lesser than that of the light-colored moths, while in the post-Industrial Revolution environment, the fitness of light-colored moths was lesser than that of the dark-colored moths. Thus, it is the combined interaction of the environment and the individual, which decides the relative fitness of the different individuals in the environment.

Thus, the idea of the theory of natural selection is intuitive and simple – individuals which 'fit' better in a particular environment (or, individuals which have a higher 'fitness' compared to others) because of a phenotype **A** will leave more offsprings as compared to the less fit individuals, which have phenotype **B**. As a result, over generations, the relative frequency of the individuals with phenotype **A** increases, while that of individuals with phenotype **B** decreases.

Before we move forward – note that – in a biological sense, individuals do not evolve. Species evolve through generations. Some evolutionary changes can take tens of thousands of generations, while others can happen relatively rapidly.

Before we move ahead, we will make one more point about selection. In the context of bacteria, we have defined fitness such that fast-dividing bacteria are fitter and slower-dividing bacteria are less fit. This is not always true. For instance, if the environment contains antibiotics, it is known that rapidly dividing bacteria are more susceptible to being killed by the antibiotic, as compared to cells which are metabolically inactive. In such a scenario, the slower you grow, the higher your fitness. Such contexts exist in biology. Hence, the idea of fitness is complex and very context-dependent. But, here, at least to start with, we equate growth rate with fitness.

1.10 TYPES OF SELECTION

In a population, when a trait (or phenotype) is linked with differential reproductive success, it is said that selection is acting on the population. Under the action of selection, phenotypes with a greater reproductive success reproduce more, as compared to those with lower fitness. This can manifest in a few ways, and in this section, we will study these cases.

1.10.1 Directional Selection

Imagine a population which exhibits a certain trait around a mean value. This distribution is as shown in Figure 1.2. Let the trait be height in a population. Let us also imagine that the reproductive success of an organism is closely linked to the height of the individual. That is, taller individuals leave behind more offsprings than

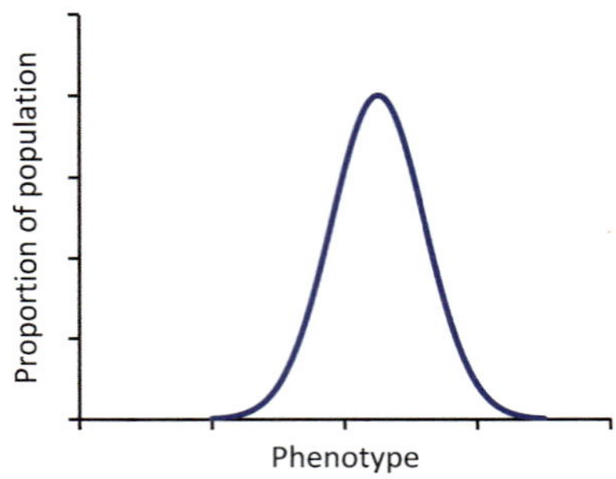

FIGURE 1.2 Distribution of height in a population. We will encounter plots like this often. The x-axis is height, and the y-axis is the percentage of the population with that height. As can be seen, there is a small percentage of the population which is short (toward the left) and a small percentage of population which is tall (toward the right). A large fraction of the population has intermediate height. Note that the y-axis represents the proportion of the population. Hence, the sum total of the y-axis (or the area under the curve) should equal one (or 100% of the population). Such distributions are called *probability density functions* (pdf).

the shorter ones. In such a scenario, what do we expect the distribution of height will look like in a few generations?

Before moving forward,

➔ Try and sketch the graph above and predict what the height distribution looks like in future time, if taller individuals leave behind twice as many offsprings and in this population, is determined genetically (all other factors, such as diet, hygiene) being constant.

As you can imagine that the population will shift toward greater height, and the distribution of the height will move toward the right. Such a change, where the population moves in a particular direction with respect to the trait, is referred to as *directional selection* (Figure 1.3).

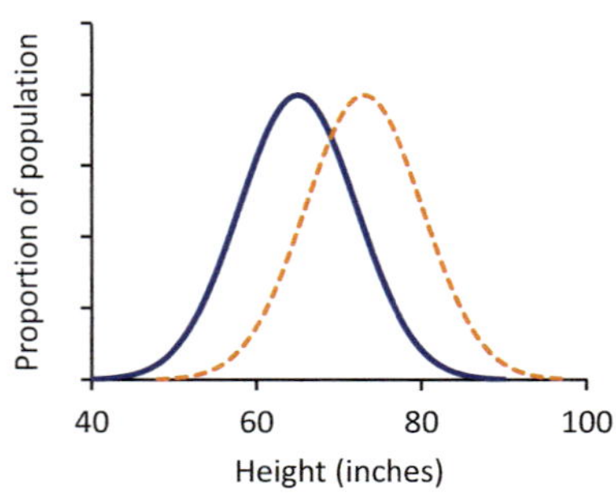

FIGURE 1.3 Under directional selection, the population moves toward the right. In each generation, the individuals toward the right of the distribution (taller) produce more offsprings compared to those to the left of the distribution (shorter). As a result, the frequency distribution of height in the population moves toward the right from the solid blue line to the dotted red.

1.10.2 Divergent Selection

Imagine a bird population in an environmental niche which has two resources, seeds and flowers. In such a setting, birds need short beaks to utilize seeds as food and need long slender beaks to use flowers as food. It can be seen here that birds with short strong beaks will not be able to reach into flowers, and those with long, slender beaks will not be able to use seeds as food.

In such a context, let us say the starting bird population has an intermediate beak size. Over the time of a few generations, this population will split into two groups of birds. One, with small, strong beaks, and the other with long, slender beaks. This starts with a unimodal distribution of beak size, the population splits into two disjointed groups (Figure 1.4).

This split happens because the environment placed divergent selection on the bird population – for short and long beaks. The population responded to this pressure and split into two groups. Thus, when environment acts to select *both* extreme phenotypes, starting from an intermediate phenotype – the population is said to be under divergent selection.

1.10.3 Purifying Selection

Consider a well-adapted population. This population has a phenotype which is optimal for the environment that it occupies. As a result, not all variations in the phenotype are desirable. Thus, selection can act to maintain the current values of the trait in the population. Any departures from the existing trait value have smaller fitness values, and as a result are weeded out from the population via the action of selection. Such action of selection is referred to as *purifying selection* (Figure 1.5).

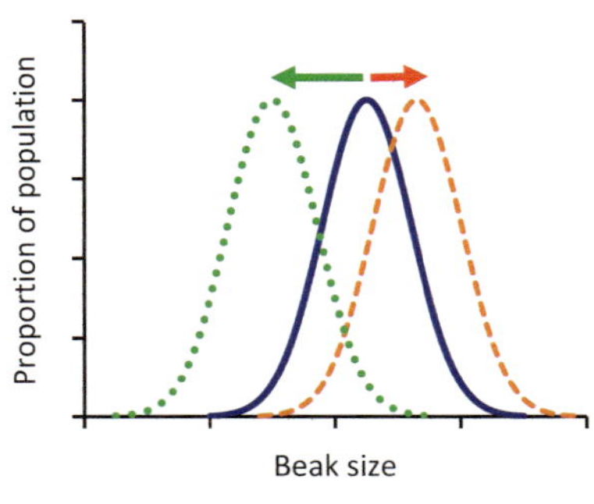

FIGURE 1.4 Under divergent selection, the population with an intermediate phenotype, splits into two groups – one with low value of the phenotype, and the other with large. A bird population starting with intermediate beak size (solid blue line) grows in an environment with two resources (seeds and flowers). Utilization of seeds requires short, strong beaks, and using flowers needs long, slender beaks. Selection thus acts so that fitness of the two extreme beak sizes is higher than the intermediate. A unimodal population thus splits into two under the action of divergent selection. Birds with smaller beak size (green dots) feed on seeds, and those with long beaks (orange dash) feed on flowers.

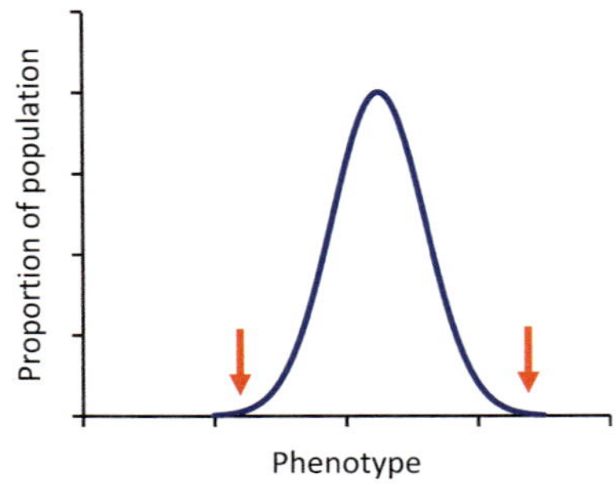

FIGURE 1.5 In purifying selection, departures from the current phenotype are rejected. The current phenotype provides a high fitness. Variants with different phenotype values have lower fitness, and are rejected by natural selection. This is shown by the red arrows. When individuals with these phenotypes arise, they are weeded out by natural selection. Hence, their frequency does not increase, and the frequency distribution of the phenotype does not change from its current distribution.

So, to summarize, evolution by natural selection takes place when,

a. Phenotypic variation exists in a population with respect to a particular trait,
b. The variation in the trait is linked with differential reproductive success, and
c. The trait is genetically dictated.

Example 1.1: Imagine a bacterial population which is susceptible to an antibiotic. When growing in an environment where there is no antibiotic, each cell divides once every hour. However, when the antibiotic is introduced into the media, the cells stop dividing. What can we say about selection in this environment?

Solution: Note that in this case, all cells in the starting population are identical. Thus, no phenotypic variation exists. As a result, all cells are susceptible to the antibiotic. Hence, when the antibiotic is introduced in the environment, fitness (which is given by growth rate) reduces to zero. Thus, in this case, selection acted to lead to extinction of the bacterial population.

Example 1.2: In the example of directional selection we saw above, taller individuals exhibited a greater fitness. What happens in the case if reproductive success is independent of height?

Solution: In such a scenario, taller/shorter/intermediate height individuals will all have the same number of offsprings. As a result, the frequency distribution of height in the population does not change from one generation to another. Hence, no evolutionary change takes place in the population.

We can also understand this from another context. In this example, phenotypic variation exists in a population and this phenotype (height) is dictated (at least partially) by the genotype. However, the example states that the trait value does not dictate reproductive success. As a result, the three tenets are not satisfied, and as a result, evolution by natural selection cannot take place with respect to height in the population.

1.11 LIMITATIONS OF DARWIN'S PROPOSAL

In *Origin of Species*, Darwin highlights several missing links from his proposal that natural selection is the agent which drives evolutionary change. We will discuss four such issues here.

Before we discuss the limitations of Darwin's proposal, it is important to take a pause here and be stunned at the intellectual leap that his work proposed. Remember that Darwin's conclusions were drawn from 'merely' observing and thinking about natural processes. As we have seen, Darwin's thoughts were crystallized soon after the completion of the *Beagle*'s journey. To admire how ahead of his time Darwin's proposal was, note that the structure of DNA was discovered in 1953 – more than a century after Darwin arrived at the idea of natural selection.

1.11.1 How Does Variation Maintain Itself?

As we have seen, for natural selection to act, there needs to be variation in a population. From among the variants, the less fit will be eliminated, and the more fit will increase in numbers. This process would, in turn, reduce the variability in the population. Hence, variation is a fuel that drives natural selection, but in the process, consumes itself. Thus, continuous action of natural selection would mean that the variation in the population would be eliminated. However, Darwin knew from observation that the amount of variation present in a population remains more or less constant, as we go from one generation to another. Hence, in the face of natural selection eliminating variation, how is variation maintained in a population?

1.11.2 Blending Inheritance

Darwin faced another conundrum while trying to explain how variation is maintained in a population. This conundrum was called blending inheritance and its impact on the amount of variation present in a population.

To understand Darwin's conundrum, imagine a human population. We measure each person's height and then ask, what percentage of the population has a height between 60 and 61 inches; what percentage of the population has a height between 61 and 62 inches? And so on and so forth. When we plot this data, the resulting graph would look something like as shown in Figure 1.6. Such graphs are called frequency distributions, and are going to be extremely useful (and frequently visited) as we move forward in this book.

As we can see, most of the population has a height between 64 and 65 inches. However, a small percentage of the population is either very tall (extreme right of the distribution) or very short (extreme left of the distribution). We also know from experience that this variation persists as we move from one generation to another. Thus, variation is preserved between generations (Figure 1.6).

However, we also know that if one parent is tall and the other short – their offspring invariably grows up to intermediate height. This phenomenon is called 'blending inheritance', where the trait value of the offspring is a blend of the two parents.

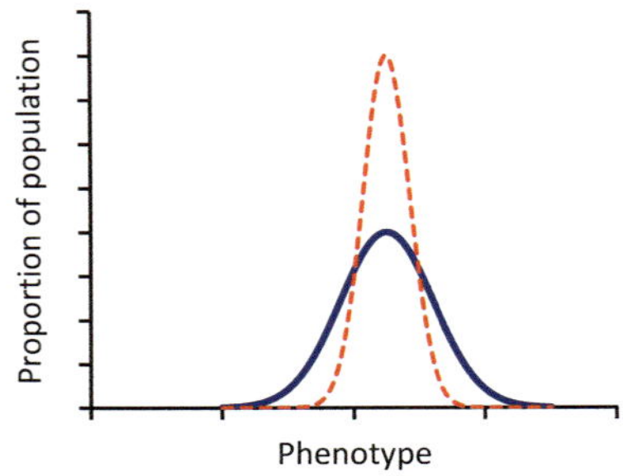

FIGURE 1.6 The problem with blending. Imagine a population with a trait spread as shown by the normal distribution above (solid blue). If mating in this population is random, and two individuals mate, blending would ensure that the offspring's phenotype is the arithmetic mean of the parent's phenotype. Should mating proceed randomly, blending inheritance implies that the mean phenotype of the population does not change with generations. However, the spread of the phenotype around the mean shrinks by a factor of two in each generation. As a result, as generations process, the distribution changes from the wider distribution (blue, solid) to a narrower (red, dashed) distribution. Thus, variation of the trait in the population decreases. However, Darwin also knew from observation that the variance of any trait in wild populations does not change with generations. How is, despite blending, variation preserved in populations was an open question in Darwin's mind.

The challenge before Darwin was explaining how, in the face of blending inheritance, variation is preserved through generations?

Using mathematical analysis, we can show that in case of blending inheritance and randomized mating – the mean height of the population, as we go from one generation to another, does not change. However, the variance of the height in the population decreases by a factor of two every generation. This implies that in the face of blending inheritance – all variation in the population would be lost.

However, variation is needed for natural selection to act, and if there were no variation in a population, evolution via natural selection would grind to a halt.

1.11.3 Lack of Mechanism

As we have remarked above, Darwin's proposal of natural selection came roughly 100 years before the structure of DNA was known. It was only in the 1970s that central dogma of molecular biology was figured out, leading us to fully understand how information regarding cellular processes is stored in DNA. Thus, it is not a surprise that Darwin did not know the mechanism which made offsprings resembled their parents. Proposals regarding how inheritance worked had been made since Pythagoras' time. Darwin also contributed to the list of such proposals via the idea of 'pangenesis' in his later book *The Variation of Animals and Plants under Domestication*. However, pangenesis was essentially Lamarckian, and was rejected soon after its proposal.

1.11.4 Altruistic Behavior

Darwin acknowledged that evolution via natural selection means that traits which enhance an individual's fitness are selected, while those traits which decrease an individual's fitness are rejected. To this effect, Darwin proclaimed that if one could observe a trait exhibited by an individual which was solely for the benefit of another individual, his theory would collapse. In such a framework, how does one explain altruistic behavior of ants and bees?

1.11.5 Long Time for Evolutionary Change

Darwin argued that evolution proceeded extremely slowly, with natural selection acting on continuous variation. Hence, hundreds of millions of years were needed to generate the variety of life as seen on the planet. This implied that the Earth had to be very old. The best estimates of the age of Earth came from William Thomson, also called Lord Kelvin.

Kelvin's estimated the age of the Earth by the following logic. Consider a large piece of meat cooked in an oven, say 200°C, for a long time. At that time, the temperature of the meat, inside and on the surface, will be 200°C. Imagine that we take the meat out and immediately transfer it to a freezer at 0°C. Immediately upon this transfer, the surface of the meat will freeze to 0°C, while the inside remains hot. With time, the temperature in the areas closer to the surface drop, and with time the meat will be at 0°C everywhere. Using Diffusion theory, we can predict the time it takes for this cooling process to occur.

Kelvin calculated the age of the Earth using the same logic. He imagined that at the time of formation, Earth was a mass of molten metals. And upon formation, the crust cooled. Hence, over time, the temperature away from the surface, deeper into the Earth's surface, will drop too. Therefore, if we know the temperature profile in the Earth's surface, we can estimate how long has Earth been cooling for. From his analysis, Kelvin estimated the age of Earth to be 20 million years.

This time was nowhere near sufficient for Darwinian evolution to take place and generate the kind of diversity of life that we see on the planet. However, Kelvin's estimate of the age of the Earth was the best at that time. Although it was later realized that Kelvin did not take into account all the forces that are responsible for heat transfer, the view at the time was that Kelvin's estimate of the age of Earth is a good one. This estimate, however, did not reconcile with Darwin's view of evolution via natural selection.

Today, we know that evolution can proceed at a rapid pace. Consider two examples.

First, when antibiotics were discovered in the first half of the 20th century, it was widely believed that microbial menace was over, since we had antibiotics at our disposal. However, in the subsequent years, it was observed that microbial populations evolved resistance to antibiotics in a relatively short span of time (see video in 'Further Readings').

Second, perhaps the longest-running evolution experiment is at University of Illinois at Urbana Champaign. In this experiment, stared in 1896, corn plants with high oil content are selected to form the next generations. Thus, each year, from a given population – only the highest oil content plants are allowed to propagate to the next generation. The remaining population is discarded (and thus, has fitness equal to zero). In the approximately 125 years since the experiment was started, the oil content has been linearly increasing. The oil content was around 10% in 1896, and it is around 30% now.

More recently, in what the world has witnessed, we have seen how variants of SARS CoV-2 evolve rapidly and spread through the world.

Thus, evolution is usually a slow process, but in certain contexts, it can be a rapid process too.

1.12 ORIGIN AND NATURE OF VARIATION

Unlike a plant/animal breeder, nature looks at the variation only in terms of the success of the organisms to survive the competition and produce more of their kind. While the idea of natural selection was generally accepted, there was considerable opposition as to how continuous variation could play such an important role in evolutionary process. The alternative view to this was that natural selection did not act on continuous variation of a trait in a population. That is, the small individual variation what Darwin referred to was irrelevant as far as evolution is concerned. Newer species arise when an individual, arising abruptly, exhibited a trait value far removed from the continuous distribution normally observed in the population. This type of variation – discontinuous in nature – was referred to as a 'sport' or 'monstrosities in the population'. One of the strongest proponents of the above were Huxley and Galton. But Darwin remained committed to the idea that small changes present in a continuous variation were the agent responsible for evolution. The critique against Darwin's idea was reinforced by Fleming Jenkin, an electrical engineer and a former student of Kelvin, who published an essay in 1867, raising questions regarding Darwin's proposal of how natural selection brings about evolutionary change. This review influenced Darwin's thinking regarding the mode of variation relevant for evolution.

1.13 JENKIN'S OBJECTIONS TO DARWIN'S IDEAS

Jenkin argued that according to Darwin, change is brought about simply by giving natural selection sufficient time to act on continuous variation in population. In the absence of a mechanism, Jenkin argued that Darwin was suggesting that merely time brings about evolutionary change. Jenkin was right in the sense that Darwin was unable to come up with a specific mechanism of variation and heredity.

Jenkin considered breeding experiments that produce faster running varieties of horses. Jenkin argued that no matter how much one tries, there would eventually be a limit in terms of how fast a horse can run. Thus, there seems to be a sphere of variation in terms of the trait value exhibited by an organism (in this case, speed of the horse). It is possible for different varieties of the species to exhibit values for that trait within the sphere. But it is quite impossible for an individual to exhibit a trait value beyond the sphere of variation. To Jenkin, behavior of organisms obeyed 'laws of matter' – which dictated that if you were closer to the boundary of the sphere of variation, you were likely to move close to the center in the next generation.

If, however, you were near the center of the sphere, the progeny in the next generation could exhibit any value of the trait. This logic agreed with the intuition of the time. Moreover, Jenkin argued that the Darwinian explanation of how evolution takes place via natural selection is only able to explain how a part becomes better in its performance via natural selection. Darwin's theory did not explain how newer parts come into being. An alternate explanation was needed to explain that facet of evolution.

1.13.1 Continuous or Discontinuous Variation

Further, Jenkin argued that blending would ensure that even these 'sports' would be unable to establish newer species. As an example, Jenkin argued, imagine an island inhabited by colored people, and if a 'sport' (a white individual) was introduced in this population. In the next generation, the white person would mate with a dark-colored individual – and blending would ensure that the offspring is gray in color. This gray offspring would then mate with another dark individual, the resulting offspring being closer to the original dark population. As this continues through generations, the 'sport' would blend into the original population. Hence, Jenkin argued, that 'sport' cannot be responsible for evolutionary change.

1.14 DARWIN'S RESPONSE TO THE CRITICISMS

This review and critique of Darwin's book was the most comprehensive in the immediate years after the publication of the *Origin*. Its effect was that it influenced Darwin's thinking on the nature of variation responsible for evolution. After publication of Jenkin's review, Darwin, in the fifth edition of the *Origin*, added a section titled 'On the great importance of individual differences, and on the unimportance of single variations'. In this section, using Jenkin's logic, Darwin argues emphatically that 'sports' cannot be responsible for evolutionary change, and it is the small, continuous variation in a population which gets acted on by natural selection. Darwin, in a letter to Alfred Wallace, at that time writes, 'the small-scale variations are of paramount importance. Jenkin's arguments have convinced me'.

Wallace agreed with Darwin's interpretation, and argued that since it was known from breeding experiments that 'sports' occurred at a frequency much lower than continuous variation, the chances that such rare 'sports' would be an exact adaptation to the environment in which the organism was living in, were next to nothing. As a result, whenever these rare 'sports' were to originate in nature, they would almost always be eliminated by natural selection. Wallace's arguments are best captured in the following section of his letter to Darwin,

> *These abnormalities are very rare in the state of nature, as compared with the ever-present individual variability ample in amount and affecting every part and organ ··· The very fixity of these abnormalities and the small number of characters affected by them, as well as their rarity, all show them to be the refuse material of nature's workshop.*

Thus, by the late 1860s, both, Darwin and Wallace had committed to small, continuous variation in a population is responsible for evolutionary change. In which direction this small change moves is mainly dictated by whether such movement confers any relative fitness advantage. However, intellectually appealing feature of large variation is that it is easy to explain the origination of new body parts. Despite the above intuitively sound arguments, Darwin stuck to his idea of small variation being constantly selected if it has an adaptive value and would eventually give rise to totally new species. He called this whole process as descent with modification.

As mentioned before, existence of variation is crucial for natural selection to operate. However, what properties of living entities lead to variation was an unknown at the time of publication of the *Origin of Species*. In a later book, *On the Variation in Plants and Animals*, published in 1868, Darwin proposed a theory of pangenesis, which sought to provide this missing mechanistic detail of variation and inheritance.

Since the publication of the *Origin of Species*, Darwin had invested considerable time and effort to explain how, inheritance and variation worked in nature. Darwin did carry out breeding experiments between different varieties of snapdragon and arrived at the 'Mendelian' 3:1 ratio, but was unable to interpret the significance of his finding. In the 1868 book, he put forward a theory, which provided a mechanistic explanation of inheritance and variation. Darwin called his theory pangenesis.

In pangenesis, each part of the body of an organism produced little particles called 'gemmules'. These gemmules then circulated in the body of the organism, from where they were grouped in the reproductive cells of the individual. When a new individual was conceived, these gemmules were transmitted from one generation to another. Via this mechanism, characters were transmitted from one generation to another. In Darwin's proposal of pangenesis, if a body part was altered (e.g., mutilation), new gemmules' which represented the severed state of the part were released. However, it was known that offspring of individuals with mutilations were not born with those parts missing. Darwin explained them by saying that prior to mutilation, or perhaps from the previous generations, the individual with the mutilation already possessed gemmules corresponding to a functional, healthy body part. Moreover, these healthy gemmules were passed onto the next generation. Through this mechanism, Darwin was able to explain much of the observed patterns in inheritance, including reversions (ancestral gemmules), organs developed in wrong place (gemmules not functioning correctly), regeneration of lost parts (ancestral/ healthy gemmules), inherited effects of use/disuse of particular organs (gemmules with acquired characters).

1.15 CONCLUSION

In view of what we now know about how inheritance works, Darwin's model looks glaringly wrong. But that is perhaps not the fairest assessment of the proposal. What Darwin's proposal of pangenesis does indicate though is how prevalent the idea of inheritance of acquired characters was, even more than 50 years after its proposal by

Lamarck. Darwin, however, does not mention Lamarck in his pangenesis book of 1868. It is in this context that texts do disservice to Lamarck. Lamarckian inheritance was very much a late 19th-century idea, and was even incorporated by Darwin in his failed attempt to explain inheritance. However, the subtle difference was that according to Lamarck, the adaptation to the environment was an inherent property of an organism which can be acquired, while according to Darwin, only those organisms that carried the beneficial variation that helped them to adapt to the environment were selected.

NOTES

Note I. Excerpt from the letter Lyell and Hooker wrote to the Linnean Society

MY DEAR SIR,—The accompanying papers, which we have the honour of communicating to the Linnean Society, and which all relate to the same subject, viz. the Laws which affect the Production of Varieties, Races, and Species, contain the results of the investigations of two indefatigable naturalists, Mr. Charles Darwin and Mr. Alfred Wallace.

These gentlemen having, independently and unknown to one another, conceived the same very ingenious theory to account for the appearance and perpetuation of varieties and of specific forms on our planet, may both fairly claim the merit of being original thinkers in this important line of inquiry; but neither of them having published his views, though Mr. Darwin has for many years past been repeatedly urged by us to do so, and both authors having now unreservedly placed their papers in our hands, we think it would best promote the interests of science that a selection from them should be laid before the Linnean Society.

Note II. Darwin and Mathew's correspondence in the *Gardner's Chronicle and Agricultural Gazette*

Letter to *Gardner's Chronicle and Agricultural Gazette* (April 1860)

In your Number of March 3rd I observe a long quotation from the Times, stating that Mr. Darwin "professes to have discovered the existence and modus operandi of the natural law of selection," that is, "the power in nature which takes the place of man and performs a selection, sua sponte," in organic life. This discovery recently published as "the results of 20 years' investigation and reflection" by Mr. Darwin turns out to be what I published very fully and brought to apply practically to forestry in my work "Naval Timber and Arboriculture," published as far back as January 1, 1831, by Adam & Charles Black, Edinburgh, and Longman & Co., London, and reviewed in numerous periodicals, so as to have full publicity in the "Metropolitan Magazine," the "Quarterly Review," the "Gardeners' Magazine," by Loudon, who spoke of it as the book, and repeatedly in the "United Service Magazine" for 1831, &c. The following is an extract from this volume, which clearly proves a prior claim.

Darwin's reply to the magazine:

I have been much interested by Mr. Patrick Matthew's communication in the Number of your Paper, dated April 7th. I freely acknowledge that Mr. Matthew has anticipated by many years the explanation which I have offered of the origin of species, under the name of natural selection. I think that no one will feel surprised that neither I, nor apparently any other naturalist, had heard of Mr. Matthew's views, considering how briefly they are given, and that they appeared in the appendix to a work on Naval Timber and Arboriculture. I can do no more than offer my apologies to Mr. Matthew for my entire ignorance of his publication. If another edition of my work is called for, I will insert a notice to the foregoing effect.

Mathew's reply:

To me the conception of this law of Nature came intuitively as a self-evident fact, almost without an effort of concentrated thought. Mr. Darwin here seems to have more merit in the discovery than I have had; to me it did not appear a discovery. He seems to have worked it out by inductive reason, slowly and with due caution to have made his way synthetically from fact to fact onwards; while with me it was by a general glance at the scheme of Nature that I estimated this select production of species as an à priori recognisable fact – an axiom requiring only to be pointed out to be admitted by unprejudiced minds of sufficient grasp.

EXERCISES

1. Summarize the three elements of the theory of natural selection? Explain why the theory of natural selection fails if any one of the three conditions is not met.
2. On a World map, draw the route that *Beagle* took around the world.
3. On a World map, draw the Wallace Line.
4. Think of an example where directional selection acting on a population selects for individuals with smaller trait value.
5. Population of bacteria A is allowed to grow in environment E1 for 1 hour. The population is then shifted to environment E2 for 1 hour. Bacteria A exhibit a growth rate of one division every 15 minutes in E1 and every 30 minutes in E2. Another bacterial species B divides every 20 minutes in E1 and E2; and is allowed to grow in each environment for one hour. Which species is fitter in (a) environment E1, (b) environment E2, and (c) environment E1 and E2?
6. A species of bacteria (A) grows at one cell division every hour in environment E1 and one cell division every ten hours in environment E2 (which contains an antibiotic). Another species of bacteria (B) divides every 20 minutes in E1 but dies instantaneously in E2. If the two species are exposed to E1 and E2 for 10 hours each in sequence, which species has the higher fitness?
   (note that fitness is sometimes just surviving).
7. On a world map, locate the Wallace line. Which two continents does this line roughly lie between?
8. How strong is the effect of blending? Do a survey to collect heights of (a) classmates, (b) their parents, and (c) their grandparents. How strongly does blending explain the height of one generation, given the parents generations' height?

9. Remember that Darwin was posed with a serious problem. He was aware that blending inheritance reduces variation in a population. However, he also knew that, with time, variation remained more or less constant in a population. Propose a mechanism that explains how diversity is maintained in a population, despite the action of blending?
10. How does Darwin's pangenesis compare with Lamarck's theory of evolution by use and disuse?

BIBLIOGRAPHY

1. Darwin C. 1859. *On the Origin of Species, Charles Darwin.* Penguin (2009).
   (In Chapters 4 and 6, Darwin lays out the structure of the theory of natural selection and highlights the shortcomings of the theory.)
2. Provine WB. 1971. *The Origins of Theoretical Population Genetics.* University of Chicago Press (2001).
   (After publication of *Origin of Species* in 1859, we typically jump to Mendel's paper, which, after publication in 1865, was rediscovered in 1900 to the proposal of the Hardy Weinberg Equilibrium in 1908. However, much intellectual creativity, and bitter scientific fights took place in the last three decades of the 19th century. Provine covers these decades in this book.)
3. Zimmer C. 2018. *She Has Her Mother's Laugh: The Powers, Perversions, and Potential of Heredity.* Dutton.
   (For a historical account of how we have understood heredity through the ages.)

2 Primer on Central Dogma of Molecular Biology

2.1 INTRODUCTION

It is said that proteins are the workhorses of a cell. This is because almost all critical functions in the cell are performed by proteins. For example, most reactions inside the cell are catalyzed by proteins – such proteins are called enzymes. As another example, uptake of sugars from the environment is also done by specific proteins. For example, there are dedicated transporters in the cell whose sole job is to bring glucose into the cell. Proteins play other roles in the cell too – like, providing structural integrity to the cell, or sensing extracellular stimuli. Thus, we can say that the identity of a cell is determined by the identity of proteins it can synthesize.

It is also often said that all information about cell's working is stored in the DNA of the cell. Or, that the DNA is the blueprint for life. This is so because it is in the DNA of the organism that information of *all* proteins it *can* synthesize is stored.

In this chapter, we will understand how the process of protein synthesis works, and how the information to synthesize proteins is stored in DNA.

2.2 STRUCTURE OF DNA MOLECULE

The structure of DNA was solved in 1953, when James Watson and Francis Crick published their results in *Nature*. This structure was deciphered with the help of X-ray crystallography images taken by Rosalind Franklin. Their proposed structure showed that DNA is a double-stranded helical molecule. We will first discuss the structure of DNA, and then move to how it stores information to encode proteins.

DNA is a polymer – a string, where monomers are linked with each other. Each monomer is comprised of three elements: (i) a sugar, deoxy-ribose, (ii) a phosphate group, and (iii) a nitrogenous base (Figure 2.1). While the sugar (deoxy-ribose) and phosphate groups are identical in every monomer, each monomer carries one of four nucleotide bases. These bases are adenine, guanine, cytosine, and tyrosine, and are simply abbreviated as `A`, `G`, `C`, and `T`. We will use these abbreviated representations of the four bases in the book. Each monomer is also referred to as a 'base'.

The carbon atoms in the sugar in each monomer are numbered one to five. Two monomers are linked together in a directional manner, where 3′ end of one monomer bonds with the 5′ end of another via the phosphate group. DNA sequences are then, read from 5′-end to the 3′-end. The sequence below is therefore read as 5′-`AGTC`-3′ (Figure 2.2). Note that sugar and phosphate groups are not read since they are present in every monomer.

DOI: 10.1201/9781003633662-2

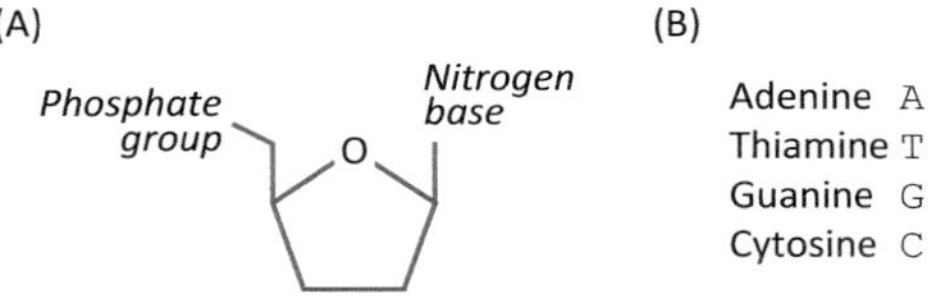

FIGURE 2.1 Nucleotide structure. (A) A nucleotide comprises of a sugar, a phosphate group, and a nitrogenous base. (B) A single nucleotide can have one of the four nitrogenous bases: Adenine (A), Guanine (G), Cytosine (C), and Thiamine (T).

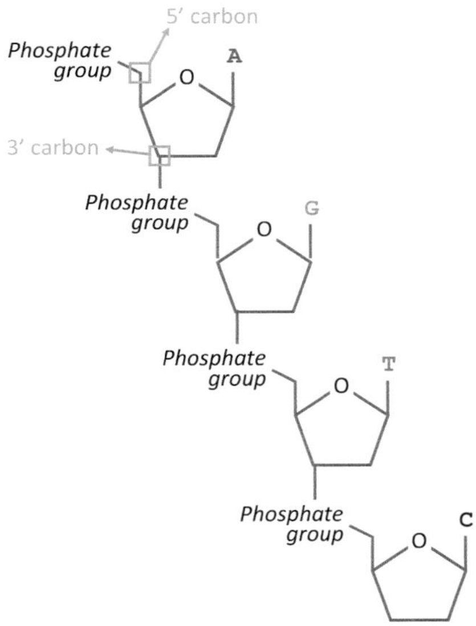

FIGURE 2.2 A single strand of DNA. DNA strand is read from the 5′ end to the 3′ end. In the figure, we start from the top nucleotide which has an unlinked 5-carbon phosphate, and end at the bottom nucleotide which has an unlinked 3′ carbon. Since the pentose sugar and the phosphate are common for each nucleotide, the identity of a nucleotide is defined by the nitrogenous base it contains. In the picture shown, the sequence of DNA is read as 5′ – AGTC – 3′.

What we have described above is a single-stranded DNA. However, note that DNA is double-stranded (Figure 2.3). The physics and chemistry of the four nitrogenous bases mean that A forms a double hydrogen bond with T, and G forms a triple hydrogen bond with C. The two strands of DNA run in the opposite direction. The nitrogenous bases of one strand pair with the nitrogen-base of the second strand. That is, wherever there is an 'A' on one strand, the complementary strand will have 'T', and wherever there is a 'G' on one strand, the other strand will have a 'C'. Each such pair is called a *base pair*.

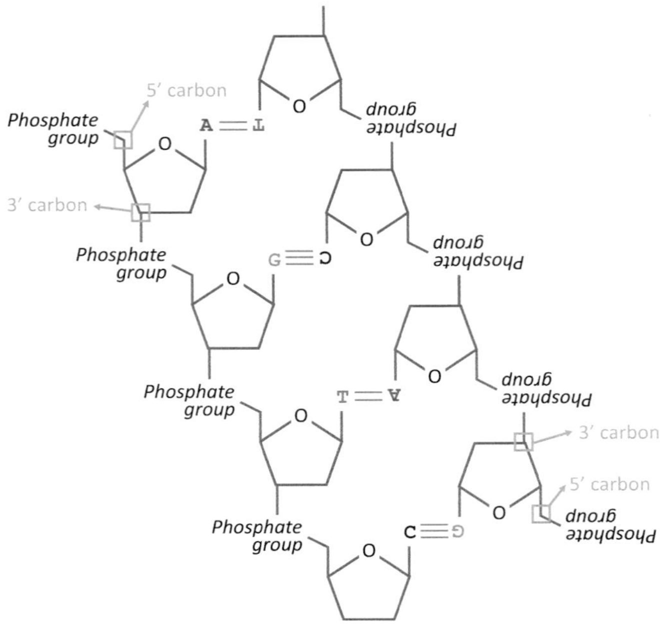

FIGURE 2.3 Double-stranded DNA structure. The strand on the left runs from 5′ (top) to 3′ (bottom) and can be read as `AGTC`. The second strand runs in the opposite direction: 5′ (bottom) to 3′ (top). The nitrogenous bases on the second strand are complementary to those of the first strand. That is, `A` on one strand is linked to `T` on the other strand via two hydrogen bonds (dashed gray lines). And, `C` on one strand is linked to `G` on the other strand via three hydrogen bonds. Thus, information about the nitrogenous base sequence on one strand is sufficient to know the sequence of the nitrogenous bases on the second strand.

Note that if are given the sequence of one strand as 5′-`ATGC`-3′, we can automatically deduce the sequence of the second strand. This is because we know that the other strand will run in the opposite orientation, and it will obey the base pairing rules such that A only pairs with T on the other strand, and G only pairs with C on the other strand. Hence, the sequence of the other strand is 5′ – `GCAT` – 3′. Thus, since the sequence of the other strand can be deciphered from one strand's sequence, DNA sequences are only reported as a single strand. Other than some viruses, all organisms have their DNA as double-stranded. Note that viruses are most diverse in terms of their material of heredity – they store information as double or single-stranded DNA, or even double or single-stranded RNA.

Example 2.1: If a strand of DNA reads 5′ – `AAAA` – 3′, what does its complementary strand read as?

Solution: Remember that A only pairs with `T` in the double-stranded DNA, thus, every molecule of `A` in our given DNA will pair with a `T`. Thus, the sequence of the complementary strand would read as 5′ – `TTTT` – 3′.

Example 2.2: If a strand of DNA reads 5′ – AATT – 3′, what does its complementary strand read as?

Solution: Remember that the two DNA strands run anti-parallel to each other. That is, the 5′ of one strand pairs with 3′ of the other. Thus, the T at the 3′ end of the given DNA sequence will pair with an A at the 5′ end of the complementary DNA. Similarly, the A at the 5′ end of the given DNA will pair with a T at the 3′ end of the complementary DNA. Thus, the sequence of the complementary strand would read as 5′ – AATT – 3′.

This base pairing rule means that a double-stranded DNA will have an equal number of A and T (and also, an equal number of C and G) nucleotides. This fact was first discovered by an American biochemist, Erwin Chargaff, in the late 1940s, and is known as the 'Chargaff rule'. Chargaff rule was a crucial input that Watson and Crick used to arrive at their structure of DNA.

Human DNA is about 3×10^9 base pair long. Each cell in our body contains this amount of DNA. Note, however, that one exception to this is the Red Blood Cells (RBCs), which do not have DNA. If the DNA in a single cell is stretched, it would be approximately 2 meters in length! How this long thread is packed in the tiny nucleus of each cell is a problem on which a lot of active research is being carried out. As a way of comparison, the bacterium *E. coli* has DNA about 5×10^6 base pair long.

Lastly, the DNA molecule is not physically present as a linear double strand (like a railroad). Instead, the two strands are curled into a right-handed helix. The problem of deciphering DNA structure was solved with input from several people. For their efforts, Watson, Crick, and Maurice Wilkins were awarded the 1962 Nobel Prize in Physiology/Medicine. Rosalind Franklin's contributions toward this effort were critical and worthy of the Nobel Prize, but she had died in 1958.

Ten years before the proposal of the DNA structure by Watson and Crick, in his 1943 book *What Is Life?*, the physicist Erwin Schrodinger had proposed that the unit of heredity or information had to be something which was repetitive (like a polymer) but in which the repeats were not identical (because then it would mean that there was very little information stored in the polymer). The discovery of DNA's structure proved that Schrodinger was correct on both aspects.

DNA is indeed a polymer with repeated units/monomers, however, the order in which the four units are linked gives rise to an astronomical number of possibilities in which the exact sequence can be laid out. For example, if we have a DNA sequence of length two (i.e., the sequence has two nucleotides), we can have 16 unique sequences (we have four options for the first base [any one of A, T, G, C], and 4 for the second [any one of A, T, G, C] – hence, the total number of possible DNA sequences with length two is 16). If we have a DNA sequence of length 3, then the total number of possibilities is 64 ($4 \times 4 \times 4 = 4^3$). Extending the same logic, if we consider a DNA sequence of length L, the total number of possible DNA sequences is 4^L. As we saw above, DNA of even a simple bacterium has L (the number of nucleotides) of the order of 10^9. Thus, the total number of unique DNA sequences of length 10^6 easily exceeds the number of atoms in the universe. The key point from our perspective is that such an astronomical number of possibilities provides an avenue to store a large amount of information in the DNA molecule.

Example 2.3: How many DNA sequences of length three nucleotides exist which begin with nucleotide C?

Solution: We are interested in the number of sequences which are $5' - \text{CNN} - 3'$, where N is any nucleotide. Which means that at position 2, we have four choices for a nucleotide (any one of A, T, G, C) and we have the same four choices for the third position. Thus, the total number of DNA sequences beginning with the nucleotide C is 16 ($= 4 \times 4$).

2.3 FROM DNA TO PROTEINS

DNA of an organism stores all information regarding which type of proteins that organism's cells can synthesize. Moreover, DNA also stores the information of when and how much of each protein will be synthesized. In the remaining part of this chapter, we will discuss these two crucially important facets of cellular functioning. First, we will study the two processes which lead to protein synthesis, while reading the DNA. This is accomplished via two steps: (i) transcription and (ii) translation.

Step 1. Transcription

Consider a stretch of DNA sequence, as represented in Figure 2.4A. In the transcription step of protein synthesis, a cellular machinery (RNA Polymerase or simply, RNAP) sits on double-stranded DNA. Part of the machinery then 'melts' the DNA (separates the two strands), and the RNA Polymerase moves from 3′ end to the 5′ end of one of the DNA strands. The 5′ → 3′ end is referred to as the coding strand. In Figure 2.4B, a single strand is shown with RNAP on the DNA strand.

As it moves along the DNA, RNA Polymerase reads the non-coding strand of DNA to assemble another polymer identical to the coding strand of DNA. The synthesized polymer is called the mRNA (messenger RNA) and is different from the coding strand of DNA in two respects. First, the sugar used in this polymer is ribose (it is deoxy-ribose in DNA). Second, the four nitrogenous bases used in RNA synthesis are adenine (A), uracil (U), guanine (G), and cytosine (C). Thus, thiamine (T) in DNA is replaced by uracil in RNA.

The RNA Polymerase moves along the DNA, and synthesizes the mRNA molecule according to the steps described above (Figure 2.4C–E). After traversing the DNA a certain distance, the RNA Polymerase is dislodged from the DNA. The two strands of the DNA are again brought back together, and the newly synthesized RNA molecule awaits its fate in the cellular environment.

RNA, because of its slightly different chemical identity, compared to DNA, is reactive and unstable.

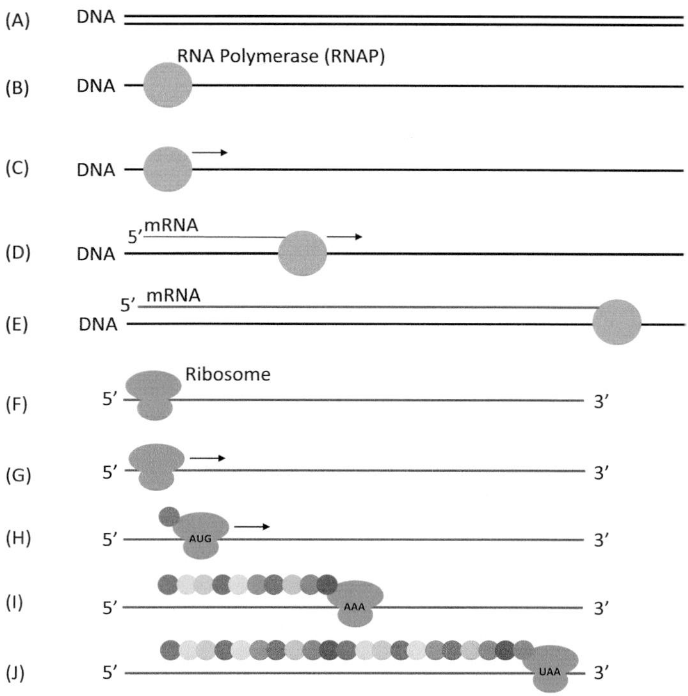

FIGURE 2.4 Central dogma. Transcription is initiated on a part of DNA (A) when an RNAP is recruited to the DNA (B). (C) Upon getting access to a site on the DNA strand, the RNAP moves along DNA, as indicated by the arrow. (D) As the RNAP moves, it synthesizes an mRNA molecule (shown as red line) which has the same nucleotide sequence as the 5′ to 3′ strand except that instead of Thiamine (T) as a nitrogenous base, mRNA uses Uracil (U). Also, mRNA uses ribose instead of deoxyribose in DNA. (E) Transcription terminates at a precise location on the DNA, and the mRNA is released into the cellular/nuclear environment. (F) The process of translation starts with the ribosome finding access to a site close to the 5′ of the mRNA. This site is referred to as the Shine-Dalgarno sequence. (G) The ribosome then moves toward the 3′ end of the mRNA, scanning the mRNA, till it encounters a start codon (AUG). (H) Upon encountering which a tRNA brings the corresponding amino acid (methionine) to the ribosome. The process of amino acid chain assembly starts here. (I) The process of amino acid chain synthesis continues as the ribosome moves three nucleotides, and assembles the corresponding amino acid to the growing chain. (J) This process continues till the ribosome encounters one of the three STOP codons (UAA in the figure). The amino acid chain (peptide chain) is then released from the ribosome. The chain then folds to its three-dimensional structure, and serves its function in the cellular physiology.

DNA is a language of four alphabets (A, T, G, and C). RNA is also a largely identical language of four alphabets (A, U, G, and C). The only difference between the two is that ‘T’ in DNA is replaced by a ‘U’ in RNA. Hence, synthesis of mRNA is simply transcribing the ‘text’ in DNA to the largely identical language of mRNA. The process is referred to as ‘transcription’.

2.3.1 Real-time Kinetics of Transcription

Recent experiments have allowed us to visualize and understand transcription in real-time. When a part of DNA is being transcribed, it is often said that transcription is in the 'ON' state. When a fragment of DNA is not being transcribed, transcription is said to be in the 'OFF' state. Two things are worth noting here.

First, not all regions of the DNA are transcribed.
Second, a given region of DNA is not transcribed all the time. A cell can tune transcription up and down, depending on the environmental context.

Some parts of the DNA only control the process of transcription and are themselves not transcribed. However, we also know that some parts of the DNA in the 'ON' state are transcribed more frequently than others.

Imagine a part of DNA which is transcribed 60 times every hour.

What is the real-time kinetics of transcription? Does transcription operate with clockwork accuracy – with one transcript every minute, or are the kinetics of transcription more chaotic. In a study in 2005, Golding and colleagues (see further readings) demonstrated that transcription operates in 'bursts' – where, lots of transcripts are generated in a short amount of time. These windows of active transcription are separated by time windows where no transcription takes place. Thus, transcription is 'bursty' and 'noisy'.

Step 2. Translation

At the end of transcription, we have an mRNA molecule. This molecule is then 'translated' leading to a protein. Let us take a look at how the events leading to protein synthesis unfold.

The mRNA is single stranded and directional. The process of translation begins when a cellular machine called Ribosome approaches the 5′ end of the mRNA and binds a specific sequence on the mRNA, referred to as the Shine-Dalgarno sequence (Figure 2.4F). The ribosome then slides across the mRNA, and typically, around six to eight bases downstream of the Shine-Dalgarno sequence, encounters a triplet of nucleotides 'AUG'. When the ribosome 'sees' an AUG, a transfer RNA (tRNA) brings an amino acid to the ribosome. However, the amino acid is not just any random amino acid. The triplet 'AUG' on the mRNA means that the amino acid Methionine will be assembled.

After this, the ribosome slides forward three nucleotides on the mRNA. Let us imagine, it reads 'GGC' as the next triplet of nucleotides. Another tRNA brings to the ribosome the amino acid Glycine, corresponding to the triplet 'GGC'. Glycine and Methionine are then joined together via a dehydration reaction (removal of water molecule), and the ribosomal machinery slides over to the next triplet of bases on the mRNA. This process continues to assemble an amino acid chain till the ribosome encounters a triplet which signals a STOP for the translation process (Figure 2.4G–J). Three triplets lead to the termination of protein assembly process. These triplets are UAA, UGA, and UAG. Upon encountering the triplet for STOP, the protein assembly process halts, and the ribosome disassembles. The amino acid chain formed prior to the STOP triplet folds, resulting in a functional protein molecule.

The region of the DNA, starting from `ATG` (which corresponds to `AUG` on the mRNA) to one of the three possible STOP codons, is called a gene. Bacteria have ~5000 genes in their DNA; humans are thought to have around 21000. Discovery of a gene, and advances in how we understand its functioning are a long, remarkable, and fascinating story.

Ribosomes read information in triplets. In all, there will be 64 possible triplets of DNA nucleotide sequence (4 × 4 × 4). Of these, 61 triplets correspond to a unique amino acid (Figure 2.5). The remaining three correspond to a 'STOP' signal. When the moving ribosomal chain encounters one of these three triplets, amino acid linkage stops, and the ribosomal machinery disassociates from the mRNA molecule. The association between the triplets (called 'codons') and the amino acids is referred to as the genetic

	Second Letter								
First Letter	U		C		A		G		Third Letter
U	UUU	Phe	UCU	Ser	UAU	Tyr	UGU	Cys	U
	UUC	Phe	UCC	Ser	UAC	Tyr	UGC	Cys	C
	UUA	Leu	UCA	Ser	UAA	STOP	UGA	STOP	A
	UUG	Leu	UCG	Ser	UAG	STOP	UGG	Trp	G
C	CUU	Leu	CCU	Pro	CAU	His	CGU	Arg	U
	CUC	Leu	CCC	Pro	CAC	His	CGC	Arg	C
	CUA	Leu	CCA	Pro	CAA	Gln	CGA	Arg	A
	CUG	Leu	CCG	Pro	CAG	Gln	CGG	Arg	G
A	AUU	Ile	ACU	Thr	AAU	Asn	AGU	Ser	U
	AUC	Ile	ACC	Thr	AAC	Asn	AGC	Ser	C
	AUA	Ile	ACA	Thr	AAA	Lys	AGA	Arg	A
	AUG	Met	ACG	Thr	AAG	Lys	AGG	Arg	G
G	GUU	Val	GCU	Ala	GAU	Asp	GGU	Gly	U
	GUC	Val	GCC	Ala	GAC	Asp	GGC	Gly	C
	GUA	Val	GCA	Ala	GAA	Glu	GGA	Gly	A
	GUG	Val	GCG	Ala	GAG	Glu	GGG	Gly	G

FIGURE 2.5 Standard Genetic Code. Every triplet of nucleotides encodes for an amino acid. The association between the triplets (called *codons*) and the corresponding amino acid is called the Standard Genetic Code, and is as shown. Note that, except Methionine (AUG) and Tryptophan (UGG), all amino acids are encoded by more than one codon. Also note that three codons (UAA, UGA, and UAG) encode for the translation process to be stopped and are hence called STOP codons. The standard genetic code is nearly universal, with a handful of exceptions. The amino acids are written as: (i) Phe – Phenylalanine; (ii) Leu – Leucine; (iii) Ile – Isoleucine; (iv) Met – Methionine; (v) Val – Valine; (vi) Ser – Serine; (vii) Pro – Proline; (viii) Thr – Threonine; (ix) Ala – Alanine; (x) Tyr – Tyrosine; (xi) His – Histidine; (xii) Gln – Glutamine; (xiii) Asn – Asparagine; (xiv) Lys – Lysine; (xv) Asp – Aspartic Acid; (xvi) Glu – Glutamic Acid; (xvii) Cys – Cysteine; (xviii) Trp – Tryptophan; (xix) Arg – Arginine; (xx) Gly – Glycine.

code and is almost universally conserved, with only a handful of rare exceptions. What this means is that the codon 'AUG' corresponds to methionine in human beings, and it also refers to the same amino acid in *E. coli*, or horse, or a dolphin.

It is interesting to note that while there are 61 codons corresponding to amino acids (the other three correspond to STOP), there are only 20 amino acids in naturally occurring proteins. What this implies is that more than one codon can correspond to the same amino acid during protein synthesis. For example, we note in the genetic code that the amino acid Serine can be encoded by six codons. Association of more than one codon for the same amino acid is referred to as degeneracy in the genetic code. On the other hand, two amino acids (Methionine or Tryptophan) are encoded by a unique codon.

Note also that a single codon never corresponds to more than one amino acid. This means that there is no ambiguity in the process of protein synthesis. A given DNA or mRNA sequence corresponds to a single, unique amino acid chain.

After the ribosome encounters a 'STOP' codon, no more amino acids are joined in the peptide chain. The ribosome disassociates, and the peptide chain folds into its three-dimensional structure. This folded structure of the amino acid chain is referred to as the protein. The protein molecule then performs its role in cellular physiology.

For example, for the amino acid corresponding to gene *lacZ* in *E. coli*, the resulting protein hydrolyzes lactose into its constituent monosaccharide sugars, glucose and galactose. The glucose and galactose resulting from the hydrolysis reaction are thereafter utilized for energy and growth by being acted upon by other proteins in the cell. A bit later in the chapter, we discuss more about how LacZ is produced in the cell.

Note that if there was no LacZ in the cell, lactose hydrolysis would not take place, and the bacterium would not be able to grow on lactose as the carbon source. Thus, LacZ has a catalytic role in the cell. Proteins which have a catalytic activity in the cell are referred to as enzymes. A key aspect of proteins as catalysts is their specificity toward their substrate. For example, LacZ will only catalyze the hydrolysis of lactose, and no other sugar. It is thought that it is for such specificity that proteins are bulky molecules, when the actual site of catalysis in them is quite small (relative to the size of the protein).

Protein molecules have other functions in the cell too – like structural strength, signaling, and transport (entry and exit) of metabolites.

Note that in the process of translation, mRNA (which is a polymer written in the language of four alphabets) was read to synthesize another polymer (amino-acid chain), which was written in the language of 20 alphabets.

2.3.2 Real-time Kinetics of Translation

Unlike transcription, translation is best approximated as a deterministic process. During translation, an mRNA molecule is occupied by multiple ribosomes – each translating the mRNA. The ribosomes are, each independently, moving along the mRNA. As you can imagine, if each mRNA molecule is occupied by multiple ribosomes, the number of ribosomes in a single *E. coli* must be very large. When in exponential phase, a single *E. coli* has $>$ 10,000 ribosomes. In fact, the number of ribosomes present in a cell is a good indicator of how fast a bacterium is growing.

2.4 CONTROL OF GENE EXPRESSION

The above discussion leads us to the following question. Although all cells in a multicellular organism contain the same DNA, they can look and function very differently. For example, a muscle cell looks very different from a skin cell on a human body, despite both containing the same DNA sequence. In fact, an adult human contains tens of trillions of cells in her body, and many of these cells look very different from each other. This dissimilarity arises despite the fact that all cells of an individual's body arose from a single cell (zygote) when the egg and sperm fused, and hence contain identical DNA sequences.

This difference in appearance of different cell types comes from the fact that the different cell types express different sets of genes. The human genome contains information for about 21,000 genes. However, not all cells in the body express all 21000 genes at a given moment in time. The identity of genes expressed in one cell type is distinct from the identity of genes expressed in another cell type. This is what gives each cell type its distinct physical and chemical properties.

How is this differential regulation maintained? There are many mechanisms that control this. Gene expression is controlled by the physical and chemical environment surrounding a cell. Dedicated proteins in the cell membrane sense the outside environment and transmit this information inside the cell. This leads to the cell tuning its gene expression appropriately.

The information regarding the extracellular environment is fed into the region of the DNA 'upstream' of `ATG` (start codon) of a gene. This region of the DNA is called the promoter region of the gene.

Let us discuss with the help of one of the best-understood models of gene regulation – the lactose utilization system in *E. coli*. Lactose, a glucose-galactose disaccharide, is internalized in the cell and is thereafter, hydrolyzed into glucose and galactose by an enzyme LacZ. When *E. coli* is fed glucose and lactose, *E. coli* preferentially utilizes glucose first, and only when all the glucose is consumed, does the organism switch to utilizing lactose. To facilitate this, genes responsible for utilization of lactose are only expressed when (a) lactose is present in the environment and (b) glucose is absent in the media.

These two conditions are encoded via the following logic (shown in Figure 2.6),

(a) When lactose is absent, a protein called LacI binds the promoter of LacZ and stops RNA Polymerase from transcribing the gene. As a result, no LacZ protein is synthesized in the cell when lactose is absent. However, in the presence of lactose, LacI binds lactose molecules, and in its bound state is unable to bind the LacZ promoter. Thus, LacI-dependent repression of *lacZ* takes place only as long as there is no lactose in the environment.

(b) When glucose is present in the media, the cellular energy state is high. The energy state of a cell is reflected in the amount of ATP in the cell. ATP (which stands for Adenine Triphosphate) is a high energy molecule which stores energy in its phosphate groups. When a cell is in a high energy state, ATP numbers are high. Conversely, in a low energy state, ATP levels drop, and ADP (Adenine Diphosphate) and AMP (Adenine Monophosphate) levels increase.

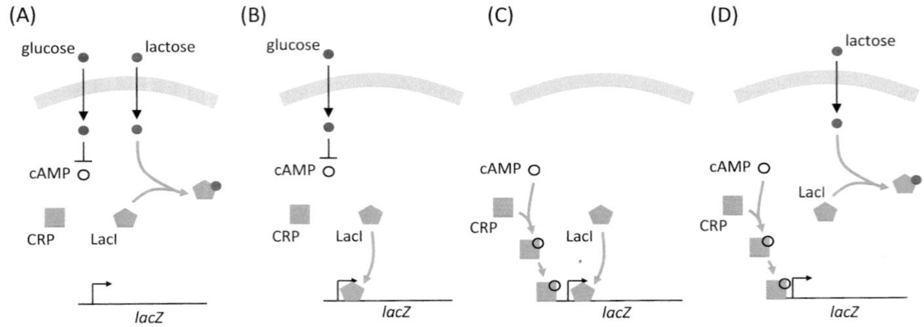

FIGURE 2.6 Lac system gene regulation. (A) When glucose and lactose are both present in the media, lactose binds LacI, and recruits it away from the *lacZ* promoter. Glucose, however, ensures that cAMP levels in the cell are low. As a result, CRP is unable to bind cAMP and positively activate the *lacZ* promoter. As a result, no transcription takes place. (B) When glucose is present in the media, CRP is unable to bind cAMP and LacI binds to the *lacZ* promoter. Both these molecular events ensure that no transcription takes place from the *lacZ* promoter. (C) When glucose and lactose are both absent from the media, LacI represses expression from the *lacZ* promoter, even though CRP bound to cAMP activates the promoter. (D) It is only when glucose is ABSENT in the media (hence, CRP-cAMP positively activates the promoter) and lactose is present in the media (thus, LacI repression is relieved) that transcription from the *lacZ* promoter takes place.

In such a state, ATP levels in the cells are high, and consequently, AMP levels are low. On the other hand, in the absence of glucose, the cell is in an energetically starved state. Hence, AMP levels are elevated, and the cyclic form of AMP (cAMP) binds a protein called CRP. Together, the cAMP-CRP complex binds the lacZ promoter and activates transcription. Thus, ensuring that *lacZ* transcription is only activated when glucose is absent from the environment. Without cAMP-CRP binding, lacZ transcription will not take place.

Thus, (a) above ensures that LacZ is expressed when lactose is present in the media, AND (b) ensures that LacZ is expressed when glucose is absent in the media (Figure 2.7). The key lesson for us here is that gene expression is highly contingent on the external environment. Cells are constantly monitoring their physical and

	Glucose Absent	Glucose Present
Lactose Absent	NO	NO
Lactose Present	YES	NO

FIGURE 2.7 The logic of the *lac* system gene regulation. Lactose gene regulation can be equated to the following logic gate, where gene expression from the *lacZ* promoter only takes place when lactose is PRESENT and glucose is ABSENT. Any other combination of the availability of the two sugars results in gene expression being repressed from the *lacZ* promoter.

chemical environments, and adjusting their gene expression in response in order to maximize their chances of survival and growth.

2.5 ALLELES

Imagine an *E. coli* population, where some cells have the following sequence of the gene *lacY*, the transporter which is responsible for bringing in lactose from the extracellular media to the inside of the cell.

Sequence I

```
ATGTACTATTTAAAAAACACAAACTTTTGGATGTTCGGTTTATTCTTTTTCTTTTACT
TTTTTATCATGGGAGCCTACTTCCCGTTTTTCCCGATTTGGCTACATGACATCAACCA
TATCAGCAAAAGTGATACGGGTATTATTTTTGCCGCTATTTCTCTGTTCTCGCTATTA
TTCCAACCGCTGTTTGGTCTGCTTTCTGACAAACTCGGGCTGCGCAAATACCTGCTGT
GGATTATTACCGGCATGTTAGTGATGTTTGCGCCGTTCTTTATTTTTATCTTCGGGCC
ACTGTTACAATACAACATTTTAGTAGGATCGATTGTTGGTGGTATTTATCTAGGCTTT
TGTTTTAACGCCGGTGCGCCAGCAGTAGAGGCATTTATTGAGAAAGTCAGCCGTCGCA
GTAATTTCGAATTTGGTCGCGCGCGGATGTTTGGCTGTGTTGGCTGGGCGCTGTGTGC
CTCGATTGTCGGCATCATGTTCACCATCAATAATCAGTTTGTTTTCTGGCTGGGCTCT
GGCTGTGCACTCATCCTCGCCGTTTTACTCTTTTTCGCCAAAACGGATGCGCCCTCTT
CTGCCACGGTTGCCAATGCGGTAGGTGCCAACCATTCGGCATTTAGCCTTAAGCTGGC
ACTGGAACTGTTCAGACAGCCAAAACTGTGGTTTTTGTCACTGTATGTTATTGGCGTT
TCCTGCACCTACGATGTTTTTGACCAACAGTTTGCTAATTTCTTTACTTCGTTCTTTG
CTACCGGTGAACAGGGTACGCGGGTATTTGGCTACGTAACGACAATGGGCGAATTACT
TAACGCCTCGATTATGTTCTTTGCGCCACTGATCATTAATCGCATCGGTGGGAAAAAC
GCCCTGCTGCTGGCTGGCACTATTATGTCTGTACGTATTATTGGCTCATCGTTCGCCA
CCTCAGCGCTGGAAGTGGTTATTCTGAAAACGCTGCATATGTTTGAAGTACCGTTCCT
GCTGGTGGGCTGCTTTAAATATATTACCAGCCAGTTTGAAGTGCGTTTTTCAGCGACG
ATTTATCTGGTCTGTTTCTGCTTCTTTAAGCAACTGGCGATGATTTTTATGTCTGTAC
TGGCGGGCAATATGTATGAAAGCATCGGTTTCCAGGGCGCTTATCTGGTGCTGGGTCT
GGTGGCGCTGGGCTTCACCTTAATTTCCGTGTTCACGCTTAGCGGCCCCGGCCCGCTT
TCCCTGCTGCGTCGTCAGGTGAATGAAGTCGCTTAA
```

Note that the gene sequence is 1,254 nucleotides long, and that the sequence starts with an ATG (*Start* codon, corresponding to amino acid Methionine) and ends with TAA (corresponding to a *Stop* signal for translation). The sequence corresponds to 417 amino acids ($417 \times 3 = 1251$; the last three nucleotides correspond to a *Stop* codon).

On the other hand, some other cells have a *lacY* sequence as shown below. Note that this sequence differs from the above sequence at precisely one nucleotide position. At position 592, the Sequence II has the nucleotide **C** (in red and highlighted in the sequence below), whereas the Sequence I had **G** at the same position. This corresponds to 198th codon in Sequence I being GCC (corresponding to the amino acid Alanine) and in Sequence II being CCC (corresponding to the amino acid Proline). Thus, these two sequences differ at precisely one amino acid (position number 198) in the LacY protein sequence that they encode for.

Sequence II

ATGTACTATTTAAAAAACACAAACTTTTGGATGTTCGGTTTATTCTTTTTCTTTTACT
TTTTTATCATGGGAGCCTACTTCCCGTTTTTCCCGATTTGGCTACATGACATCAACCA
TATCAGCAAAAGTGATACGGGTATTATTTTTGCCGCTATTTCTCTGTTCTCGCTATTA
TTCCAACCGCTGTTTGGTCTGCTTTCTGACAAACTCGGGCTGCGCAAATACCTGCTGT
GGATTATTACCGGCATGTTAGTGATGTTTGCGCCGTTCTTTATTTTTATCTTCGGGCC
ACTGTTACAATACAACATTTTAGTAGGATCGATTGTTGGTGGTATTTATCTAGGCTTT
TGTTTTAACGCCGGTGCGCCAGCAGTAGAGGCATTTATTGAGAAAGTCAGCCGTCGCA
GTAATTTCGAATTTGGTCGCGCGGATGTTTGGCTGTGTTGGCTGGGCGCTGTGTGC
CTCGATTGTCGGCATCATGTTCACCATCAATAATCAGTTTGTTTTCTGGCTGGGCTCT
GGCTGTGCACTCATCCTCGCCGTTTTACTCTTTTTCGCCAAAACGGATGCGCCCTCTT
CTGCCACGGTT**C**CCAATGCGGTAGGTGCCAACCATTCGGCATTTAGCCTTAAGCTGGC
ACTGGAACTGTTCAGACAGCCAAAACTGTGGTTTTTGTCACTGTATGTTATTGGCGTT
TCCTGCACCTACGATGTTTTTGACCAACAGTTTGCTAATTTCTTTACTTCGTTCTTTG
CTACCGGTGAACAGGGTACGCGGGTATTTGGCTACGTAACGACAATGGGCGAATTACT
TAACGCCTCGATTATGTTCTTTGCGCCACTGATCATTAATCGCATCGGTGGGAAAAAC
GCCCTGCTGCTGGCTGGCACTATTATGTCTGTACGTATTATTGGCTCATCGTTCGCCA
CCTCAGCGCTGGAAGTGGTTATTCTGAAAACGCTGCATATGTTTGAAGTACCGTTCCT
GCTGGTGGGCTGCTTTAAATATATTACCAGCCAGTTTGAAGTGCGTTTTTCAGCGACG
ATTTATCTGGTCTGTTTCTGCTTCTTTAAGCAACTGGCGATGATTTTTATGTCTGTAC
TGGCGGGCAATATGTATGAAAGCATCGGTTTCCAGGGCGCTTATCTGGTGCTGGGTCT
GGTGGCGCTGGGCTTCACCTTAATTTCCGTGTTCACGCTTAGCGGCCCCGGCCCGCTT
TCCCTGCTGCGTCGTCAGGTGAATGAAGTCGCTTAA

Such variants of the same gene are referred to as *alleles*. Sequences I and II are said to be two different alleles of the gene *lacY*.

Note that every time a mutation happens in the coding region of a gene, a new allele is created. A newer allele might have,

a. the same functional efficiency as the original allele (this would be the case when the mutation did not affect the function of the gene),
b. its performance compromised as compared to the ancestral allele, or
c. better performance as compared with the ancestral allele.

Any of the three possibilities can manifest, depending on the gene and the precise mutation that takes place in its sequence.

Mutations resulting in different alleles are responsible for various disease conditions. For example, sickle cell anemia is caused when an individual carries an allele of beta globin gene which has an A replaced by a T at position 17 in the gene sequence. In another example, the disease Cystic Fibrosis is caused when three nucleotides, from positions 1522 to 1524, are deleted from the sequence of the gene Cystic Fibrosis Transmembrane Conductance Regulator (CFTR). This means that the 508th amino acid, which in the original allele encodes for Phenylalanine is missing in the mutant sequence. And this missing amino acid in the mutant allele makes the protein non-functional, leading to the disease condition.

2.6 CONCLUSION

In this chapter, we have studied the process of protein synthesis in a cell. The process proceeds in two steps: transcription and translation. These processes are universally conserved and are essential (and the only way!) to produce proteins in all life forms. We also saw that the process of protein production is regulated – i.e., *E. coli* only makes proteins needed for utilization of lactose when lactose is present in the environment and glucose is absent. This ability to discern environment and regulate gene expression is critical for cellular functioning.

From the context of this book, this discussion gives us enough background in biology to start discussing evolution in detail. We next study our choice of organism to study evolutionary change.

NOTES

NOTE I

How did we find out that the molecule responsible for the storage of information is DNA? This was uncovered via a series of experiments in the 1940s. In this work, Avery, McLeod, and McCarty used two strains of the bacteria *Streptococcus* – one pathogenic, and the other non-pathogenic. The pathogenic strain was able to kill a mouse, and the non-pathogenic variant was unable to. Also consistent with intuition, when the mice were fed liquid where the pathogenic strain was heat-killed, the mice survived. However, when the mice were fed liquid containing live non-pathogenic strain and heat-killed pathogenic strain – the mice died, and live pathogenic strain was isolated.

DNA as a molecule for storage of information was proposed after this experiment. It was hypothesized that when DNA fragments of pathogenic bacteria were taken up by the non-pathogenic variants, the non-pathogenic variants acquired the ability to cause infection.

Prior to this work, DNA was thought not to be the molecule which stores information as it was known to be a repetitive molecule (with little chance to store large complex information, as would be needed to define life) with little tendency to react with anything (hence, chemically inert, and likely without any enzymatic activity).

NOTE II

The race to decode how DNA stores information for protein synthesis is a fascinating story in science. In 1961, Francis Crick and Syndey Brenner reported that the genetic code was a non-overlapping triplet code (meaning that ribosome moved three bases to 'read' the next codon, and not one base at a time). There is a beautiful story of the two arriving in lab one night to check the results of a critical experiment. On seeing the results of their experiments, the two men noted that they had discovered that the genetic code was a non-overlapping triplet, and that in that moment, they were the only two people on the planet who knew that. Brenner won the 2002 Nobel Prize in

Physiology/Medicine for his work on establishing *C. elegans* as a model system to study development.

The same year, 1961, Marshall Nirenberg demonstrated, in a biochemistry conference in Russia, that the codon 'UUU' corresponded to the amino acid Phenylalanine. This was despite the best attempts of the illustrious members of the 'RNA Tie Club' to solve the mystery of the genetic code via the sole power of thought and logic. As Nirenberg demonstrated, sometimes, you just cannot replace experiments!

NOTE III

The universal conservation of the genetic code has huge implications for biotechnology. A gene which encodes for a particular amino acid sequence in bacteria, corresponds to the same amino acid sequence in human beings, too. Thus, the universality of the genetic code meant that genes could be moved around species, and would correspond to the same amino acid. One of the first such demonstrations of the implications of this was in the 1970s when Insulin was produced by cloning the gene for insulin in the bacterium *E. coli*. Prior to that, the biotechnology industry relied on grinding pounds of pig liver to isolate insulin.

When the technical expertise to clone genes was first developed in the 1970s, there was a major concern regarding the ethics and biosafety associated with such a technology. Two Asilomar Conferences, led by Paul Berg, were held to this effect in the 1970s. While they pushed the issue of ethical implications of potential human cloning to a future date, how the concerns regarding biosafety were addressed makes for an extremely interesting reading. Paul Berg was, in 1980, for his role in the development of cloning technique, received the Nobel Prize in Chemistry (along with Walter Gilbert and Fredrick Sanger – for their role in DNA sequencing).

EXERCISES

1. Consider the codon CCC.
   a. Which amino acid does it encode for?
   b. There are 12 ways to introduce a single chance of nucleotide in this codon. List them all.
   c. In how many of the 12 changes in (b) the resulting codon encodes for the same amino acid as in (a)?
2. Repeat the question (1) for all codons in the genetic code.
3. Based on your calculations for the above question, what is the percentage of mutations in all codons which DO NOT result in a change of amino acid? (as we will see later in the book, such mutations are called synonymous mutations)
4. Which is the (a) most and (b) least frequently used amino acid in an organism? Check for *E. coli* and *H. sapiens*. Does the answer change depending on the organism?
5. What is the speed with which transcription proceeds? (in terms of nucleotides per second) If there is gene of length 1,200 nucleotides, how many seconds are needed for the gene to be transcribed?

6. What is the speed with which translation proceeds? (in terms of amino acids assembled per second) If there is a transcript of length 1,200 nucleotides, how many seconds are needed for this transcript to be fully translated?
7. *E. coli* has ~5000 genes. How many transcripts does an *E. coli* cell have? How many ribosomes are there in a cell at any given time?
8. Sickle cell anemia is caused by an A to T mutation at position 17 in its sequence. Find out the corresponding change in the amino acid which is caused by this nucleotide change.

BIBLIOGRAPHY

1. Watson JD, Crick FH. 1953. Molecular structure of nucleic acids; a structure for deoxyribose nucleic acid. *Nature* 171:737–8.
2. Watson JD, Crick FH. 1953. Genetical implications of the structure of deoxyribonucleic acid. *Nature* 171:964–7.
3. Maddox B. 2003. The double helix and the 'wronged heroine'. *Nature* 421:407–8.
   (Publications regarding the structure of DNA.)
4. Mukherjee S. 2016. *The Gene: An Intimate History*. Allen Lane.
   (A marvellous account of the search for a "gene", and what we understand from the term.)
5. Schrodinger E. 1992. *What is Life?* Cambridge University Press.
   (This is a short book based on collection of lectures Schrodinger gave. The book is insightful regarding how to think about an abstract problem.)
6. Avery OT, Macleod CM, McCarty M. 1944. Studies on the chemical nature of the substance inducing transformation of pneumococcal types: Induction of Transformation by a desoxyribonucleic acid fraction isolated from pneumococcus type III. *J Exp Med* 79:137–58.
   (This paper describes a critical experiment which showed that DNA was the material basis of heredity. Prior to this work, most researchers thought that material of inheritance was proteins.)
7. Cobb M. 2017. 60 years ago, Francis Crick changed the logic of biology. *PLoS Biol* 15: e2003243.
   (The discovery of how information travels from DNA to RNA to Protein was a fascinating journey. A key contributor in this direction was Francis Crick. Matthew Cobb (2017) *PLoS Biology* writes a summary of Crick's contribution.)
8. Golding I, Paulsson J, Zawilski SM, Cox EC. 2005. Real-time kinetics of gene activity in individual bacteria. *Cell* 123:1025–36.
   (This is a marvelously simple and elegant paper to study how transcription takes place in real-time).

3 Model Organism to Study Evolution

3.1 INTRODUCTION

As we have seen in the previous chapter, the DNA of an organism contains all the necessary information regarding which proteins an organism can synthesize? The DNA of an organism also controls the timing and amount of a particular protein that will be made in any particular cell of an organism. If mutations in DNA take place, the information regarding the type of protein (amino acid sequence), its timing of expression, and the amounts in which a protein is synthesized can change, compared to the original sequence. This change in protein quality or quantity or timing of expression can lead to a change in phenotype (behavior or physical manifestation) of an organism. Natural selection can thereafter act on this phenotypic variation.

The goal of this book is to learn how to think about and develop frameworks which allow us to think how mutational changes can lead to evolutionary change. For this purpose, we need model systems in which we study these processes.

We can study these using two types of model systems.

First, asexually reproducing organisms, like bacteria.

Second, sexually reproducing organisms such as mice, fruit flies, or chimpanzees.

Our inquiry and the resulting analysis depend on which of the above two model systems we use. In this brief chapter, we will discuss how these two types of model systems are fundamentally different when it comes to studying evolutionary change. We will then pick one of the two systems and study it for the rest of the book to study and develop models to understand evolution.

3.2 EVOLUTION IN BACTERIA

Bacteria divide asexually, and have one copy of the genome (DNA). During their life cycle, the DNA is replicated, and when a cell divides into two, each offspring inherits a single copy of the DNA. Hence, with every generation, DNA is passed from one generation to the next, from one parent to the offspring.

3.2.1 Generation of Diversity

Imagine a particular species of bacteria that divides every 30 minutes. This time is referred to as *generation time*. For a division time of 30 minutes, bacteria can process 48 generations in a single day! If we started this experiment with a single

 DOI: 10.1201/9781003633662-3

bacterium, after one generation, we would have two individuals. After two generations, we will have 4 (2^2) bacterial cells, and so forth. After g generations, the population size would be 2^g (i.e., after one day of growth, or after 48 generations, the population size would be 2^{48}).

In this time, evolutionary change is dictated by newer mutations that occur in the process of DNA replication. Thus, if we start with a population where every individual has identical DNA sequence (i.e., the population is isogenic population), every individual in the population will have the same phenotypic manifestation.

As reproduction proceeds, and DNA is replicated over and over again (remember, that after g generations, there are 2^g cells – and cell division requires that DNA is copied). During this process of replication of DNA, errors in copying DNA will be made. No machine is 100% efficient – i.e., every machine makes mistakes, however infrequently. So is the case with the molecular machine that copies DNA in a bacterium. While copying DNA, it makes errors in copying. Thus, newer mutations arise and create genetic diversity in the population.

Some of these mutations will lead to a change in the bacterium which decreases fitness. These mutations are called deleterious mutations. On the other hand, some mutations will not lead to any change in the fitness (these are referred to as neutral mutations). From the perspective of adaptive evolutionary change, we are most interested in mutations which increase fitness – i.e., beneficial mutations.

It is evident that when studying evolution via bacterial populations, we are interested in novel (or new) mutations occurring in the population and lead to genetic diversity. Natural selection then acts on the phenotypic diversity so generated leading to adaptive change. Remember that for natural selection to act, diversity or variation is key. The variation generated via mutations is going to be dictated by the error rate of DNA Polymerase (DNAP). Let us quantify these ideas with actual numbers.

3.2.2 Waiting Time for New Mutations

The time we have to wait for these new mutations to come up is called *waiting time*. This time, for bacterial populations, is often small. In other words, novel variation arises in a bacterial population rapidly. This can be seen with the help of an example, which we discuss next.

Example 3.1: In nutrient-rich media (like Luria-Bertani Broth), a 1 ml of LB culture contains 10^8 bacteria. Every member of this population undergoes one cell division. The mutation rate (the rate at which DNA Polymerase makes error while copying DNA) in *E. coli* is 10^{-3} per cell per division. How many mutants are generated in one generation for this population?

Solution: Since every cell in the population divides in the culture, the total number of cell divisions taking place is 10^8. The mutation rate of *E. coli* is 10^{-3} per cell per generation. That is, an error is made in DNA replication once every 1,000 cell divisions. In other words, out of 1,000 cell divisions, 999 are without errors and only one progeny ends up with an error in its DNA. Thus, the total number of mutants generated in the population is $10^8 \times 10^{-3}$. Or, in an *E. coli* population of size 10^8, 10^5 mutants are generated in a single generation.

The important point for us to appreciate is that in such a short span of time of one generation, a huge amount of genetic diversity is generated in a bacterial population.

Thus, if we are to study evolution using bacterial populations, we have to understand that genetic (and therefore phenotypic) variation is generated via new mutations in the population. Bacteria are studied in a large number of laboratories across the world to study evolutionary processes. We will see many such studies in the section on experimental evolution later in the book.

In addition to the vast amount of diversity generated in a short time, working with bacteria has other advantages, too. Let us consider them next.

3.2.3 Short Generation Time

To study evolutionary change using bacteria in a laboratory setting, we evolve bacterial populations in environmental conditions of interest for a certain number of generations. For example, in a famous example, *E. coli* has been evolved for over 80,000 generations in a laboratory in an environment which contains limited glucose, as an energy source. The experiment started in 1988, and since then *E. coli* has been propagated in this environment. More importantly, this experiment tells us about the pace of an evolution experiment, when we are working with bacteria.

Example 3.2: The *E. coli* experiment has been going on for the last 37 years (there have been few short breaks in between when the experiment was halted, but we will ignore them for the time being). In this time, 80,000 generations have been processed. How many generations of *E. coli* are processed in this experiment in a single day?

Solution: Each year is 365 days. Thus, the experiment has lasted for ~13,500 days. Thus, on an average, the experiment has processed ~6 generations in a single day!

The key point to note for us here is that, using bacteria, we can design experiments such that the number of generations processed in a given time is large. Remember, evolutionary change occurs over generations. I, as an individual, do not evolve (at least not biologically!).

3.2.4 Genome Sequencing

After evolving the population of bacteria for a certain number of generations, researchers then sequence the DNA of the evolved bacteria and compare with the DNA sequence of the bacteria they started the experiment with. Upon comparison of the two DNA sequences, we can identify the genetic changes that take place in the population in the time of the experiment. Clearly, it must be because of these mutations, that the population evolved to become fitter in the environment in which they were evolved. Molecular biologists then try and make sense of the mechanisms (at the level of protein activity, expression) via which the mutations increased fitness of the population in the given environment.

As shown in the Figure 3.1, when the DNA sequence of the evolved bacteria is compared with that of the starting population, we note that three nucleotides have

```
Ancestor Sequence:      5' - ATGCTCGCTCGATATGCTC - 3'
Evolved Sequence:       5' - ATGGTCGCCCGATATGATC - 3'
                                ↑    ↑       ↑
```

FIGURE 3.1 Comparison of the ancestor and evolved sequence reveals mutations. As shown (indicated by arrows), the comparison of sequences identifies three mutations in the evolved sequence, in the region of the DNA shown. At position 4, nucleotide A has changed to G; at position 9, T has changed to C and at position 17, C has changed to an A.

changed (highlighted in blue). Molecular biology techniques are then used to decipher the precise role that each of these mutations plays in dictating evolutionary change.

3.2.5 Frozen Fossils

Another advantage of working with bacteria is that we can store them in deep freezers (−80°C) for an indefinite amount of time. Imagine a population which has been evolved for 2,000 generations. Should we want to directly compare the ancestral bacteria (that we started the experiment with) with the evolved ones, how do we do this? For instance, I cannot compare myself to my ancestors from 2,000 generations ago!

Such a comparison is, however, easily possible in bacterial populations. At the start of the experiment, as the population is allowed to propagate in the environment of choice, some members of the isogenic population are stored at −80°C in a freezer. These bacteria are metabolically dormant and alive at that temperature for an indefinite amount of time. To compare the evolved bacteria with the ancestral ones, we simply have to revive these metabolically dormant bacteria from the freezer into a test tube with appropriate nutrients and allow them to grow at a conducive temperature.

For example, in the *E. coli* experiment of 80,000 generations, the ancestor bacteria (from the 1980s) is routinely compared with the evolved bacteria, even after 37 years of experiments.

All these features of working with asexually reproducing organisms make them an attractive proposition to study evolution. Let us now look at why, working with sexually reproducing organisms, to study evolution is a fundamentally different task than what we have seen in the sections above.

3.3 EVOLUTION IN SEXUALLY REPRODUCING ORGANISMS

Reproduction and evolutionary change in sexually reproducing organisms are more complex than in bacteria in two separate aspects.

3.3.1 Biparental Inheritance

Note that, in bacteria, the genome of the offspring (barring errors that take place during the process of DNA replication) is identical to the genome of the parent. This is not true for species which reproduce sexually, such as us. In humans, half our DNA comes from our mother, and the other half from father. Thus, inheritance of DNA in sexually reproducing organisms is biparental (i.e., an organism's DNA

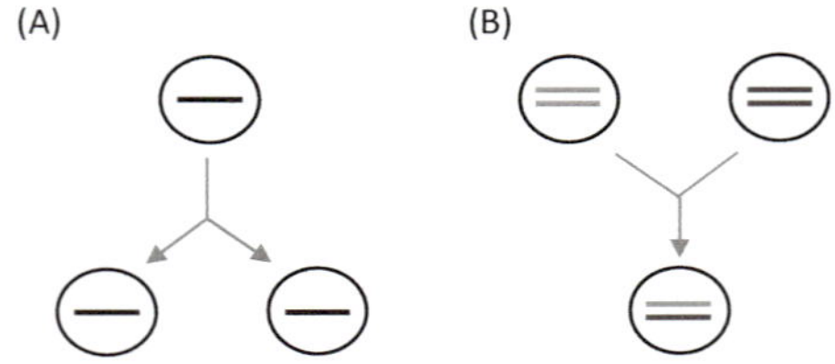

FIGURE 3.2 Asexually reproducing organisms have uniparental inheritance, and sexually reproducing organisms have biparental inheritance. (A) Bacteria divide asexually, and progeny inherit their entire DNA from a single parent. (B) Sexually reproducing organisms reproduce such that the offspring's DNA comes from two parents. Note that the offspring DNA has a 50% contribution from each parent. For simplicity, the two copies of DNA in the parent are shown as identical.

comes from two parents); compared to bacteria, where inheritance of DNA is uniparental (an organism's DNA comes from one parent) (Figure 3.2).

3.3.2 Recombination

Second, let us take a closer look at how sexually reproducing organisms inherit DNA from parents. For instance, taking myself as an example, half my DNA comes from my father. My father, in turn, has two copies of chromosome (one from his mother, and one from his father), and he passes off one copy to me. However, which copy does he pass to me?

The answer to this question is shown in Figure 3.3. At the time of production of sperm, a hybrid between the two copies that my father is carrying is generated. Another hybrid is, similarly, generated in my mother's egg. Thus, my DNA is a combination of two hybrids – acquired from my parents.

Of course, the two copies of DNA that my parents have are a combination of hybrids generated from their parents. And so on. This process of generating hybrids is called recombination. The same process happened for every other chromosome that I inherited from my parents (except chromosome Y, which I inherited without recombination, from my father, since only males carry Y chromosome).

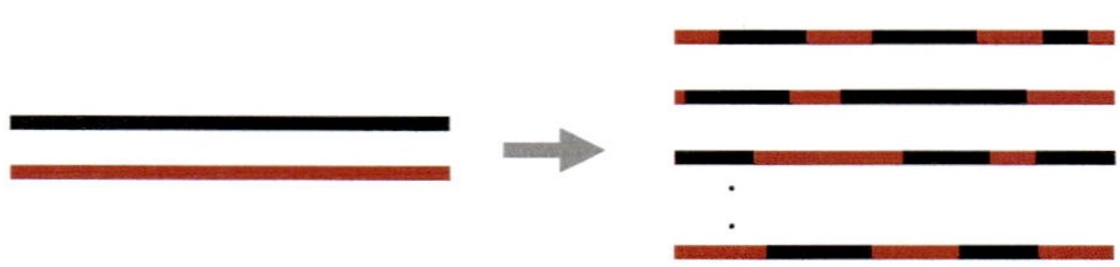

FIGURE 3.3 Recombination generates variation in sexual reproduction. An individual carries two copies of chromosome *I* (indicated by red and black). The individual only passes one copy to the offspring. Which copy is passed to the offspring? The individual generates a large number of variants of chromosome *I*, each carrying a unique combination of the two existing copies. Four such chromosome *I* are indicated in the figure. Note that each is a unique combination of the red and black copies of chromosome *I*. One such copy, randomly chosen, is passed to the offspring.

These two processes:

(a) Recombination in a parent to generate newer genotypes. For example, every sperm carries a novel hybrid of DNA and hence is genetically distinct from other sperms in the same individual.
(b) Biparental inheritance. The hybrid DNA so generated is combined with another hybrid DNA from another individual to produce an offspring.

generate diversity in sexually reproducing populations. Note that genetic diversity, in this case, is predominantly generated not by novel mutations (errors during the replication process) but by, via recombination and biparental inheritance, generating genomes which carry novel DNA sequences. Recombination means that my genetic contribution to my every progeny would be different, and biparental inheritance decides the other 50% of my progeny's DNA, irrespective of my contribution to the progeny's DNA.

3.3.3 Illinois Corn Oil Experiment

To get a sense of the genetic diversity that is generated via the process of recombination and biparental inheritance, consider the following experiment. Corn plants are grown in a field, and every year, each plant's oil content is measured. Of all the plants, only those which are among the top 10% in oil content are allowed to mate and form the next year's crop. This process is repeated every year.

From this experiment, if we are to plot oil percent (y-axis) as a function of time of experiment (in years, on x-axis), what would be our expectation from such an experiment? Figure 3.4 is a blank graph. Before moving ahead, use your intuition to sketch what you think would be a qualitative outcome of this experiment.

Before moving ahead,

➔ Sketch the graph below.

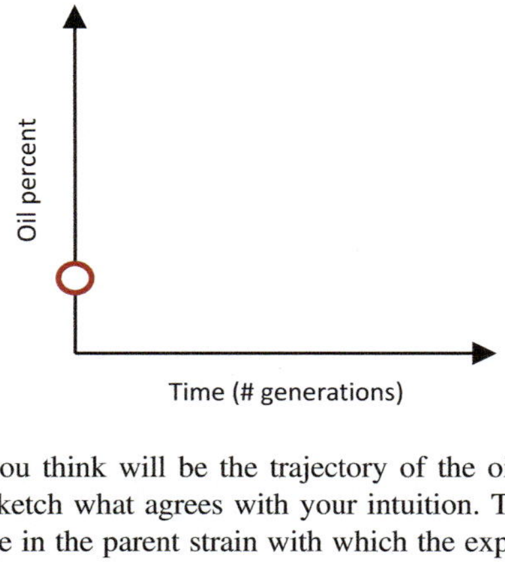

FIGURE 3.4 What do you think will be the trajectory of the oil percent as a function of number of generations? Sketch what agrees with your intuition. The red circle on the graph indicates the oil percentage in the parent strain with which the experiment was started.

Scenario I

Consider the possibility that oil content of a plant is decided by a single locus on the DNA – and in the population there are several alleles present at that particular locus. As the experiment proceeds, the allele, which corresponds to the highest oil content, is going to get selected and, therefore, will increase in frequency in the population. As a result, the other alleles will be eliminated from the population or be reduced in frequency.

Thus, evolutionary change can be measured as the rate at which allele frequency changes in the population. However, if oil content was decided by one locus only, then once every plant in the field carries the allele that corresponds to the highest oil content, further increase in oil content can only take place if a newer allele is introduced in the population, via mutation. This would mean a waiting time, when prior to the arrival of this new allele, no increase in oil content takes place. In such a scenario, the graph we imaged will appear as Figure 3.5.

Scenario II

On the other hand, consider the possibility that oil content is dictated by a hundred loci, spread through the genome. At each of these loci, let us assume there are two alleles present in the population. Let us call the alleles at the ith locus A^i and a^i. This means that three genotypes are possible at each locus (because at this locus, an individual could be any of the three genotypes A^iA^i, a^ia^i, or A^ia^i). If two different alleles exist at each of the 100 loci, then over 100 loci, 3^{100} unique genotypes are possible, as far as oil content determination is concerned. 3^{100} is an astronomical number (3^{100} is approx. 10^{47}. Compare this with the fact that the entire universe is thought to contain around 10^{80} atoms).

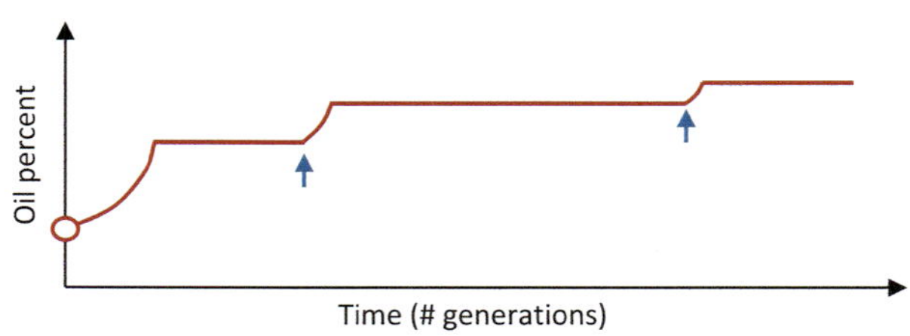

FIGURE 3.5 Oil content increases in a step-like function. The initial population has several alleles at the locus which dictates oil content. The allele which corresponds to the highest oil content is selected. After a while, indicated by *to* in the figure, all plants are carrying this allele. After this, oil content only increases when a mutation is acquired by an individual. The arrival of these mutants is indicated by blue arrows. Thereafter, the new allele spreads in the population in the subsequent generations, till every individual is carrying it. The periods between the mutations are the waiting times associated with the arrival of a new allele, which confers a higher oil content. Note that actual trajectories will have noise (e.g., due to measurement error). These trajectories are indicated as straight lines for clarity.

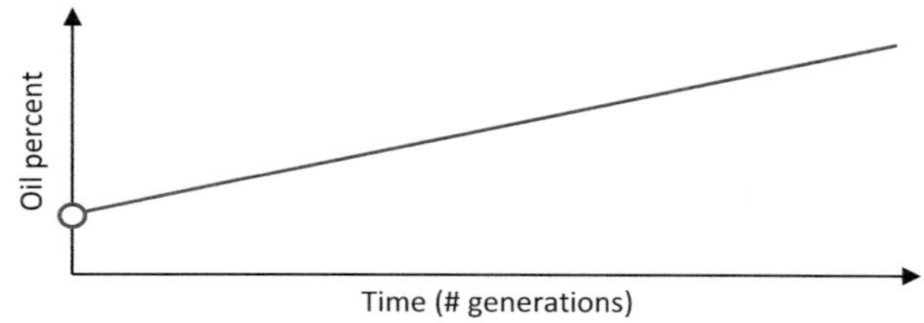

FIGURE 3.6 Recombination improves oil percentage as a (roughly) linear increase. If oil content was dictated by hundreds of loci spread in different parts of the plant genome, and each locus contained several alleles, recombination would keep generating newer allele combinations corresponding to higher oil content. In such a scenario, increase in oil content is because of variation generated by recombination (and not new mutations). Note that the actual trajectory will have noise (e.g., measurement error). The trajectory is shown as a straight line for clarity.

Thus, recombination and biparental inheritance will keep generating newer combinations and genotypes every generation, but still only be able to scan an extremely small fraction of this total number of possible genotypes. Thus, recombination and biparental inheritance can create genetic diversity for an extended amount of time, and natural selection can act on the diversity thus generated. Thus, in our experiment, oil content will continue to increase in every generation as these two forces create newer genotypes. The trajectory of oil content with time of experiment will, in this case, be a more or less linear increase (Figure 3.6).

Example 3.3: Which of the two scenarios looks more realistic to you, as far as the corn oil experiment is concerned? Before you read ahead, think about this question and write a short paragraph on why you think one scenario is more appealing than the other.

Solution: The experiment described above is being carried out since 1896 in the University of Illinois at Urbana Champaign, USA. A sketch of how the oil content has actually changed with time is very similar to what we discuss in Scenario II. The data has two clear trends. First, the oil content is constantly increasing. This means that there are newer genotypes constantly being created which have oil content higher than the parental generation. This genetic diversity is being achieved via recombination and biparental inheritance. Second, there is no time during the course of the experiment when the oil content was constant with time. This lack of waiting time for increase in oil content suggests that the increase is not due to newer mutations (also see item [2] in Bibliography).

3.3.4 Evolution as Change in Allele Frequency

Just as we measure evolutionary change as the new mutations that arise in the population in sexually reproducing organisms, evolutionary change can be measured by change in frequency of an allele. For example, if there is a locus with two alleles *A* and *a*. Allele *A* corresponds to high oil content and allele *a* corresponds to low oil content. If at the start of the experiment, half the population had a genotype *aa* and the other half *AA*, then the allele frequency of *a* was 0.5, and that of *A* was also 0.5 – both were present in equal amounts in the population. However, as the experiment proceeds, we would expect that the frequency of allele *A* increases, and that of allele *a* decreases. This change in allele frequency (at one locus or several loci) can be quantified as evolutionary change.

Example 3.4: A drosophila population was started where half the population was genotype *AA* and the remaining half was *Aa*. After 30 generations, it was found that 10% of the population was *AA*, 30% of the population was *Aa*, and 60% of the population was *aa*. What is the frequency of the two alleles at the beginning and after 30 generations of the experiment?

Solution: Imagine a population size of 100. Then, at the start of the experiment, 50 individuals were genotype *AA*. These individuals carried 100 copies of the *A* allele. The other half, 50 individuals, carried one copy of *A* allele. Hence, total number of *A* alleles at the start of the experiment was 150. The total number of *a* allele at start of experiment was 50. Thus, allele frequency of *A* at the start was 0.75 (150/200), and that of *a* was 0.25.

After 30 generations, the number of *A* alleles was 50 ($2 \times 10 + 1 \times 30$), and that of *a* allele was 150 ($1 \times 30 + 60 \times 2$). Thus, allele frequency of *A*, at the end of the experiment, was 0.25 (50/200) and that of *a* was 0.75.

Thus, over a period of 30 generations, allele frequencies changed significantly. That's evolutionary change.

3.3.5 Number of New Mutations Depends on Population Size

The above discussion is not to say that new mutations do not happen in sexually reproducing organisms, or that they are not relevant for their evolution. Genetic diversity, generated via any mechanism, is very relevant for evolutionary change. But the molecular mechanisms of recombination and mutation mean that most of diversity generated in sexually reproducing organisms is via recombination and because of biparental inheritance. And hence, over the course of short term (~100 generations), recombination is going to be the more relevant mechanism for generating diversity.

What adds weight to this argument is the fact that the newer mutations are more likely if the population size is large. A flask with *E. coli* growing in 100 ml rich media contains 10^{11} cells. On the other hand, the entire human population of human beings on the planet is ~10^{10}.

3.3.6 Natural Selection in Nature

The oil experiment described above corresponds to artificial selection. By artificial selection, we mean that the selection pressure was imposed by humans, and was not necessarily imposed by the natural habitat. That is, the design that only plants with high oil content propagate to the next generation is an artificial selection imposed by the experimenter. As against this, natural selection's results can also be seen in wild populations, which are under purely ecological pressure.

A few years ago, scientists studied the coat color of mice in Nebraska, USA. The terrain in the question was largely light colored, and was formed a few thousand years ago. This light-colored terrain is surrounded by dark soil. In such an environment, what would be the coat color of the mice inhabiting this area? The coat color of the mice living in the two conditions can be linked with natural selection quite easily. You can imagine that against a light-colored background, the light color mice would camouflage better. On the other hand, against a dark background, mice with a darker coat would camouflage better. The camouflage would provide the mice protection against predators, as they would be harder to detect against the background.

This is exactly what was observed. Scientists noted that the mice inhabiting the light terrain have light-colored coat, while those living in dark soil areas have a darker coat. Scientists were also able to pin down the change in the coat color to the change in DNA and protein sequence (see chapter reference list).

Before moving ahead,

➔ Is this by chance? Or has selection played any role in this choice? What do you think? Do you see a similarity between this example and one with moths in 18th-century England?

Similar to the example above, mice living on a Florida beach and inland have different coat color, and the coat color in each region matches the background color.

A number of other such examples are also known from around the world. Thus, we can be confident in saying that it is not by chance that the coat color matches the color of the surroundings. There appears to be selection going on for a long period of time, and being camouflaged against the background color provides an individual greater fitness.

It is now known that many loci are involved in determining the coat color. Each locus in turn can have many alleles in the population. Assuming that these alleles function in an additive manner, one can, in principle, generate a wide variety of coat color. This raises a number of questions for us to consider. For example,

- What was the color of mice living in each terrain?
- What were the frequencies of the different alleles in this population?
- What will happen if we try to replace the mice from one terrain to the other?
- If selection is the driving force, then over a period of time the population of mice with compatible color would populate the region. Suppose we were given the initial equilibrium allele frequency in the two populations of mice, can we predict how fast will these alleles' frequency, and consequently, the mean phenotype of the population, change?

All these are questions that population geneticists studying evolution of sexual reproduction study and try to decipher. Note the additional complexities associated with the study of sexual reproducing organisms compared to asexual populations. This makes our choice of model organisms to study evolution crucial.

3.3.7 Heterozygosity

Before we move ahead in our analysis, we should acknowledge one more factor which makes studying evolutionary change in sexually reproducing organisms much more challenging than in asexually reproducing populations. Since inheritance of DNA is biparental, it is quite likely that the genotype of the offspring at a particular locus is such that a unique allele is inherited from each of the two parents. Imagine a scenario where one parent had a genotype *AA* at a particular locus, the other parent had a genotype *aa*. In such a case, the genotype of the offspring will be *Aa*.

Let us consider the case that the locus in question controls a quantitative trait. If a genotype *AA* corresponds to a trait value 1, and genotype *aa* corresponds to trait value 0.5, then what does the genotype *Aa* correspond to? The answer to this question depends on the relationship between the alleles *A* and *a* is concerned, with respect to the phenotype in question.

For instance, if, phenotype of *Aa* is,

- equal to that of *AA*: *A* is completely dominant over *a*,
- greater than 0.75 but less than 1: *A* partially dominant over *a*,
- equal to 0.75: No dominance relationship between *A* and *a*,
- greater than 0.5 but less than 0.75: *a* is partially dominant over *A*,
- equal to that of *aa*: *a* is completely dominant over *A*, and
- greater than 1: Case of overdominance.

It is difficult to a priori comment on the dominance relationships that two alleles at a particular locus might share. Moreover, alleles at every locus will have a unique dominance relationship. Hence, study of evolution in sexually reproducing organisms becomes that much more challenging.

3.4 OUR CHOICE OF MODEL SYSTEM

Given the above discussion, we have a choice to make at this point. Do we study evolution of a microbial population; or a sexually reproducing population? Studying each requires a different set of tools, approaches, and intuition. Several excellent texts already exist which study evolution from the context of sexually reproducing organisms. This study area is referred to as population genetics.

Going forward, we will consider evolution in microbial populations in this book. It is important to note that while the fundamental principles of evolution remain the same, our choice of model system dictates which factors are likely to be more relevant than the others in dictating evolutionary change. In turn, that decides what are going to be the relevant tools, analysis, and experimental techniques relevant for us.

3.5 CONCLUSION

It is clear from the discussion we have had thus far, a population is always evolving and, as a consequence, the environment does not remain static either. Thus, the population goes through evolutionary changes in a dynamic fashion, albeit imperceptibly, because the timescales of such a change is too long for us to observe. If we have to capture such a dynamic process that has occurred for millions of years, we need to develop new theories and test them by doing experiments either in a laboratory setting or in a more natural setting. Of course, the other option is to observe as Darwin observed and then see whether the predictions made from such observation is compatible with theory. This process has to go through many iterations before we can understand the underlying features of an evolutionary process. Darwin's theory of natural selection was quantified into mathematical equations roughly 60 years after the publication of the *Origin of Species*. Darwin himself was not proficient in mathematics, but realized the importance of mathematical analysis in evolutionary processes. He remarked,

> *I attempted mathematics··· but I got on very slowly···. I have deeply regretted that I did not proceed far enough at least to understand something of the great leading principles of mathematics; for men thus endowed seem to have an extra sense.*

In fact, mathematical descriptions of processes and phenomenon can lead us to insights, which simple experiments cannot. Under the correct assumptions, mathematical analysis can lead us to capture trends and help us design experiments to prove/disprove ideas. Along with mathematical representations of ideas, we must also discuss geometric/graphical representations of ideas. Thinking about biological/ evolutionary processes in a graphical manner, clears concepts and helps develop an intuitive understanding of the underlying fundamentals.

In principle, the time evolution of an inanimate system is no different than the time evolution of a biological system. Just as the ideal gas law links Pressure, Volume, number of moles, and Temperature via a mathematical relationship, we aspire to develop the same quantitative framework to study evolution. Darwin's theory of natural selection only tells us that allele frequency will increase or decrease depending upon the selection. But from Darwin's qualitative descriptions, it is impossible to predict the rate of such evolutionary change.

But the problem we are trying to tackle here is much more complex than the analogy of ideal gas law given above. This is largely because of the role chance plays in dictating evolutionary outcomes. Ideal gas law is also dictated by chance events (like collisions between molecules) but because the number of participating molecules is very large (remember a mole of a gas has ~10^{23} molecules), the chance events get averaged out. When number of participating players/molecules is small, chance events are much more relevant, as we will see.

Consider a coin toss. We know that the coin lands on Heads with a probability 0.5, but for each coin toss, we cannot say with certainty whether it will land on Heads or Tails. Thus, a coin toss is an example of a process whose fate is dictated by chance. Such a process, whose outcome cannot be said as a certainty a priori, is said to be a stochastic process. Chance events play an important role in dictating evolutionary processes. For example, which one of two alleles, at a locus, I inherit from my father is dictated by chance. Hence, the prediction of the future population structure cannot be made with deterministic approach, as discussed above for the ideal gas.

In this book, using simple algebra, we develop quantitative relationships which can provide us with some insights into how evolutionary change takes place.

EXERCISES

1. What is the average number of nucleotide positions by which you and a stranger in your city differ? Does this number surprise you?
2. From our discussion of the Illinois corn oil experiment, it seems that the oil content is a trait which is dictated by hundreds (if not more) loci on the genome. How many loci in humans dictate height of an individual?
3. The corn oil experiment, because of involvement of a large number of loci, shows gradual increase in oil content every generation. Why did Mendel not see this gradual change in height in his pea plant experiment? We are told that Mendel saw short and long plants only.
4. A population has the following structure at a locus *i*. Forty percent individuals are genotype *AA*, 25% are genotype *Aa*, and the remaining are *aa*. What is the frequency of allele *A* in the population?
5. Suppose in the population, all individuals of the genotype *aa* migrate to another location. What is the frequency of the allele *A* in the remaining population?
6. After such a migration, what are the possible implications for the population left behind?

BIBLIOGRAPHY

1. Endersby J. 2007. *A Guinea Pig's History of Biology: The animals and plants that taught us the facts of life*. William Heinemann.
   (Our knowledge of biological systems stems from a handful of model systems. In fact, we have no idea how to work with most organisms. How are these model systems chosen? In this entertaining book, Endersby discusses how certain organisms ended up being model systems, and how work on them has enhanced our understanding about them and biology in general.)
2. Anonymous. 2025. Illinois Long-term Selection Experiment Accessed 25-05-25.
   (The Illinois corn oil experiment is more than 125 years old. Its history is available at this link: http://mooselab.cropsci.illinois.edu/longterm.html.)
3. Barrett RDH, Laurent S, Mallarino R, Pfeifer SP, Xu CCY, Foll M, Wakamatsu K, Duke-Cohan JS, Jensen JD, Hoekstra HE. 2019. Linking a mutation to survival in wild mice. *Science* 363:499–504.
   (This paper describes the mouse coat color study done in Nebraska, US.)

4 Growth Models

4.1 INTRODUCTION

A key aspect of evolution is that mutations happen as bacteria divide. Thus, growth or cell division is an important aspect that enables evolution of species. Once a mutation happens, it influences the genotype and the resulting phenotypes of the organism. The fundamental phenotype of importance in evolutionary biology, from the context of microbes, is growth rate. Or, how fast goes a bacterium carrying a particular genotype divide.

In this chapter, we will study some fundamental models to represent microbial growth quantitatively. *Escherichia coli* (or *E. coli*) has been a workhorse to study microbial physiology in thousands of laboratories across the world. Hence, it is the bacteria about which we know the most! Hence, we will consider many aspects of microbial physiology and evolution, while putting into practice lessons from *E. coli*. However, focusing on *E. coli* does, in no way, diminish the generality of the principles we discuss. Our conclusions and results from the discussions in this and subsequent chapters will be equally applicable to all microbial species.

Before we begin, let us get an intuition about a bacterium *E. coli*. These intuitions or quantitative understanding of *E. coli* is also going to be true for most other microbes. When we develop these numbers, we are only interested in order-of-magnitude estimates.

4.2 *E. COLI*

4.2.1 Size

How large is *E. coli*? *E. coli* is a rod-shaped bacterium which is about 2–3 μm in length, and 1 μm in width. Which means that if you line up around 300–500 *E. coli* cells end-to-end, their combined length will be 1 mm. The diversity in the morphology of bacterial species that exist on the planet is huge, and many exceptions exist (in biology, exceptions always exist!). For example, in 2022, a report in *Science* described a bacterial species *Candidatus* (*Ca.*) *Thiomargarita magnifica*, which has cells of size 9,000 μm! The individual bacteria of this species are of the size which is visible to the naked eye. Nevertheless, most bacterial species are of this approximate size, and 1 μm (remember, we are interested in order of magnitude estimate) is a good approximation for the size of a bacterium.

4.2.2 Weight

How much does an *E. coli* weigh? That sounds like a very abstract question, and something that seems impossible to solve without knowing more about the bacterium. However, note that, in biology, when we ask a question such as this, we are

DOI: 10.1201/9781003633662-4

often only interested in an order of magnitude estimate of the quantity at hand (a bacterium's mass, in this case). So, how would we approach this question? We already know the bacterium's size, and hence, its volume (~20 μm^3, simply using the formula for volume of a cylinder, given its radius and height).

We also know that complex organisms have density not too different from that of water (we learned in school that 70% of human body mass is water; in the case of watermelon, the figure is 95%). Hence, it seems like a fair estimate that the density of a living being or cells in general is not too different from that of water. Hence, to a first approximation, if we assume that *E. coli*'s density is close to that of water, then a single cell of *E. coli* weighs, to an order of magnitude approximation, ~10^{-15} kg.

4.2.3 Cell Division

E. coli divides by growing to a certain size, and then splitting through the middle into two cells. It is critical that during cell division, the DNA of the organism (which is circular in *E. coli*'s case) is copied and each of the two progeny receives one copy each. The rest of the cellular contents (RNA Polymerases, Ribosomes, all other proteins, mRNAs etc.) are divided randomly among the two progenies. Since division takes place roughly along the center of the cell's length, each progeny receives roughly half the cellular contents.

With these broad estimates of a few aspects of *E. coli*'s physiology, let us move ahead and develop growth models of bacteria in a variety of contexts (see Note 1).

4.3 GROWTH IN A BATCH CULTURE

In a batch culture, no material exchange takes place with the surroundings. That is, no member of the population leaves the culture environment, nor does any material exchange take place with the environment. Such conditions are mimicked in a test tube or a flask in a laboratory environment (Figure 4.1). We will begin by developing some quantitative models to capture growth in such batch conditions.

4.3.1 Exponential Growth in a Flask

Imagine a single *E. coli* in a flask containing 100 ml nutrient media. In this media composition, when grown at 37 deg C, *E. coli* divides every 30 minutes. Thus, after 30 minutes, there will be two bacteria in the flask; and after one hour, there would be four. Using this logic, we can keep track of the number of bacteria with time. We can plot the number of bacteria with time, and get an exponential curve as shown in Figure 4.1.

Before moving ahead,

➔ In the figure above, we assume that bacteria divide like clockwork, where cell division takes place exactly every 30 minutes. Is this what you expect to happen in an actual test tube? Or, you would expect some cells to divide faster and some slower than 30 minutes – averaging to 30 minutes? What does your intuition tell about what would the actual cell division statistics look like, for a real culture?

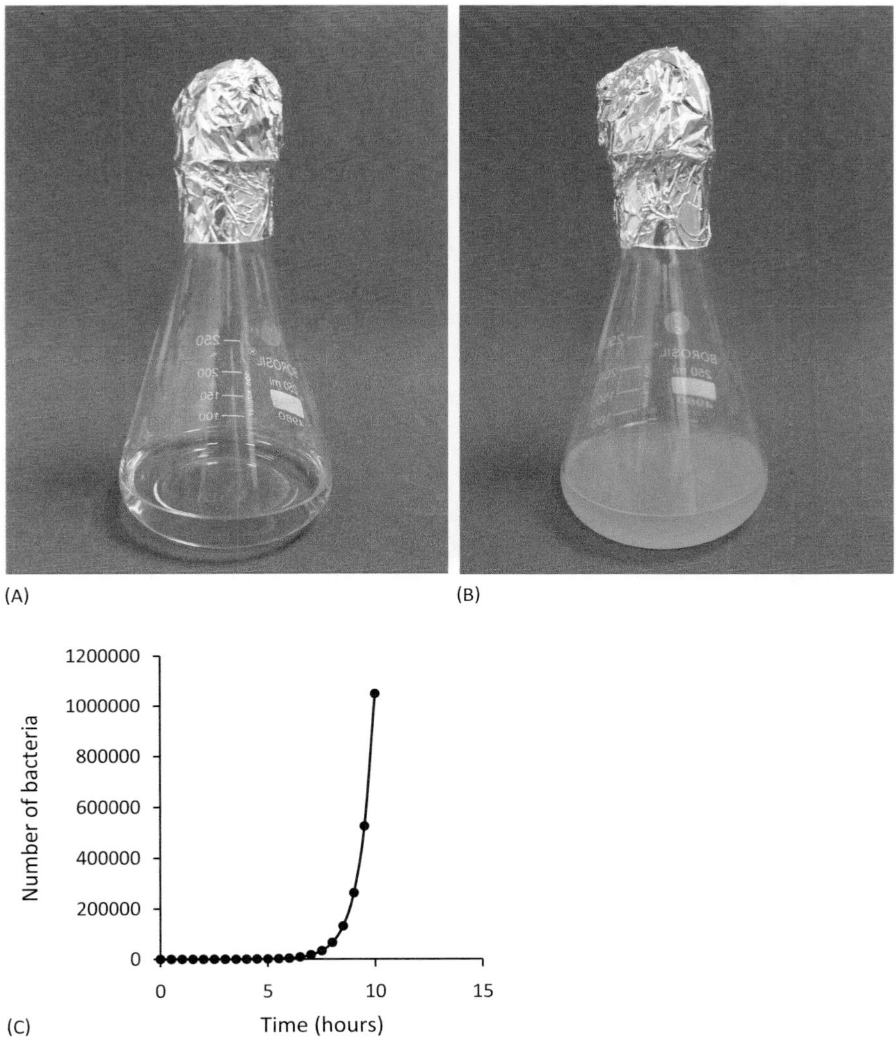

FIGURE 4.1 Growth profile of a bacterial population in a batch culture. (A) A flask containing fresh culture media is seeded with a few bacteria. Note that the culture media is transparent. (B) After 24 hours of growth, the culture media becomes turbid due to bacterial growth. (C) Starting a culture with a single bacterium in a test tube, we can track the number of bacteria in the tube. In this case, if bacteria undergo cell division every 30 minutes, after 10 hours of growth, the bacterial count in the tube will be about 1 million.

In other words, we can quantify the growth dynamics as,

$$N_{t+1} = 2\,N_t \tag{4.1}$$

This equation can be modified slightly to represent exponential growth as the following equation,

$$\frac{dN}{dt} = rN \tag{4.2}$$

For our purposes, we will treat both the above representations as qualitatively same.

Where, N_t is the number of bacteria in the flask after t rounds of division, and N_{t+1} is the number of bacteria in the flask after $t + 1$ rounds of division.

However, a closer scrutiny of the graph shows that there is a serious flaw in measuring bacteria count in this fashion. This is illustrated in the next example.

Example 4.1: In a flask with 100 ml liquid media, what would be the mass of the bacteria after two days of growth according to the model represented by equation (4.1)?

Solution: After 2 days (or 48 hours) of growth, there would have been 96 rounds of division. Which means, the number of bacteria in the flask media, using our method, would be around 2^{96} (this is about 10^{28}).

But we should note that since we know that each bacterium weighs about 10^{-15} kg, the mass of the bacteria after 48 hours, as predicted by our model, would be 10^{13} kg ($10^{28} \times 10^{-15}$)!

It should strike you that 100 ml media should weigh roughly 100 grams (using the approximation that the media is largely water, at least at the level of order of magnitude). Thus, growth in 100 grams of media cannot lead to bacterial mass of 10^{13} kg. Moreover, after growth for two days, we are quite easily able to lift the flask with our hand – which would hardly be possible, if the flask weighed 10^{13} kgs!

Thus, clearly, our analysis went wrong somewhere. What did we do wrong?

The problem with the analysis is that we assumed that the bacteria were going to keep dividing every 30 minutes through the course of two days. In the beginning of our experiment, that is indeed what will happen. The single bacterium divides in 30 minutes. The resulting two bacteria divide 30 minutes after that. This phase of growth is referred to as exponential phase of growth. However, as the bacterial count in the flask increases, the nutrients in the flask are being consumed. After a few rounds of division, there will not be sufficient nutrients left in the flask to support exponential growth. At such a time, growth halts, and the number of bacteria in the flask does not change with time. This phase of growth is referred to as stationary phase of growth.

Therefore, while our model says that bacteria keep dividing every 30 minutes, in a real flask culture, that would not be the case for an extended period of time. Growth would slow down because of (a) increased competition for resources, (b) the nutrient concentration decreasing with time, (c) cellular waste products secreted into the media. This growth to the bacterial count in the flask would grind to a halt in the stationary phase.

Thus, we need to adjust our model to accommodate the fact that exponential growth slows down rapidly in a test tube. To incorporate this aspect of growth dynamics in a flask (batch culture), we can tweak our model to build the logistic model, as we discuss next.

4.3.2 Logistic Equation

In this model, we represent growth rate as product of two terms, as shown below,

$$\frac{dN}{dt} = rN\left(1 - \frac{N}{K}\right) \tag{4.3}$$

where,

> N is the number of bacteria at time t, r is the growth rate when the nutrients are not limited (i.e., at the beginning of the experiment), and K is the carrying capacity of the flask. By carrying capacity, we mean the total number of bacteria that the flask can support growth of, given the amount of resources present in it. This equation is simulated for a parameter set and the resulting growth trajectory is shown in Figure 4.2.

We know from experiments that K, for a 10 ml culture volume, in rich media, is of the order of 10^{10} for *E. coli* (see Notes II and III). Thus, at the start of the experiment, the second term on the right-hand side of equation (4.2) $\left(1 - \frac{N}{K}\right)$ is nearly one (as $N \sim 1$ and $K \sim 10^{10}$). Thus, $\frac{dN}{dt} \sim rN$ in this regime. However, as the bacterial count N begins to increase in the flask, $\left(1 - \frac{N}{K}\right)$ is no longer close to one. In fact, as N increases, $\left(1 - \frac{N}{K}\right)$ decreases, and is a number between 0 and 1. This means that the growth rate is no longer $\sim r$ but is smaller than that. As N increases, the effective growth rate keeps decreasing. Eventually, when the population in the flask reaches carrying capacity, i.e., $N = K$, $\frac{dN}{dt} = 0$. Which means, the bacterial count N does not change with time, and growth rate is zero. Equation (4.3) is known as the logistic equation and can be used to represent the growth dynamics in a batch culture.

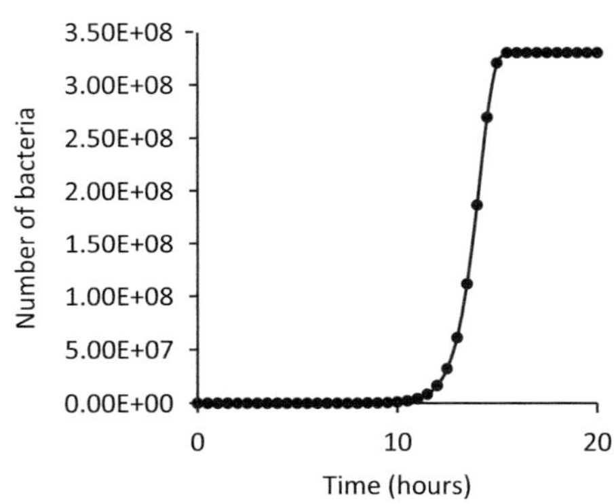

FIGURE 4.2 Bacterial growth model according to the logistic equation. The carrying capacity of the flask in the equation (4.2), K, is set to 10^9. As a result, the number of bacteria increases and then saturates at K.

4.3.3 Competition between Two Genotypes in a Batch Culture

Imagine that we start a bacterial culture with two different genotypes. Bacteria with genotype A have a growth rate r_1 and those with genotype B have a growth rate r_2. Let us also imagine that $r_2 > r_1$. If at the start of the experiment, the flask has an equal number of bacteria with genotypes A and B, what would be the numbers of the two genotypes when the population reaches the carrying capacity of the flask?

Before we develop a quantitative solution for this problem, let us first try and understand what will happen in the flask. Since $r_2 > r_1$, the individuals with genotype B divide faster than those with genotype A. This implies that despite starting with an equal number of individuals with genotypes A and B, soon, the culture flask will contain more individuals of genotype B than those of genotype A. Since the environment (culture flask) can only support a total of K number of individuals, growth continues till the combined number of individuals with genotypes A and B reaches K.

Mathematically, this idea can be quantified using the following differential equations,

$$\frac{dN_A}{dt} = r_1 N_A \left(1 - \frac{N_A + N_B}{K}\right) \tag{4.4}$$

$$\frac{dN_B}{dt} = r_2 N_B \left(1 - \frac{N_A + N_B}{K}\right) \tag{4.5}$$

Given that, at the start of the experiment, $N_A = N_0$ and $N_B = N_0$. A solution to equations (4.4) and (4.5) is shown in Figure 4.3.

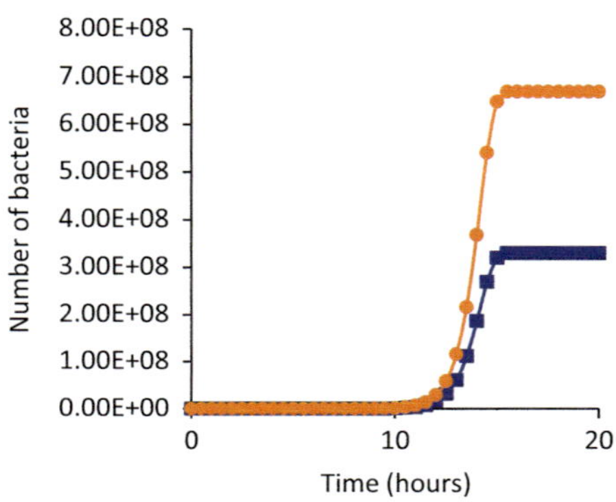

FIGURE 4.3 Bacterial growth model according to the logistic equation, when two strains are co-cultured in the same growth. In the figure, strain 1 (blue, squares) has a growth rate of 2 hour^{-1}, and strain 2 (orange, circles) has a growth rate of 2.1 hour^{-1}. Note that despite the difference in growth rate of the two strains being 5%, the number of cells of the two genotypes differ by a factor of two, when the carrying capacity of the strains is reached. In the simulation above, at t equal to zero, starting number of cells of each type was equal to one.

By extension of the logic in equations (4.4) and (4.5), we can examine how the relative ratios of the number of individuals with any number of genotypes changes in a batch culture in a test tube or a flask.

4.4 CHEMOSTAT

Batch cultures are convenient (growing bacteria in a test tube is easy!) and are often used in laboratory conditions. However, ecologically relevant niches are rarely batch-like.

Let us revisit the flask experiment and examine the growth conditions more carefully. In this growth set-up, once the experiment (growth) starts, no material exchange takes place with the environment. No individual of the population exits the environment, nor does a foreign individual enter the system. Similarly, no resources leave or enter the system once growth starts. This is a very unnatural condition for examination of growth (of bacteria or any other species).

Let us examine an ecological niche within our bodies where trillions of bacteria reside – our intestines. Every day, we take in resources (food), which reach the intestines. Among other things, a part of these nutrients is consumed by the bacteria in the intestine to grow in numbers. The waste products of the bacteria, indigestible constituents of our food, and bacteria themselves are also shed regularly from our intestines to the outside environment.

Thus, our intestines represent a system where material and bacteria are exchanged with the environment at regular intervals. Nutrients (and occasionally bacteria too!) are supplied to the 'flask' (intestine) regularly, and waste (which includes secretions of cells, undigested food, and also bacteria) are removed from the system regularly. If we examine carefully, most niches in an ecological setting resemble the intestinal example much more closely, as compared to the batch culture flask example.

Also note that over a long time, the number of bacteria in the intestine of an adult stays constant. This implies that the number of cell divisions taking place in the intestine must be equal to the number of bacteria shed from the intestines. If this balance is not maintained, then the number of bacteria in the intestine must increase or decrease with time. Hence, for steady-state operation of the intestine, bacterial growth has to be balanced by their exit via excretion.

In a laboratory setting, we mimic systems such as the intestine using a chemostat (Figure 4.4).

In a chemostat, growth is supported in a chamber of fixed volume V. However, contrary to the batch flask example, fresh media is constantly supplied to the chemostat at a rate v_o time^{-1}. The inlet stream contains no bacteria. To ensure that the total volume of the liquid does not exceed V, spent media is removed from the chemostat at the rate v_o time^{-1}. Note that the spent media contains: (a) unused nutrients in the chemostat, (b) chemicals/metabolites secreted by the cells during growth in the chemostat, and (c) bacteria present in the chemostat.

You should be able to draw an analogy between the intestinal example and that of the chemostat – they are virtually the same. Most niches on the planet, which support life, are chemostats of some sort. Thus, chemostats are an excellent tool to study evolution in real time (we will study more about this in the Chapter 12).

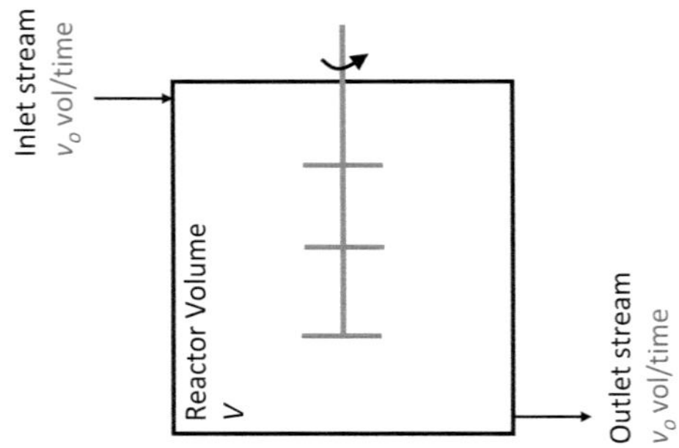

FIGURE 4.4 A chemostat to monitor growth and evolution of a microbial population. Liquid with fresh media is fed into the reactor at rate v_o vol/time. Spent media, which contains unused nutrients, waste, and cells, is removed from the reactor at v_o vol/time. The total reactor volume is V. The reactor is stirred continuously to ensure that the contents of the reactor are homogeneous with respect to space.

Suppose we have two genotypes (A and B) with growth rates r_1 and r_2, respectively, coexisting in a chemostat. Suppose we seed the chemostat with ten bacteria of each of the two genotypes. Both start dividing in the chemostat, and while this is happening, the inlet stream is supplying fresh resources, while the exit stream is taking out spent resources, unused resources, and also some of the bacteria in the chemostat.

However, when the culture density in the chemostat is dilute, addition of bacteria to the chemostat via cell division (which depends on the resources available) is faster than the rate of removal of the bacteria from the chemostat (which depends on the density of the culture). Thus, the number of bacteria in the chemostat increases with time. This continues till we reach a state where the density of bacteria is so high such that the rate of addition in bacterial numbers (because of cell division) is exactly balanced by the number of bacteria removed from the chemostat via the exit stream. This is the equilibrium setting of the chemostat.

4.4.1 Competition of Two Strains in a Chemostat

Imagine that the chemostat is operating at its full capacity and that individuals of both genotypes are present in equal numbers. Thus, the starting frequencies of the two genotypes are 0.5 each. That is, 50% of the bacteria are of one genotype, and the remaining 50% of the other. How do these frequencies change with time?

As in the case of the batch culture, let us first try and understand intuitively the growth dynamics in the chemostat. Once we develop that intuition, we will develop the quantitative framework for the same. As we saw above, at steady state, the rate of removal of bacteria from the exit stream of the chemostat is exactly balanced by the rate of generation of bacteria via cell division in the chemostat.

In our case, when we start with an equal number of A and B type bacteria – the exit stream will contain equal numbers of A and B. At any given point in time, any individual bacteria is equally likely to be washed away from the chemostat. Since,

A and B have equal numbers – statistically speaking, each type of bacteria will have an equal number washed away.

On the other hand, the rate of generation of bacteria in the chemostat depends on the growth rate of the individual genotypes. In our example, genotype B will increase in numbers faster than the genotype A.

When we combine our thoughts from the above two paragraphs, we get the following: genotypes A and B are being removed from the chemostat at the same rate, and genotype B is being generated faster than genotype A. As a result, the frequency of genotype B individuals increases and that of genotype A individuals decreases with time.

That is, the higher fitness genotype (genotype B) replaces the lower fitness genotype (genotype A) in the chemostat.

Let us now quantify this idea,

The rate of change of the two genotypes can be represented as,

$$\frac{dN_1}{dt} = r_1 N_1 - \text{Ø} N_1 \tag{4.6}$$

where the first term on the right-hand side of equation (4.6) represents the division of A type genotype individuals, and the second term on the right represents the rate at which genotype A individuals exit the chemostat. In this equation, Φ is the proportionality constant, which we do not know at this point. Let us try and figure this out.

Similarly, growth of genotype B in the chemostat can be represented by,

$$\frac{dN_2}{dt} = r_2 N_2 - \text{Ø} N_2 \tag{4.7}$$

In addition, since the chemostat is operating at steady state, the number of individuals in the chemostat is fixed with time, we have the following,

$$N_1 + N_2 = K \tag{4.8}$$

Where, K is the carrying capacity of the chemostat. If we divide equations (4.6) and (4.7) by K, we get,

$$\frac{dx_1}{dt} = r_1 x_1 - \text{Ø} x_1 \tag{4.9}$$

and

$$\frac{dx_2}{dt} = r_2 x_2 - \text{Ø} x_2 \tag{4.10}$$

where x_1 is the fraction of all individuals which are genotype A $\left(x_1 = \frac{N_1}{N_1 + N_2}\right)$, and x_2 is the fraction of all individuals which are genotype B $\left(x_2 = \frac{N_2}{N_1 + N_2}\right)$. This implies, $x_1 + x_2 = 1$.

To find the expression for Ø, let us add equations (4.8) and (4.9), we get the LHS as,

$$\frac{d\,(x_1 + x_2)}{dt} = \frac{d(1)}{dt} = 0 \tag{4.11}$$

The RHS of addition of (4.8) and (4.9) we get,

$$(r_1x_1 + r_2x_2) - Ø\,(x_1 + x_2) = (r_1x_1 + r_2x_2) - Ø \tag{4.12}$$

When we equate (4.10) and (4.11), we get,

$$Ø = (r_1x_1 + r_2x_2) \tag{4.13}$$

Example 4.2: A culture consists of two genotypes, A and B, in equal frequency. The two strains, A and B, have fitness 1.1 h^{-1} and 1.3^{-1}, respectively. What is the mean fitness of the culture?

Solution: Since the two strains are in equal frequency, the fraction of each strain is 0.5. Thus, the mean fitness of the culture, Ø is

$$Ø = 1.1\,x\,0.5 + 1.3\,x\,0.5 = 1.2\,h^{-1}$$

Example 4.3: A culture consists of three strains, A, B, and C, with frequencies 1:1:3. The fitness of the three strains are 1 h^{-1}, 1.2 h^{-1}, and 1.4 h^{-1}. What is the mean fitness of the culture?

Solution: The frequency of the three strains, A, B, and C, are $\frac{1}{1+1+3}$; $\frac{1}{1+1+3}$; $\frac{3}{1+1+3}$. Thus, the frequency of A is 0.2, B is 0.2, and C is 0.6. Thus, the mean fitness of the culture, Ø is

$$Ø = 1\,x\,0.2 + 1.2\,x\,0.2 + 1.4\,x\,0.6 = 1.28\,h^{-1}$$

Thus, now that we have found a quantitative expression for Ø. What does equation (4.13) mean? The quantity Ø, equation (4.13) tells us, represents the mean fitness of the culture in the chemostat, which is calculated by taking a weighted average of the two strains, where weights are the frequency of each genotype.

If we replace this expression for Ø in equation (4.6), we get,

$$\frac{dx_1}{dt} = [r_1 - (r_1x_1 + r_2x_2)]\,x_1 \tag{4.14}$$

On the right-hand side of the equation (4.14), x_1 is frequency and hence, is always greater than zero. It is always positive. Notice the term in the bracket. It represents the difference between the fitness of genotype A and the mean fitness of the chemostat culture. Thus, the term in the bracket can be positive or negative. If this term is positive, it means that $\frac{dx_1}{dt} > 0$ and hence, as time increases x_1 increases.

On the other hand, if the term in the bracket is negative, then $\frac{dx_1}{dt} < 0$ and hence, as time increases, x_1 decreases. The frequency of the three strains, A, B, and C are 1/(1 + 1 + 3), 1/(1 + 1 + 3), 3/(1 + 1 + 3). Thus, the frequency of A is 0.2, B is 0.2, and C is 0.6.

Equation (4.14) also means that the larger the advantage of genotype A over the mean fitness of the chemostat culture, the faster the rate at which its frequency increases. On the other hand, if the fitness of genotype A is lesser than the mean fitness of the chemostat culture, $\frac{dx_1}{dt} < 0$, i.e., the frequency of genotype A decreases with time.

Thus, if we solve (4.9) and (4.10) together, we will note the dynamics via which the fitter genotype (the one with higher growth rate) replaces the genotype with lesser fitness (Figure 4.5).

Depending on the context, we will keep using one of the two formulations discussed above – batch growth or chemostat. It is easy to imagine how an evolution experiment can be done using a chemostat. We seed the chemostat with bacterial one/more bacterial strains, and let the system develop, with inlet and outlet streams. These streams can continue for an indefinite amount of time, and hence, we can monitor the system for any duration of time we like.

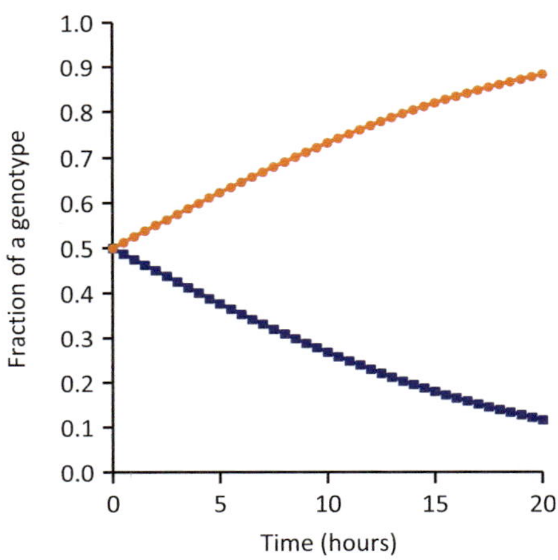

FIGURE 4.5 Change in frequency of the two genotypes in a chemostat with time. Starting with an equal number of the cells of the two genotypes, the more fit strain (represented by orange circles) replaces the less fit strain (represented by blue squares). The process continues till the less fit strain is completely eliminated from the reactor. Note that in a real scenario, while the two genotypes are competing and the more fit genotype replaces the less fit, newer mutations will arise in the population. Thus, the number of genotypes in the chemostat at any given point in time, in such a context, will be greater than two. For the simulations showed above, the starting frequency of the two genotypes was 0.5 each. The more fit genotype (represented by orange) has a fitness of 2.1 time^{-1}, while the less fit genotype (represented by blue) has a fitness of 2 time^{-1}.

On the other hand, it is not obvious to think how evolution experiment can be conducted in a batch culture. This is so because after a phase of growth, the nutrients in the batch flask will be all used up, and growth will come to a halt. How, then, can we study evolution experiment using batch cultures? As we will see later in the book, an overwhelming majority of evolution experiments in laboratories around the world are carried out using batch cultures.

4.5 CONCLUSION

In this chapter, we studied growth models of microbial species for two systems. In the first, growth in batch cultures is represented as a differential equation. The key aspect of mathematical modeling which makes it realistic is incorporating a term which accounts for the carrying capacity of the environment. In the second, we model growth in a chemostat where continuous growth occurs because of constant supply of nutrients. In such a case, growth is best modeled via monitoring the frequency of the different species or genotypes in the chemostat. The principles of this chapter are the core of developing a quantitative framework of microbial growth. And it is these principles which we rely on for developing a framework for evolutionary dynamics.

NOTES

Note I

E. coli's DNA is copied by a machine called DNA Polymerase (DNAP). Two DNAPs start copying the DNA from one end of the circular DNA, and move in opposite directions. They meet at the diagonally opposite end of the DNA, hence copying the entire DNA content of the organism. The speed at which DNAPs copy is 1,000 bases/second. By this account, since two DNAPs are working to copy DNA, it should take ~40 minutes to copy the genomic DNA of *E. coli* (which is 4.5×10^6 bases long). However, experimentally it has been observed that under nutrient rich conditions, *E. coli* can divide in 20 minutes. Given that DNAP speed is a constant, and that only two DNAP machines work to produce another copy the genomic DNA.

How then is division in 20 minutes possible?

Note II

Stationary phase of growth should not be thought of as a phase in which 'nothing happens'. Stationary phase is a dynamic phase of growth where the growth and death rate of the bacterial population are matched with each other. As a result, the over cell count does not change. However, since there is active cell division taking place in the stationary phase, newer mutations (which enable better survival in stationary phase) get selected. An article summarizing evolution in stationary phase of bacterial growth is given in the further readings for this chapter.

The stationary phase does not last indefinitely. After stationary phase, the nutritional stress on the population means that the death rate exceeds the growth rate, and the number of viable bacteria in the flask decrease with time.

NOTE III

To be able to use equation (4.2), we need an estimate of K. How does one estimate K? Imagine a dense culture which has reached its carrying capacity. If we take 10 µl of the liquid from this flask and spread on a solid agar media, the individual bacteria in the 10 µl volume would be spread over the plate surface. Of course, these bacteria would be too small for us to see and know their location. After spreading on the solid agar plate, if we leave the plate overnight in an incubator, the individual bacteria spread over the place will grow and divide. The next morning, each of these growth phases can be observed as what is referred to as a 'colony'. So, if there are 200 colonies on the plate the next morning, we know that each of those colonies originated from a single bacterium that was present in the 10 µl culture that we had spread. This implies that 10 µl of the culture contained 200 cells, or 1 ml of the culture in the flask contained 2×10^4 cells. In reality, the typical number of cells per ml of saturated culture will be 10^9–10^{10} per ml, depending on the precise constitution of the media used for the experiment.

EXERCISES

1. We discussed that the mass of an *E. coli* is ~10^{-15} kg. Show all calculations which lead to this number.
2. Using the logic that we used for an *E. coli*, can you estimate your mass? By how much is your estimate off from your actual mass?
3. The actual distribution of division time for *E. coli* in LB can be estimated to be a normal distribution around 30 minutes. How does this change the growth kinetics graph we see in Figure 4.1?
4. What is the answer to the above question if we start the culture with 10 cells of strain A and 5 cells of strain B?
5. Two strains with growth rates 1.1 h^{-1} (strain A) and 1.3 h^{-1} (strain B) are added to a flask containing 100 ml fresh media. The carrying capacity of the flask is 10^{10}, and the starting numbers of each strain is 10. What is the ratio of the number of bacteria of each strain when the number of total bacteria in the flask reach,
   a. Carrying capacity, K,
   b. Half the carrying capacity.
6. Three strains with growth rates 1.1 h^{-1} (strain A), 1.3 h^{-1} (strain B), and 1.25 h^{-1} (strain C) are added to a flask containing 100 ml fresh media. The carrying capacity of the flask is 10^{10}, and the starting numbers of each strain is 10. What is the ratio of the number of bacteria of each strain when the number of total bacteria in the flask reach,
   a. Carrying capacity, K,
   b. Half the carrying capacity.
7. See python code I. In this you can simulate growth of a single species. Run the code five times, each with a different value of r and K. Identify the change in the trend of the graph as the two parameters change.
8. See python code II. Using this code, you can simulate growth of two species in a batch culture. Run this code five times using different values of r and K for the two strains. What are the trends in the graphs that you observe?

9. See python code III. This code simulates growth of two strains in a chemostat. Pick growth rates of the two strains and simulate the code. Does the answer of the code agree with your intuition about what is likely to happen in the chemostat?
10. Extend code III to simulate competition between three genotypes in a chemostat.
11. Starting with a population of size 100, assume division every 30 min. Plot number of cells with time (exponential phase only). Compare this growth kinetic with the case where division time is a normal distribution centered at 30 min, and standard deviation of 5 min. Use code IV to run this simulation. What do you observe?
12. What happens to the result you note in question (4.11), as you increase the standard deviation in the division time? (Use code IV to answer this.)

BIBLIOGRAPHY

1. Volland JM, Gonzalez-Rizzo S, Gros O, Tyml T, Ivanova N, Schulz F, Goudeau D, Elisabeth NH, Nath N, Udwary D, Malmstrom RR, Guidi-Rontani C, Bolte-Kluge S, Davies KM, Jean MR, Mansot JL, Mouncey NJ, Angert ER, Woyke T, Date SV. 2022. A centimeter-long bacterium with DNA contained in metabolically active, membrane-bound organelles. *Science* 376:1453–8.

   (This paper describes the mm long bacterium. Thus, while bacteria are typically a few µm in length, exceptions always exist in bacteria.)
2. Zambrano MM, Kolter R. 1996. GASPing for life in stationary phase. *Cell* 86:181–4.

   (Stationary phase is usually taken to be a phase in growth where nothing happens. However, we are discovering that a lot of activity goes on in the stationary phase. Bacteria are dividing, mutations occurring. This early review of discovery of the activity in stationary phase nicely introduces this aspect of bacterial physiology.)

5 Type of Mutations and Selection Coefficients

5.1 INTRODUCTION

Natural selection needs phenotypic variation to act on. If all members of a population exhibited identical phenotype (and hence, identical fitness), natural selection would have nothing to act on. The primary underlying cause of phenotypic variation is genotypic variation. In this chapter, we will study how precisely genetic variation is generated in microbial populations. How can we quantify the amount and nature of variation that will arise in a microbial population? We will also study a key quantity in evolutionary biology called selection coefficient (s). These two quantities will allow us to develop our quantitative framework in which to visualize an evolutionary process.

5.2 MUTATION RATE, μ

Remember that DNA is copied prior to cell division in bacteria. The process of copying DNA is done by a molecular machine called DNA Polymerase (DNAP). Like any machine in biology or elsewhere, DNAP also has a finite accuracy. While copying DNA, DNAP, every once in a while, makes an error copying DNA.

For the most part, the replication process proceeds without any errors – i.e., the DNA copy is an identical copy of the template. As far as machines go, DNA Polymerase is an incredibly accurate machine. However, at times, errors are made while copying DNA – as a result of which the DNA of the two offsprings post cell-division is not identical. The rate at which DNAP makes errors in copying DNA is called the *mutation rate*, and is represented with the Greek letter μ in evolutionary biology literature.

Mutation rates are extremely important from the context of evolutionary biology – not only because they lead to generation of diversity, which is acted upon by natural selection. But also because they give rise to variations which are responsible for many disease conditions in humans and other organisms. From the context of our discussion, we will study mutations as agents responsible for providing the variation in a population on which natural selection acts. If mutations did not arise in a population, then there would be no genetic variation in a population, and evolution would grind to a halt.

5.3 MUTATIONS ARE RARE

So, how often does DNAP make errors?

Let us do some simple calculations to understand the implications of mutation rates on diversity in a population. The genome of *E. coli* is roughly 5×10^6 base pairs (there is significant variation in the size of the genome of different *E. coli*

DOI: 10.1201/9781003633662-5

strains, but 5×10^6 is a good measure for most strains that researchers study in laboratories). This genomic size means that for every cell division, 5×10^6 bases have to be copied. Each cell division also equates to one generation for the bacterium.

The rate at which *E. coli*'s DNAP makes error is 10^{-9} per base per generation. Which means that the DNAP makes *one* error in copying every 10^9 bases copied. Note that 10^9 is much bigger than the genome of the organism (5×10^{11}). Hence, errors are made at a rate which is lower than one error per replication. Let us look a bit closely regarding the frequency of mutations.

Given the above information, how do we calculate the probability that no error is made when DNA is copied by *E. coli*?

For the entire genome to be copied without error, the first base must be copied without error. This should be followed by the second base copied without error, and so on and so forth, eventually ending with the necessary condition that the last base should be copied without error. Note that, for every base, the probability that it is copied correctly is simply given by $(1–10^{-9})$.

This means that the probability of no error is equal to the probability that *every* one of the 5×10^6 bases is copied accurately. This probability can be computed as follows,

$$\begin{aligned} P(\text{no error in progeny}) &= [P(\text{no error at position } 1).P(\text{no error at position } 2)\cdots \\ &\quad P\left(\text{no error at position } 5 \times 10^6\right)] \\ &= [P(\text{no error at one position})]^{\text{Genome Length}} \\ &= \left(1 - 10^{-9}\right)^{5 \times 10^6} \end{aligned}$$

$$P(\text{no error in progeny}) \sim 0.995 \tag{5.1}$$

This suggests that most progenies of *E. coli* are born with a DNA sequence which is identical to that of the parent. In fact, from these numbers, we note that ~0.005 ($\sim 10^{-9} \times 5 \times 10^{11}$) errors are made at every cell division. Hence, it would take approximately 200 cell divisions for one error (mutation) to take place.

Hence, mutations are rare!

Example 5.1: A bacterial population grows from 200 to 2 billion in a day. Approximate the number of mutations that take place in this time?

Solution: Note that each division increases the size of the population by exactly one. Thus, for the population size to increase from 200 to 2×10^9, the number of cell divisions that take place is simply $(2 \times 10^9 - 200)$. Note that this number is approximately equal to $\sim 2 \times 10^9$. We saw that one mutation takes place every 200 cell divisions, the number of mutations that take place in the flask is simply, $\frac{2 \times 10^9}{2 \times 10^2}$, which is 10^7.

Does the mutation rate appear too small for generation of variation in a population? Note that if the variation is introduced slowly in the population, natural selection will also be slow to act – since there is little variation to act on. In fact, in an important result in Population Genetics, the British statistician Ronald Fisher proved that the speed of action of natural selection is proportional to the variation that exists in the population. This result is known as Fisher's Fundamental Theorem.

Let us take a look at the mutation rate in another way.

Example 5.2: Imagine a 100 ml culture which is started by inoculation of a single bacterium (see Note I). The flask is then allowed to grow overnight at 37°C in an incubator. When we note the turbid flask the following morning, the liquid culture will contain approximately 10^9 bacteria per ml. Thus, the total number of bacteria in the flask is 10^{11} (100 ml × 10^9 bacteria/ml). How many cell divisions happened in this flask? How much genetic diversity is present in this flask?

Solution: Since every cell division increases the population size by exactly one (10^{11} – 1), cell divisions needed to have taken place for the population to reach 10^{11}, starting from a single bacterium. Note that (10^{11} – 1) is effectively 10^{11}. Thus, overnight, ~10^{11} cell divisions took place in the flask. This is assuming no deaths take place in the flask.

From our discussion above, we know that one error in DNA replication takes place every 200 cell divisions. Thus, the total number of errors in DNA replication (or equivalently, the number of mutants that are present in this population of 10^{11}) that happened in the flask is $5 \times 10^8 \left(= \frac{10^{11}}{200}\right)$. That is, 500 million genetic variants exist in this flask, after one day of growth.

Thus, even in a culture that we assume to be isogenic, huge genetic diversity exists.

Example 5.3: Can we estimate how large is this number of mutations in the previous example, compared with the number of mutations that *can* take place in an *E. coli* genome?

Solution: To appreciate how large this number is, consider the following: the size of *E.* coli's genome is 5 × 10^{11}. At every nucleotide, there are three mutations possible (an Adenine (`A`) residue can change to a `T`, `G`, or `C`). Thus, the total number of possible point mutations (in which only one nucleotide is changed to another nucleotide) in the genome is 1.5 × 10^7 (3 × 5 × 10^{11}). Thus, the variation generated in the flask is greater than all mutations that can take place in an *E. coli* genome.

This number of distinct mutations that *can* take place is considerably smaller than the number of mutations that happened in our flask! Thus, in a single overnight growth experiment, the amount of genetic diversity generated is more than all possible genetic diversity (in terms of point mutations) that could be generated!

Natural selection, thus, has plenty of variation to act on, and select the fittest genotypes from a population.

At first glance, the mutation rate of *E. coli* might have appeared to be a small number. However, because of the large size of microbial populations, the number of mutations that happen in a short span of time is very large.

The important point to note here is that mutations are the key to generating diversity for selection to act on, and hence, mutation rate (μ) is a critical quantity in evolutionary biology (see Note II).

5.4 NUMBER OF GENERATIONS IN A SINGLE DAY

In an evolution experiment, the relevant time scale is the number of generations processed. This is because mutations are generated every time a cell divides. Thus, from an experimental context, it makes sense to design evolution experiments with a species which has a short generation time. We saw in the previous section that, overnight, a single bacterium can divide and the population size can increase to 10^{11}. But let us take a look at how many generations does this correspond to.

Example 5.4: How many generations were processed in this flask as the population size transitioned from one to 10^{11}?

Solution: Starting with a single bacterium, in one generation, the bacterium divides once, and we get two bacteria. Thus, after one generation, the population size is two. After another generation, the two bacteria each divide, and we get a population size of $4(2^3)$. Thus, after n generations, the population size in the flask is 2^n. Since we know that the population size in the flask after reaching saturation is 10^{11}, n can be determined by solving,

$$2^n = 10^{11},$$

Solving for n by taking logarithm of both sides, we get

$$n \sim 36 \tag{5.2}$$

Thus, in a single culture, roughly 36 generations of the bacterial population were processed in the conditions we mention in our experiment.

Studying a culture growth for a population in a flask has other interesting features too. Note that in the first generation, only one cell division took place. Hence, the probability that a mutation took place in the first generation is extremely low. However, if a mutation did take place in the first generation, every subsequent division of the progeny carrying the mutation also carries the mutation. Thus, half the population would carry the mutation that occurred at the time of first cell division. The mutation itself occurred only once, but its early timing ensured that subsequent generations simply inherited it from the parent mutant. Hence, early mutations are rare but they spread in a population.

On the other hand, half the total number of cell divisions (5×10^{10}) took place in the last generation. Thus, the probability that mutations occurred in the last generation is very high. However, since there were no more divisions after the last generation (as the resources in the flask were consumed fully), the mutations that occurred late will not have a chance to spread in the population. Thus, late mutations occur with high frequency but they do not spread in the population. This is shown in Figure 5.1.

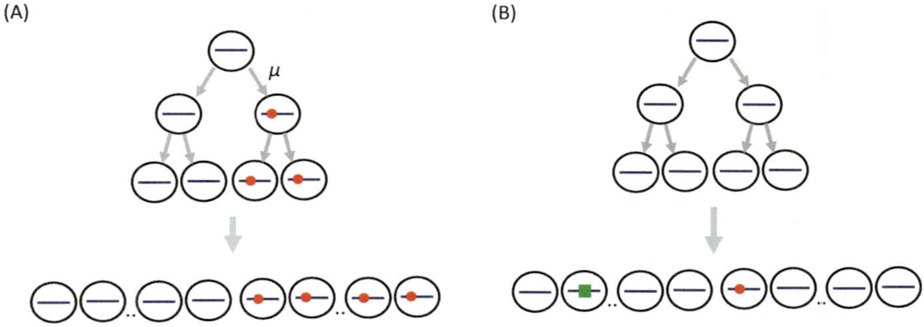

FIGURE 5.1 Spread of a mutation in a population is dependent on the time at which it occurs. (A) An early mutation occurs with a very low probability but will spread to high frequencies in the population. In the figure, a mutation (indicated by a red circle) occurs at the time of first cell division, and thereafter, at every cell division of the mutant, the progeny simply inherits the mutation. Hence, 50% of the population will have this mutation. (B) On the other hand, at a later time in the culture, a lot more cell divisions take place. As a result, the probability of mutations happening will be much greater. However, since the culture is close to carrying capacity, the mutants that so arise will not divide further. Hence, their frequency in the culture media remains small. In the figure, two mutants are indicated by a green square and a red circle.

5.5 TYPES OF ERRORS, AND HOW DO THESE ERRORS EFFECT CELL FUNCTION/FITNESS?

In the discussion in this chapter, we have assumed that errors are made in DNA replication when one nucleotide is incorrectly copied as another. However, errors in DNA replication can take place via a number of other mechanisms too. In this section, we will study these and other types of mutations that can take place as DNA is copied.

5.5.1 *Point Mutations* (Single Nucleotide Polymorphisms, SNPs)

A major class of mutations is called point mutations, where a nucleotide at a particular location in the genome is incorrectly copied as another nucleotide. This is the type of mutation that we have been considering so far in this chapter. For example, in a DNA sequence, an 'A' can change to a 'C'. Such mutations are also referred to as Single Nucleotide Polymorphisms (SNPs) (pronounced as 'snips').

What can a point mutation do? If a point mutation occurs in a gene, and this mutation changes a codon (like, `ATT` to `CTT`) – the mutation will change the amino acid encoded in the protein sequence. In this example, instead of the amino acid Leucine (encoded by `ATT`), amino acid Isoleucine (encoded by `CTT`) gets encoded in this case.

Such mutations, which lead to a change in amino acid sequence of a protein, are called 'non-synonymous' changes. Such a change can enhance or decrease protein functionality. Alternatively, it is also possible that the non-synonymous change occurs in a part of protein such that the protein functionality is not affected. Alternatively, changes in the sequence of gene via a SNP can change the structure and stability of the mRNA so produced, leading to lesser/more translation.

Alternatively, an 'A' to a 'C' change in the sequence of a gene can lead to a codon change CGA to CGC. Both these codons encode for the same amino acid, Arginine. Thus, in this case, while the gene sequence changed, the resulting amino acid sequence does not change. This is because of the redundancy in the genetic code (more than one codon encodes for the same amino acid). Such mutations are referred to as 'synonymous' mutations. Intuitively, we would imagine that synonymous mutations will not change protein functionality. However, we know of a number of cases where synonymous mutations can lead to changes in protein amounts, and even structure (and hence, function) (see Note III).

Alternatively, point mutations can alter the sequence in the non-coding regions of the DNA. This could mean changes in the promoter regions of genes, and as a result of a mutation, the level of expression of the transcript can change (Figure 5.2). Alternatively, via mutations in the promoter region, the control of gene expression, which links transcription to specific environmental or cellular conditions, might be lost.

These mutational events, starting from a sequence as shown in Figure 5.3A, are pictorially represented in Figure 5.3B.

5.5.2 Insertions and Deletions (indels)

Another class of mutations is insertions or deletions (collectively referred to as 'indels'). In this class of mutations, nucleotide(s) are added or deleted from the organism's DNA. The insertion or the deletion could be as small as a single nucleotide, or very large (up to hundreds of thousands of bases). The implications of any insertion or deletion are varied. First, let us consider an insertion or a deletion in a gene sequence. If the insertion or deletion is a multiple of three nucleotides and is appropriately inserted – then, the amino acid sequence of the original protein is conserved. In this case, however, additional amino acids are inserted in the new

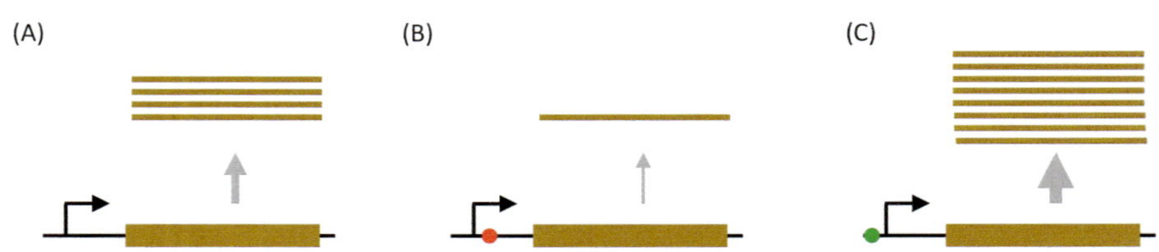

FIGURE 5.2 Mutations in promoter region of a gene can change the level of transcript production. (A) A promoter sequence transcribes a gene. (B) A mutation (indicated by red circle) in the promoter region of the gene decreases the amount of transcript produced. (C) Mutation (indicated by green circle) in the promoter region can increase the transcript amount.

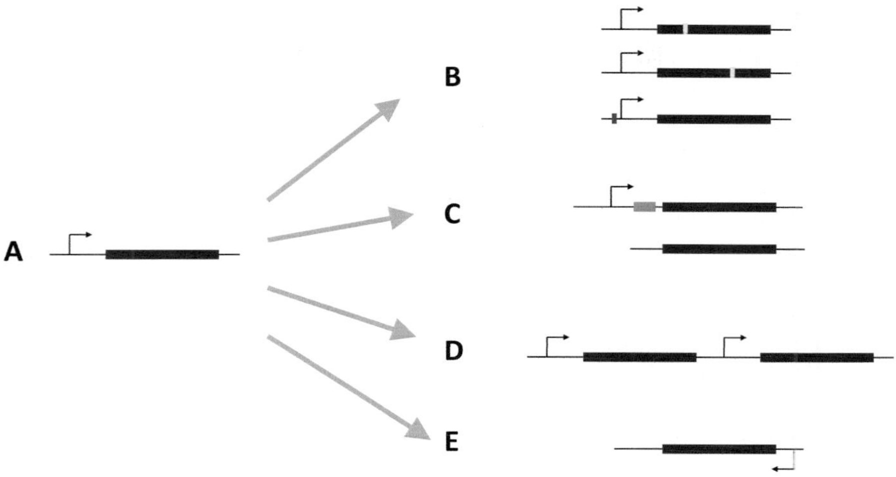

FIGURE 5.3 Type of mutational events that can take place during DNA replication. (A) Consider a region of the genome which contains a gene (purple) and its promoter region (arrow). (B) Point mutation (SNP). In this mutational event, a single nucleotide is incorrectly copied by the DNAP. The change in nucleotide can lead to a change in the amino acid of the protein sequence (in which case the mutation is referred to as a non-synonymous change), or it may encode for the same amino acid (in which case the mutation is called a synonymous mutation), or the mutation may be outside the coding region of the gene (bottom panel of B), in which case the mutation may alter the timing and level of transcript (and consequently protein) being produced in the cell. (C) Indels (Insertion-Deletions). While DNA is copied, additional nucleotides may get inserted in certain regions (e.g., green region in top panel of C), or parts of DNA might get deleted (the promoter region is deleted in the bottom panel of C). (D) Duplication. During the process of DNA replication, parts of DNA might get copied twice. In the example shown, the promoter region and gene are copied twice. (E) Inversion. In this mutational event, the region of the DNA flips, that is – certain sections of the DNA change their strands. As a result, the promoter is on the bottom strand of the DNA, and the gene sequence is from the right to left on the bottom strand.

sequence in the case of insertions, and one/more amino acids removed in the case of deletion. Such an insertion or deletion is referred to as ‘in-frame’. Such an insertion or deletion may or may not lead to an impact on protein functionality. Factors such as which, how many, and the precise location of the amino acids inserted/deleted in the peptide chain combine together to dictate the impact of the insertion/deletion mutation.

On the other hand, if the number of nucleotides inserted or deleted is not a multiple of three (or is inserted at a location to alter the reading frame of a gene) – then the resulting amino acid chain from translation is going to have a completely different identity. In such a scenario, the protein functionality will be completely lost.

Additionally, indels can also occur in non-coding regions of the genome. One such schematic of an insertion or a deletion occurring in the promoter region of a gene is schematically shown in (Figure 5.3C).

5.5.3 Duplication

In another class of mutations, a region of DNA is copied twice by DNAP, thus creating two copies of that part of the DNA. Two copies of one/more genes can have interesting evolutionary implications for a species. It is a subject that we will revisit later in the book.

An extreme example of the impact of a duplication event is the baking yeast, *Saccharomyces cerevisiae*, which underwent a whole genome duplication (WGD) event 80 million years ago. This event created an organism with two copies of every gene (*S. cerevisiae* has about 6000 genes). The gene pairs have had interesting evolutionary dynamics in the time since then. While most duplicates have been lost by the *S. cerevisiae* genome since the WGD event, about ~500 such duplicates still persist in its genome. The evolutionary history of these genes tells us how redundancy in genes can lead to evolution of novelty and complexity in a species' evolutionary trajectory (Figure 5.3D).

5.5.4 Inversion

Lastly, in 'inversions', a segment of the DNA has its orientation reversed. That is, a fragment of DNA is flipped so that the sequence on one strand is shifted to the other (and vice versa). In such a case, one or many gene(s) present on one strand is shifted to the other strand.

The genic content of the organism does not change via this mutational event. However, the orientation of the genes on the chromosome, the genic neighborhood of the regions at the edge of flipped region changes. These events can have profound consequences on the organism's fitness. In an extreme manifestation of such an event, about one-third of the entire genome of the organism was switched in its orientation (Figure 5.3E).

Having studied the types of mutations, we next move to study two extremely important concepts in evolutionary biology. These concepts are called *fitness* and *fitness effect of a mutation*. These two concepts are ubiquitous in all of evolutionary biology, and hence, their understanding is critical to development of our understanding of evolution.

5.6 FITNESS OF A GENOTYPE

Imagine an *E. coli* with a genotype g in a particular environment, where glucose is the only carbon source. Let us imagine that we measure the growth rate of this genotype in the given environment and find it to be 1 h^{-1}. If we grow another *E. coli* strain with genotype g' in the same environment, we find that its growth rate is 1.5 h^{-1}. This means that the second strain (with genotype g') is more suited to growing in this environment, as compared to the first strain (genotype g).

The suitability of a genotype in a particular environment is quantified in evolutionary biology as *fitness* of the organism in a particular environment. In the example discussed above, we are equating growth rate of the bacteria as its fitness. Thus, fitness of genotype g is 1, and that of genotype g' is 1.5.

The idea of fitness is, thus, quantified. We will use this quantified idea of fitness in much of our discussions throughout the book.

It is important to note that fitness can have different meanings in different environmental contexts. For *E. coli* in a flask with abundant glucose, the growth rate (or how fast the bacterium divides) is an appropriate measure of fitness of a strain. This is so because any strain that divides faster than other strains in that particular environment will outcompete them and take over the environment.

However, imagine *E. coli* in a stressful environment (chemical [pH], physical [high temperature], biological [predators] stresses) with limited resources for growth. In such a scenario, the bacterium is not going to be able to divide very fast. In such an environment, the ability to survive stress longer becomes an ecological measure of fitness. This is so because growth rate of the population is minimal given the environmental stressors, however, death rate in the population due to these stresses is very high. Hence, the ecological determinant of which strain takes over the environment is going to be the ability of the strain to simply survive in these stressful conditions. Hence, fitness is not growth rate but the ability to survive.

Note also that a mutation that enhances growth rate in nutrient-rich media (and hence, increase fitness) can decrease the ability of the cell to survive nutritional (or other) stress. Hence, in poor environmental conditions, such a mutation would decrease fitness.

Remember that fitness is not a function of a genotype alone. It is a property of a genotype in a given environment.

5.7 WHAT IS THE FITNESS EFFECT OF MUTATIONS?

As described above, mutational events can occur in many ways. A mutation may or may not have an impact on the fitness of the organism. As evolutionary biologists, we are interested in deciphering the impact of these mutations in dictating changes in fitness. Broadly, mutations can be divided into three types, depending on their effect on fitness. These three are,

a. Deleterious mutations – mutations that decrease fitness,
b. Neutral mutations – mutations that have no effect on fitness, and
c. Beneficial mutations – mutations that increase fitness.

We discuss these three types of mutations below.

a. *Deleterious mutations*.

Imagine that the sequence of Hemoglobin gene in a human being acquires a point mutation, `C255T` (this means that the 255th nucleotide in Hemoglobin's sequence changed from a '`C`' to a '`T`'). This mutation changes the 85th amino acid in Hemoglobin's protein sequence from Valine to Serine – this is a non-synonymous change.

Biochemists have worked out that this mutation leads to a decrease in the ability of Hemoglobin to carry oxygen to the body's tissue. The decreased ability to carry oxygen leads to loss of fitness. Hence, C255T in Hemoglobin is, thus, a deleterious mutation – a mutation that decreases fitness of the individual carrying it.

Consider another example, in yeast *S. cerevisiae*, the gene GAL2 encodes for a membrane protein which transports galactose from outside the cell to inside. The internalized galactose can then be processed to yield energy. The GAL2 protein is 450 amino acids long, and thus, its gene sequence is 1353 (450 × 3 + 3 [for stop codon]) bases long. If the GAL2 protein acquires a mutation G300A, Cysteine at the 100th residue changes to a STOP codon. The individual with this mutation no longer produces a full GAL2 protein. As a result, this individual cell cannot bring in galactose from the extracellular environment into the cell, and hence, its fitness in an environment where galactose is the sole carbon source for the cell is zero. The mutation G300A, thus, is a deleterious mutation in such an environment.

The above two are examples of deleterious mutations – mutations which, in certain environmental contexts, lead to a decrease in fitness of the organism.

b. *Neutral mutations*

Some mutations have no impact on the fitness of the organism. For example, a G300A mutation in the GAL2 gene, as discussed above, can arise in an individual during growth on glucose. In such a context, a mutation in GAL2 is irrelevant. This is because of two reasons. First, as the cells are growing on glucose, whether a cell is synthesizing a functional GAL2 or not is irrelevant. Second, it turns out that during growth on glucose, yeast switches the transcription of GAL2 'OFF'. Hence, since GAL2 DNA is not transcribed, and no GAL2 mRNA transcripts are made. Which means that in environments with glucose, GAL2 protein is not produced in the cell. Thus, the G300A mutation in GAL2 sequence does not have any impact on cellular fitness.

Such a mutation is a neutral mutation. Note that the same mutation, which was deleterious in the section above, is now neutral in another environmental context. This is another illustration of the concept that the effect of mutations is not just dictated by the identity of the mutation, but also the environment in which this change takes place.

Mutations in DNA regions between genes can also be neutral. Microbial genomes are quite compact, i.e., the region of the DNA which encodes for proteins can be as high as 70–80% of the entire genome. On the other hand, in genomes of complex organisms, only a small fraction of DNA encodes for proteins (for human beings, the coding region is ~2%).

Note that a mutation in the non-coding region does not mean that it *must* be a neutral mutation. As we saw earlier in this chapter, a mutation in the coding region could impact the timing and level of protein production, and therefore, affect the organism's fitness.

In this discussion, we only make the claim that, statistically speaking, a mutation in the non-coding region is more likely to be a neutral mutation as compared to a point mutation in the coding region of the DNA.

Sometimes, a point mutation in the coding region of a protein can also be a neutral mutation. This can happen when the mutation is synonymous (i.e., does not lead to a change in the amino acid sequence), or even when an amino acid change is incorporated in a part of the protein which does not alter the function or stability of the protein.

We should note from this example that the effect of a mutation on the organism's fitness cannot be commented on without knowing the precise environmental context in which this mutation took place in the genome of the organism.

c. *Beneficial mutation*

Enzyme β-lactamase confers resistance to a class of antibiotics, like penicillin. Imagine a population of bacteria which carries a particular sequence of β-lactamase gene. This particular sequence confers resistance to the antibiotic penicillin up to a concentration of 1 μg/ml. This concentration of the antibiotic is referred to as the Minimum Inhibitory Concentration (MIC), below which bacterial growth is positive. Which means that in order to completely halt bacterial growth, antibiotic penicillin should be used at a minimum concentration of 1 μg/ml.

One individual in the population acquires a mutation `G444T` in the β-lactamase gene sequence. The new variant of the β-lactamase enzyme produced in this individual confers resistance to penicillin up to a concentration of 2 μg/ml.

Thus, if this population of bacteria were exposed to a penicillin concentration of 1.5 μg/ml, only the individual carrying the mutant β-lactamase gene would be able to survive and grow. Thus, in such an environmental context, the `G444T` mutation in the β-lactamase gene is a beneficial mutation.

The above example represents one class of beneficial mutations, where a change in the nucleotide sequence of a gene leads to enhanced activity of the resulting enzyme. The enhanced enzyme activity leads to increased fitness of the organism.

Another mechanism to increase fitness can be by increasing the amount of protein (enzyme) synthesized. Such a change can be accomplished by a mutation in the promoter region of a gene, which leads to an increase in the rate at which transcription takes place.

Thus, all mutations can be classified into the above three categories: deleterious, neutral, and beneficial.

Before moving ahead,

➔ Of all the mutations that are possible in a gene sequence, what, according to your intuition, is the percentage of (a) deleterious mutations, (b) neutral mutations, and (c) beneficial mutations?

➔ How, according to you, does the above answer change if we were talking about the entire genome of the organism and not a single gene.

5.8 SELECTION COEFFICIENT

Categorizing mutations into three categories (deleterious, neutral, and beneficial) is helpful in understanding how mutations can impact evolutionary trajectories. However, are all beneficial mutations equally beneficial? For example, imagine a scenario where a mutation *A* increases growth rate of a bacterium from 1 h^{-1} to 1.1 h^{-1}, i.e., an increase of 10% in the growth rate. However, if another mutation *B* were to take place in the original genotype, the fitness of the bacterium would increase from 1 h^{-1} to 1.3 h^{-1}, i.e., an increase of 30%. Thus, while A and B are both beneficial mutations, their effect on fitness are not the same. Hence, beneficial mutations are not all equal. They differ in the amount of benefit they confer.

The same argument also holds for deleterious mutations. Deleterious mutations differ in by how much do they decrease fitness.

Thus, we would like a framework which would allow us to quantify the increase in fitness that a beneficial mutation confers. Or, a decrease in fitness that a deleterious mutation confers.

In order to develop a quantitative understanding of the process of evolution, we need mathematical constructs to refine our understanding of mutations and their impact on evolution. For this purpose, in this section, we define 'selection coefficient' (represented in evolution literature by s).

Every mutation has a selection coefficient associated with it. Imagine a bacterium with fitness f_0. Suppose, this bacterium divides and one of the progenies acquires a mutation. Because of this mutation, the fitness of the progeny changes to f_1. The selection coefficient associated with this mutation (in the given environment) is quantified as,

$$s = \frac{f_1 - f_0}{f_0} \tag{5.3}$$

In words, selection coefficient s of a mutation is the fractional change in fitness brought about the mutation.

It should be immediately apparent from equation (5.3) that,

Beneficial mutations have selection coefficient $s > 0$,
Deleterious mutations have selection coefficient $s < 0$, and
Neutral mutations have selection coefficient $s = 0$.

Selection coefficient is a fundamental quality in evolutionary biology literature, and its importance cannot be exaggerated. Equation (5.3) and the discussion above will form the core of many of our discussions in the book. It would make sense to ensure that the above discussion makes sense quantitatively and intuitively, before moving ahead.

Example 5.5: A mutation increases growth rate of a bacteria from 1 h^{-1} to 1.02 h^{-1}. What is the selection coefficient of this mutation? What is the nature of this mutation?

Solution: Since the mutation increases the organism's fitness, it is a beneficial mutation. We know that the selection coefficient s of a beneficial mutation is greater than zero. By using equation (5.1), we get selection coefficient s as,

$$s = \frac{1.02 - 1}{1} = 0.02$$

Thus, the mutation has a selection coefficient of 0.02.

Example 5.6: A deleterious mutation which decreases growth rate from 0.9 h^{-1} to 0.78 h^{-1}. What is the selection coefficient associated with this mutation?

Solution: Using equation (5.1), we can calculate the selection coefficient s of this mutation as,

$$s = \frac{0.78 - 0.9}{0.9} = -0.13$$

has a selection coefficient of −0.02. All neutral mutations, since by definition they do not change the fitness value, have a selection coefficient of zero.

Defining a selection coefficient allows us to go beyond simply categorizing all mutations in three baskets (beneficial, deleterious, and neutral). Selection coefficient allows us to differentiate between a mutation that is weakly beneficial (for instance, s equal to 0.001) and a strongly beneficial mutation (say, s equal to 0.1).

As we will see in the chapters coming up – the fate of a mutation is not just dependent on the nature of the mutation (whether it is beneficial/deleterious/neutral) but is also strongly dependent on its magnitude.

5.9 CONCLUSION

With this discussion, we are now ready to dive deep into the nuts and bolts of evolutionary biology. Remember that concepts discussed in this chapter are not just ubiquitous in evolutionary biology literature, but are also critical to developing an understanding of the subject. We will be using fitness and selection coefficients throughout the remaining part of the book.

NOTES

Note I

It is quite impossible to, in practice, start a culture with a single bacterium – but for the point we are trying to make, it does not make a difference. Typically, in a laboratory experiment, we start a culture with about 10^{11}–10^{7} bacteria.

Note II

There are experiments where bacterial populations are evolved in a certain laboratory environment. One of the crucial observations in one such experiment was that mutations which enhanced the mutation rate (μ) were selected. Why did this happen? Because an increase in mutation rate meant errors happened more frequently, thus providing a higher genetic diversity for natural selection to select from.

Note III

How do synonymous mutations effect fitness. In recent years, a number of mechanisms have established that synonymous mutations are not necessarily neutral. These mechanisms are briefly described below.

First, a synonymous mutation changes the nucleotide sequence in the mRNA. mRNA, in general, is an unstable molecule. A change in a nucleotide can lead to change in stability of the mRNA. As a result, the amount of protein translated from the mutant transcript may be lesser or greater than the original mRNA sequence. Change in protein amount can have an effect on fitness.

Second, synonymous mutation can also change the rate at which translation occurs on the mRNA. It can change the mRNA structure to facilitate or hinder ribosome access and movement on the mRNA, while translating. As a result, the protein amounts can change, leading to a possible effect on fitness.

Third, among synonymous codons (which encode for same amino acid), not all are translated at the same rate. As a result, when a transcript contains a codon which is translated slowly, the already formed amino acid chain (of the mRNA already transcribed) folds into a local structure. When the slow codon is translated, the rest of the mRNA is also then translated. The resulting amino acids then fold into their local energy minima structure. This structure can be different from the global energy minima structure for the entire amino acid chain. Thus, when the entire transcript is translated rapidly, the 3D structures that the amino acids fold into is the global minima. Thus, a synonymous mutation can lead to a change in protein structure, which impacts protein function and hence fitness.

Note IV

When do mutations occur? For the long time – this was an open question, and two thoughts prevailed. The first argued that mutations occur all the time, and selection acts on the variation that is present in the environment at that particular time. The second idea argued that mutations are induced in response to the environmental stress. This debate was resolved in a classical paper in 1940 by Luria and Delbruck, where they demonstrated that the first idea is indeed correct, and mutations occur quite independent of selection pressure. Luria and Delbruck came up with fluctuation test, as a test between the two competing ideas.

EXERCISES

1. If *E. coli*'s genome was the size of a human genome, on an average, how many cell divisions would it take for one mutation to occur?
2. If *E. coli*'s mutation rate was ten-fold higher, on an average, how many cell divisions would it take for one mutation to occur?
3. What is the mutation rate in our species? How does it compare with *E. coli*'s mutation rate? How does it compare with the mutation rate in an elephant?
4. We all start with one cell (zygote) and grow up to, let us say, 40 trillion cells. How many mutations are present in our body? (use the mutation rate of humans to calculate this).
5. In Example 5.1, we assume that $2 \times 10^9 - 200 \sim 2 \times 10^9$. By what percentage does the answer of Example 5.1 change if we do not make this assumption?
6. Given below is the start of sequence of gene *lacI* in *E. coli*.

   5′ GTGAAACCAGTAACGTTATACGATGTCGCAGAGTATGCCGGTGTCTCTT ATCAGACC3′

a. What is the amino acid sequence corresponding to this DNA sequence?
b. What is the amino acid sequence if an 'ATG' is inserted after three nucleotides in this sequence?
c. What is the amino acid sequence if the 'ATG' was inserted after four nucleotides?
d. Which amino acid sequence (between b and c) is likely still functional?

Note that *lacI* is one of the few genes in *E. coli* which does not start with an 'ATG'.

7. What is the selection coefficient of a neutral mutation?
8. Among beneficial mutations, which, according to your intuition, is more frequent:
   e. Mutations with selection coefficient between 0 and 0.001
   f. Mutations with selection coefficient between 1 and 1.001

   Why do you think so?

BIBLIOGRAPHY

1. Li CC. 1967. Fundamental theorem of natural selection. *Nature* 214:505–6.
   (A paper describing Fisher's Fundamental Theorem. Fisher is quite hard to read himself, and this paper does a nice job explaining the theorem.)
2. Wolfe KH, Shields DC. 1997. Molecular evidence for an ancient duplication of the entire yeast genome. *Nature* 387:708–13.
   (One of the more dramatic cases of duplication is in yeast *S. cerevisiae* which underwent a whole genome duplication event.)
3. Parmley JL, Hurst LD. 2007. How do synonymous mutations affect fitness? *Bioessays* 29:515–9.
   (A review paper on how synonymous mutations need not be always neutral.)
4. Shen X, Song S, Li C, Zhang J. 2022. Synonymous mutations in representative yeast genes are mostly strongly non-neutral. *Nature* 606:725–31.
   (A recent paper in *Nature* from 2022 which claims that, contrary to the popular opinion, synonymous mutations are mostly strongly non-neutral.)
5. Bailey SF, Alonso Morales LA, Kassen R. 2021. Effects of synonymous mutations beyond codon bias: The evidence for adaptive synonymous substitutions from microbial evolution experiments. *Genome Biol Evol* 13.
   (Synonymous mutations and their fitness effects.)
6. Luria SE, Delbruck M. 1943. Mutations of bacteria from virus sensitivity to virus resistance. *Genetics* 28:491–511.
   (A classical paper. It was not clear in the early 1940s whether mutations were spontaneous, i.e., occurred randomly, or if they happened in response to environmental stress.)

6 Fitness Landscapes

6.1 INTRODUCTION

While natural selection is an intuitive idea, it is difficult to visualize geometrically. This changed in 1930s, when an American geneticist, Sewall Wright, in a seminal work, proposed the idea of fitness landscape to visualize an evolving population.

Since their proposal, fitness landscapes have been a subject of intense study in the last 90 or so years. While till the 1980s, much of the progress in understanding them was theoretical and computational, a lack of experimental data prevented us from understanding the structure of actual or empirical fitness landscapes. In the last two decades, this is changing fast. High throughput experimental techniques have facilitated construction of empirical fitness landscapes.

Before we introduce fitness landscapes, we will discuss two concepts: sequence space and Hamming distance. Having understood these two, we will then be ready to define fitness landscapes.

6.2 SEQUENCE SPACE

Let us start with the following question: how many unique DNA sequences are there of length two nucleotides?

The sequence can be thought of as two blanks (_ _), which can be filled up using nucleotides. For the first position, we have the option of filling it with any of the four bases (`A/T/G/C`). And for the second position, we, again, have the option of filling it with any of the four bases (`A/T/G/C`).

Thus, the total number of unique sequences of length two that we can write is $4 \times 4 = 16$.

In this counting, we have made two implicit assumptions,

First, the actual number of sequences will be half of this, since DNA is double-stranded, and this means that the sequence $5' -$ `AA` $- 3'$ is the same as the sequence $5' -$ `TT` $- 3'$. For the purpose of our argument, however, we will continue to work with the analysis above – assuming DNA is single-stranded.

Second, we have assumed DNA to be a linear molecule. Most bacterial genomes are circular, and this means that for a given DNA of length L nucleotides, there are fewer unique sequences in a circular arrangement as compared to the linear one.

However, for the purpose of our presentation, we will ignore the above two inaccuracies and proceed. Making these two assumptions does not make any qualitative change in the argument we propose when discussing landscapes. These two assumptions do, however, make the counting in this permutation problem a lot easier.

So, for length L equal to two, the total number of possible sequences is 16. Similarly, for a DNA sequence of length three, the total number of possible

 DOI: 10.1201/9781003633662-6

5′ – AA – 3′	5′ – GA – 3′
5′ – AT – 3′	5′ – GT – 3′
5′ – AG – 3′	5′ – GG – 3′
5′ – AC – 3′	5′ – GC – 3′
5′ – TA – 3′	5′ – CA – 3′
5′ – TT – 3′	5′ – CT – 3′
5′ – TG – 3′	5′ – CG – 3′
5′ – TC – 3′	5′ – CC – 3′

FIGURE 6.1 Sequence space for DNA strings of length L nucleotides equal to two. There are 16 unique sequences of single-stranded DNA for L equal to two. Using the same logic, sequence space for a DNA string of any length L can be defined. Note that the sequence space for a DNA string of length L nucleotides is 4^L.

sequences is $4 \times 4 \times 4$, i.e., 64. Extending the same argument, we note that for a DNA sequence of length L, the total number of sequences will, therefore, be 4^L.

The set of all possible sequences of a given length L is referred to as the sequence space. A sequence space for L equal to two is shown in Figure 6.1.

6.3 HAMMING DISTANCE (H)

Hamming distance is defined as the number of nucleotide positions where the two DNA sequences are different from each other.

For example, consider sequence A (5′ – ATGCGCGC – 3′) and sequence B (5′ – ATGGGCGC – 3′). Both sequences have a length of eight nucleotides. The two sequences are identical at all other seven places, except for position number four, where sequence A has a 'C', and sequence B has a 'G'. Thus, the Hamming distance between the two sequences is 1. This difference is represented as,

$$H_{AB} = 1 \tag{6.1}$$

Note that for two given sequences H_{AB} equals H_{BA}. Also note that Hamming distance is only defined for sequences which are of the same length.

Example 6.1: What is the Hamming distance between sequences C (5′ – ATTTGGGCCC – 3′) and sequence D (5′ – ATTGGGGGCC – 3′)?

Solution: Both the sequences have length 10 nucleotides, hence Hamming distance is defined between them. The two sequences are identical except at position four (where sequence C has a 'T' and sequence D has a 'G') and at position eight, where sequence C has a 'C' and sequence D has a 'G'). Thus, the Hamming distance between the sequences is 2. Or,

$$H_{CD} = 2 \tag{6.2}$$

Identifying the Hamming distance between sequences becomes easier if one is written directly below the other (as shown below):

Sequence C 5′ – ATT**T**GGG**C**CC – 3′
Sequence D 5′ – ATT**G**GGG**G**CC – 3′

The two positions where the sequences contain non-identical bases are immediately apparent. Note that while writing DNA sequences, we use a font (Courier New). This is because in this font, each alphabet is written using the exact same width. That is, the letter '*i*' occupies the same width as the letter '*O*', thus making it a convenient choice for writing DNA sequences one over the other, and convenient for bioinformatics and sequence analysis-related work.

Example 6.2: Compute the Hamming distance between sequences P (5′ – ATTTGGGCCC – 3′) and Q (5′ – ATTGGGC – 3′)?

Solution: Note that the two sequence are of unequal length. Sequence P contains ten bases and Q contains only seven bases. Since Hamming distance is only defined for sequences of equal length, H_{PQ} is not defined.

In a similar manner, we can quantify Hamming distance between any two sequences given to us.

Note that,

- Hamming distance is only defined between two sequences of equal length,
- Hamming distance is defined pairwise – i.e., it is only defined between a pair of sequences. Thus, Hamming distance is not defined for three (or more) sequences.
- Hamming distance cannot be negative. The minimum value Hamming distance can take is zero, when the two sequences are identical. It cannot be less than zero.
- Hamming distance cannot be greater than the length of sequences under consideration. For example, if the length of the two sequences is L (equal to 10), the Hamming distance cannot be greater than 10. In this case, Hamming distance between the two sequences would be 10, when they are different from each other at all 10 places on the sequence.

6.4 SEQUENCES WITH HAMMING DISTANCE EQUAL TO ONE ARE OF SPECIAL INTEREST

As should be apparent, that for sequences of length L, the minimum Hamming distance is zero (when the two sequences are identical) and the maximum Hamming distance is L (when the two sequences are different at each of the L positions).

For example, the Hamming distance between sequences,

P (5′ – ATGCATGC – 3′) and,

Q (5′ – ATGCATGC – 3′)

is zero.

$$H_{PQ} = 0 \tag{6.3}$$

and, the Hamming distance between the following sequences

$$R\,(5' - \mathtt{ATGCATGC} - 3') \text{ and,}$$

$$S\,(5' - \mathtt{GCATCGAT} - 3')$$

is eight.

$$H_{RS} = 8 \tag{6.4}$$

In between these two extremes, we can have Hamming distance between two sequences anywhere between 0 and 8. Of all the possible values of Hamming distance between two sequences, a case of Hamming distance equal to one is of most interest to us.

Let us see why this is so.

What does a Hamming distance between two sequences equal to one mean? If two sequences (A and B) have Hamming distance 1, it means that they differ from each other at only one position. Thus, sequence A via acquisition of a single mutation can become identical to sequence B.

For instance, a sequence $5' - \mathtt{AAAA} - 3'$ can acquire a single mutation (A to G at position four) and become sequence $5' - \mathtt{AAAG} - 3'$.

If Hamming distance between two sequences (C and D) was 2, then it would need two mutations in C to become identical to sequence D.

A typical bacterium like *E. coli* has a genome size of $O(10^6)$. The mutation rate associated with the bacterium's DNAP (the molecular machine which copies DNA) is 10^{-9} base^{-1} division^{-1}. Based on this value, what is the probability that DNA replication will lead to a progeny which has identical DNA as the parent? That is, the Hamming distance between the parent and progeny is zero. We saw this calculation earlier in the book, but let us go over it one more time.

For this to happen, no error must be made at any of the 5×10^6 bases (the typical size of an *E. coli* genome). The probability of such an event is,

$$\begin{aligned} P(\text{no error}) &= (\text{Probability of no error at one base})^{\text{length of sequence}} \\ P(\text{no error}) &= (1 - \text{Probability of error at one base})^{\text{length of sequence}} \\ &= \left(1 - 10^{-9}\right)^{5 \times 10^6} = 0.995 \end{aligned} \tag{6.5}$$

Thus, there is a 99.5% chance that the progeny, post-cell division, will have identical DNA sequence as the parent. From an evolutionary context, such an event is not of much interest. This is so because an individual of the DNA sequence already existed in the population (the parent). Thus, no new variation was created in the process of birth of an individual with identical DNA sequence.

Let us next ask, what is the probability that the progeny is born with a Hamming distance equal to one?

Imagine that the one place where the progeny and the parent DNA differ at the first position in the DNA sequence. This means, that the DNA was copied incorrectly at the first position, AND correctly at every other sequence. The probability of such an event is,

$$P(\text{error at position 1}) = \left(10^{-9}\right)\left(1 - 10^{-9}\right)^{5 \times 10^{6}-1} \sim 10^{-9} \tag{6.6}$$

By the same token, the one error can take place at any of the 5×10^6 positions in the DNA sequence. To get the overall probability that the progeny will have exactly one error (but at any place in the genome), we simply add the probability of error at each position. Hence, the probability that the progeny differs from the parent at exactly one is,

$$P(\text{Hamming dist b/w parent and progency is 1}) = \left(5 \times 10^{6}\right)\left(10^{-9}\right) \sim 5 \times 10^{-3} \tag{6.7}$$

From the perspective of evolutionary change, sequences corresponding to H equal to 1 is of interest to us. This is because progeny is different from its parent, and genetic variation thus introduced in the next generation is critical for evolutionary change.

You will also note that the probability of H equal to zero and the H equal to one, as calculated above, add upto ~ 1. However, we know that higher values of H are also possible. What is the probability of those events?

Let us calculate the probability that the Hamming distance between the progeny and parent is two.

$$P(H = 2) = \left(10^{-9}\right)^{2}\left(1 - 10^{-9}\right)^{5 \times 10^{6}-2} \sim 10^{-18} \tag{6.8}$$

The above equation computes the probability that two errors are made in replication of a genome of size 5×10^6. However, it does not contain the possibility that the two errors could be at any two places in the genome. In other words, of the 5×10^6 sites in the genome, which two got mutated? Thus, we need to compute the number of ways in which we can pick two sites out of 5×10^6. Remember that the number of ways to pick k items out of N non-identical sites is given by,

$$\text{Number of ways to choose } k \text{ out of } N = \binom{N}{k} \tag{6.9}$$

Thus, the number of such pairs in the DNA sequence is,

$$\textit{Number} \text{ of ways to choose two positions in genome} = \binom{10^{6}}{2} \sim 10^{12} \tag{6.10}$$

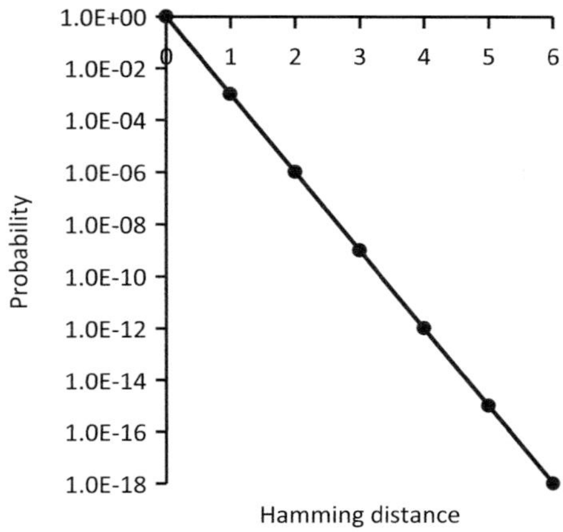

FIGURE 6.2 Hamming distance and probability. Post-cell division, the chances that the progeny has identical DNA as parent is ~0.999. The chances that the progeny and parent DNA sequence vary at exactly one position (i.e., H equals one) is ~0.001 and so on. H equal to zero is not of interest from the context of evolutionary change. H equal to one once every 1,000 divisions. While H equals two occurs once every million divisions. Higher values of H occur even more rarely. Thus, from an evolutionary context, we are only interested in non-zero values of H which occur most frequently (i.e., H equals one).

Thus, the probability that the Hamming distance between the progeny and the parent is two is equal to,

$$P(H = 2) \sim 10^{-18}\, x\, 10^{12} = 10^{-6} \tag{6.11}$$

From an evolutionary perspective, the above event is of great interest. However, since the mutation rate of DNAP replication are so small, the likelihood of H equal to 2 between a parent and an offspring is extremely small. Compared to Hamming distance equal to 1, the probability of Hamming distance equal to 2 is extremely unlikely.

Similarly, the probability of Hamming distance greater than two is smaller than the probability of H equaling two. Hence, from an evolutionary perspective for the bacterial population, those events are increasingly rare.

The result of the above discussion is that while, to study evolutionary change, we are interested in all sequences which acquire mutations, we need to focus only on Hamming distance of one sequence (Figure 6.2).

6.5 CONNECTING SEQUENCES WITH *H* EQUAL TO ONE

We now go back to the sequence space diagram discussed earlier in this chapter. For a sequence length L equal to 2, we had 16 possible sequences (Figure 6.3). We will now connect all nodes which have a Hamming distance equal to one. That is, sequences 5′ – AA – 3′ and 5′ – AT – 3′ are connected with each other (blue line),

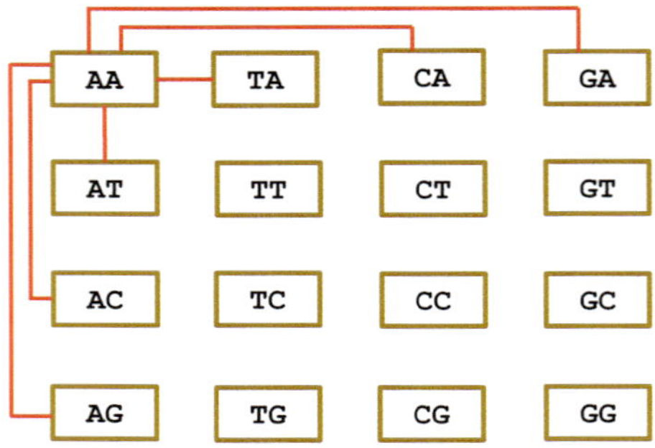

FIGURE 6.3 Sequence space and Hamming distances. Given above are 16 nodes representing all sequences of length L equal to two. For each node, all other nodes which are at a Hamming distance equal to one is connected. For example, in the figure, all nodes which are at Hamming distance equal to one from the node AA are connected by a blue curve. Note that there are six nodes which are at a Hamming distance equal to one from the node representing AA. Three of them differ from AA at position 1, and the other three differ from AA at position 2. Similarly, each node in the sequence space will be connected with six other nodes.

since the Hamming distance between them is equal to one. On the other hand, sequences 5′ – AA – 3′ and 5′ – GG – 3′ are not connected, since the Hamming distance between them is two.

When we make all such connections, we get a structure called a 'graph'.

This graph can be for small DNA sequences – like in Figure 6.3, where the sequence space is only 16 nodes. The graph can also be constructed for somewhat larger sections of the genome – say, a gene (typical length of a gene is ~1000 bases). But in this case, the sequence space will be 4^{1000} nodes. On the scale of an entire organism, the sequence space will be of the order of $4^{10\wedge 6}$ nodes. Thus, as the length of the sequence we are examining increases, the complexity of the sequence space increases exponentially. So much so that at the scale of the organism, the number of nodes in the sequence space exceeds the number of atoms in the universe!

For a particular node, the one-distance neighbors which differ from it at position one is three (that is because the nucleotide present at position one can change to any of the other three nucleotides). In our example above, one distance neighbors of sequence 5′ – AA – 3′, which differ at position one, are three (5′ – TA – 3′; 5′ – GA – 3′; and 5′ – CA – 3′). Similarly, there are three one-distance neighbors for this node, which differ from it at position *i*. Thus, the total number of one-distance neighbors for every node in the sequence space is *3L*.

The total number of nodes in the sequence space is 4^L. Thus, as L increases, the fraction of the nodes that any particular node is connected to is p, and can be quantified as,

$$p = \frac{3L}{4^L} \tag{6.12}$$

As we can see from the figure, as L increases, the connectedness of any node decreases rapidly. This is because the numerator in equation (6.12) is increasing linearly with L but the denominator is increasing exponentially with increasing L.

6.6 PUTTING TOGETHER CONCEPTS TO UNDERSTAND *FITNESS LANDSCAPE*

Let us now put together what we have learned in this chapter to define all elements of a fitness landscape. Let us do this considering the sequence space of length two. That is, in all, there are only 16 sequences possible.

1. First, we make nodes – each representing one of the 4^2 possible sequences.
2. We join all pairs of nodes which differ from each other at one nucleotide position (i.e., have Hamming distance equal to 1). This sequence space graph lies in the x-y plane.
3. Next, for each node, imagine an organism with the sequence corresponding to the node. The organism carrying that particular sequence will have a particular fitness value. We lift each node in the z-direction, by a distance equal to the fitness corresponding to that particular node.

Thus, on our diagram, the x-y plane presents the sequence space and the Z-axis corresponds to the fitness.

We do this for every node in the sequence space. The final resulting structure we get is referred to as a 'fitness landscape'.

In the toy example we discussed above, the sequence space is very small. As we move toward bigger sequences, we will immediately realize that the sequence space grows astronomically (4^L for a sequence of length L). Thus, with increasing L, constructing fitness landscapes for actual sequencing and testing them in organisms becomes a challenge very soon.

Till date, the most complete fitness landscape that we have available to us is for a nine-base sequence in a gene called *folA* in *E. coli*. This landscape, therefore, has fitness values of 4^9 (approx. 250000) sequences in *E. coli*. Thus, while we have known of fitness landscapes for nearly 100 years, empirically, we know little about what exactly do they look like.

This problem was touched upon by a review article in 2009 by Frances Arnold, where she highlights that real fitness landscapes could look like one of many possibilities (highlighted in Figure 6.4). She speculated that large parts of the fitness landscape would have a fitness equal to zero (indicated by black regions in Figure 6.4A). In between, there likely exist small islands with non-zero fitness. The structure of these islands could be any of the possibilities shown in the figure. One of the challenges before the field of evolutionary biology is deciphering more accurate and larger maps of fitness landscapes. This is important, because as we will see, the precise structure of the islands in the landscape has a large bearing on how populations can evolve.

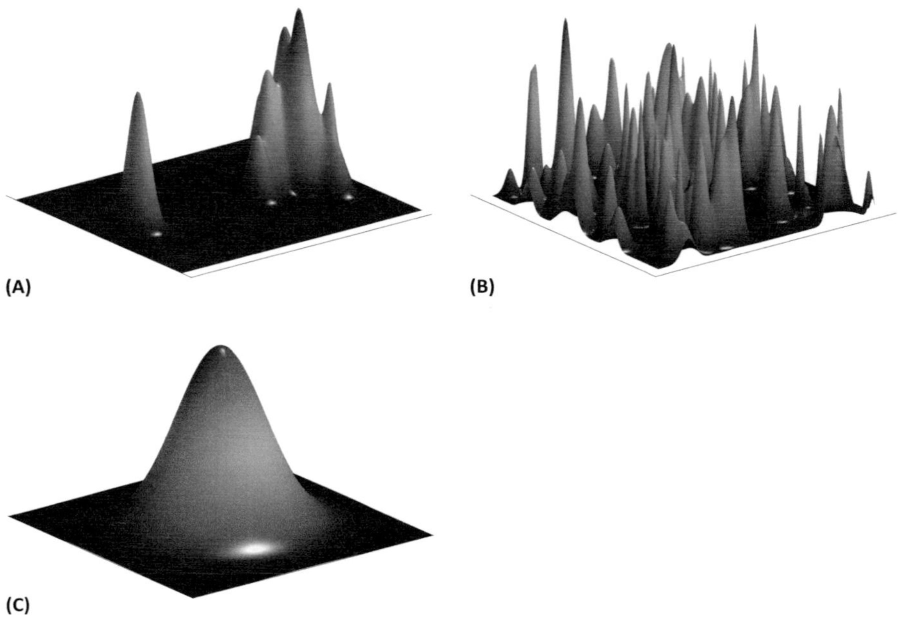

FIGURE 6.4 Fitness landscapes and evolution. (A) What does the fitness landscape look like? In this figure from a review paper by the Nobel Laureate Francis Arnold, the structure of fitness landscape is viewed. On the x-y plane is the sequence space. On the z-axis is the fitness of an organism corresponding to every sequence on the x-y plane. The figure illustrates that the majority of sequences on the x-y plane correspond to zero fitness. In this sequence space, there are islands of sequences which correspond to non-zero fitness. The local structures of the landscape where the fitness values are non-zero can be rugged (B) or smooth (C).

6.7 HOW DOES A FITNESS LANDSCAPE HELP VISUALIZE ADAPTATION?

Imagine an isogenic population of bacteria. Since all individuals in the population have identical sequence, the location of the population can be represented by a single node in the fitness landscape. The fitness corresponding to the node where the parent population lies is f_o. As cells in this population divide, newer progeny is produced. We want to locate the progeny in the fitness landscape (Figure 6.5).

If a progeny is born without any mutations – then, its location in the fitness landscape is represented by the same node as the parent population. Thus, from an evolutionary perspective, this progeny does not change anything.

However, if a progeny is carrying a mutation, its location on the landscape is represented by one of the one-distance neighbors of the node representing the parent population. Let the fitness of the mutant progeny be f_1. Now, depending on the

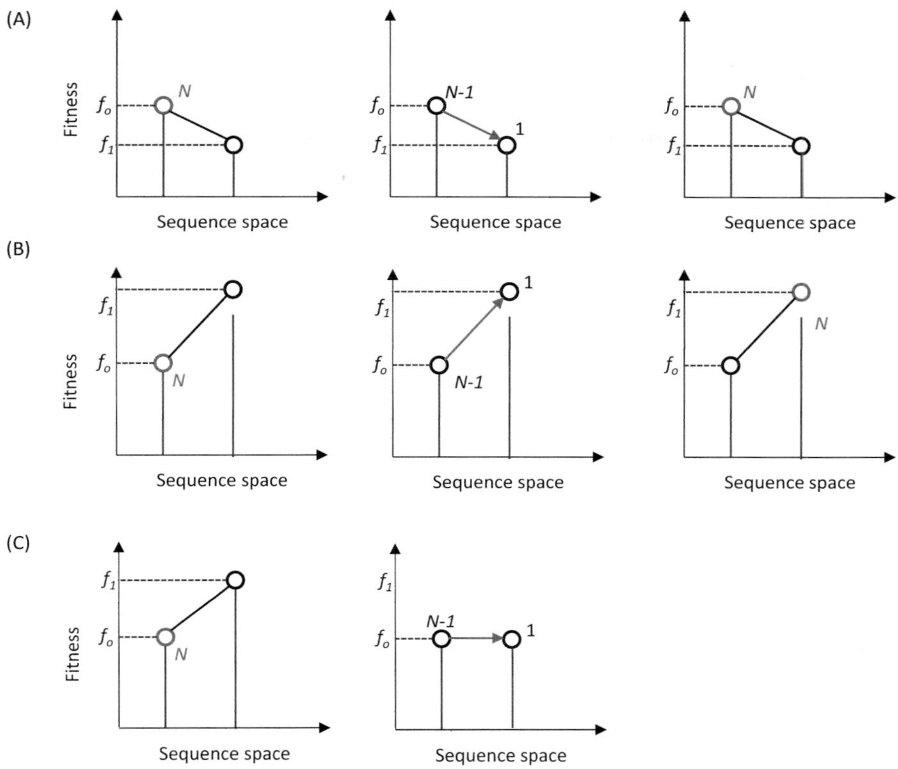

FIGURE 6.5 Imagine population at a point on the sequence space, which corresponds to fitness f_o. The population size is N. (A) One individual in the population acquires a mutation. As a result, this individual is represented by another point in the sequence space, which corresponds to fitness f_1 (middle panel). Since the mutant has a fitness lower than the ancestral population, selection eliminates the mutant and the population remains at the original place in the sequence space (right panel). (B) Starting from a point in the sequence space which corresponds to fitness f_o, one individual acquires a mutation and moves to another point on the sequence space corresponding to fitness f_1. Since the mutant individual is at a higher fitness than the ancestral population, selection ensures that the offsprings of the mutant outcompete the ancestral population. As a result, over evolutionary time, the population moves on the landscape from a point corresponding to fitness f_o to f_1. (C) The figure shows the scenario where one individual in the population acquires a neutral mutation. The fate of the mutation in this scenario is dictated by chance only, as all individuals have identical fitness.

fitness corresponding to the node at which this mutant progeny lies, three possibilities arise:

Case I. $f_o > f_1$ (Figure 6.5A). In this case, the fitness of the progeny is less than that of the parent population. Such a mutation is referred to as deleterious mutation. Hence, the one-distance neighboring node which represents the mutant lies at a lower fitness on the landscape, as compared to the node representing the ancestral population. Natural selection then acts and eliminates the less fit individual (mutant) from the population. The population, therefore, remains at the original node.

Case II. $f_o < f_1$ (Figure 6.5B). If the fitness of the mutant is higher than that of the ancestor, then the mutant is represented by a node which is of higher fitness than that of the ancestor, and the mutation is referred to as a beneficial mutation. In this case, the mutant, owing to its higher fitness, outcompetes the ancestral population. As a result, after a while, the population is represented by the node corresponding to the mutant. This movement corresponds to an 'uphill' movement of the population on the fitness landscape. Note that once the entire population has moved to the node corresponding to the higher fitness, the whole process repeats itself. Thus, the population, as we progress in time, keeps moving uphill on a fitness landscape. It is this movement of a population toward higher fitness values, which leads to the analogy between evolution and climbing a mountain.

Case III. $f_o = f_1$ (Figure 6.5C). There also exists the case where the fitness of the mutant is the same as that of the ancestor. When this happens, the mutation is said to be a neutral mutation. In this case, while genetic variation exists in the population, at the level of fitness, no difference exists between members of the population. In the absence of phenotypic (fitness) difference, natural selection does not act. The evolutionary fate of the population is decided by drift (or randomness). We will discuss the role of drift in dictating evolutionary change in Chapter 8.

6.8 WHAT IS THE MODE VALUE OF FITNESS ON A LANDSCAPE?

Imagine a thought experiment. We know that *E. coli* has a genome of size 10^6. This corresponds to $4^{10\wedge 6}$ unique sequences. Let us number these sequences S1, S2, ··· , $S4^{10\wedge 6}$. If *E. coli* with each of these sequences existed, each would have a fitness value (growth rate). Let us call the corresponding fitness values as f1, f2, ··· , $f4^{10\wedge 6}$. What is the mode value in this list of fitness? Think about this for a few minutes before moving on to the next paragraph.

Before moving ahead,

➔ If we list the sequences of possible sequence space numbering $4^{10\wedge 6}$ for *E. coli*, at what point do we call it another species and not *E. coli*?

The mode value in this list will be zero!

This is because most of these sequences of length 10^6 would simply correspond to a polymer, and not have sufficient meaning encoded in them to be biologically meaningful. For example, a strain of 10^6 'A's would not correspond to an actively dividing bacterium. Thus, fitness landscape in this view would have large sections of the sequence space with fitness value corresponding to zero (see Figure 6.4A again to see this point). In this large space, we will likely have small sections interspersed with sequences which correspond to non-zero fitness of bacteria carrying that species. Thus, fitness landscapes likely look something like the Figure 6.4A. We say 'likely' because exploring fitness landscapes is an exceptionally difficult task. As mentioned below, the number of nodes in the sequence space is greater than the atoms in the universe! We will look at experimental explorations of the movement of populations on a fitness landscape in Chapter 14.

6.9 CONCLUSION

In this chapter, we study the geometric construct called fitness landscape. The construct allows us to visualize evolution as a geometric process, akin to a mountain climber. To define a fitness landscape, we define sequence space and Hamming distance. While theoretical and computational investigations of landscapes have been carried out for a hundred years, what do true, empirical fitness landscapes look like has been an open question. It has only been in the last few years that large sequence spaces have been investigated experimentally to determine the structure of fitness landscapes. The key lessons learned from these empirical fitness landscapes are discussed in Chapter 14. Interested readers can therefore go straight to Chapter 14, before returning to Chapter 7. Alternatively, to continue the discussion of conceptual ideas in evolution, we move next to Chapter 7 in the book.

NOTES

NOTE I

Fitness landscapes are enigmatic structures. We have heard of both Sewall Wright, who proposed fitness landscapes, and the British statistician, Ronald Fisher. Both together were instrumental in developing the quantitative theory of evolutionary biology. As is often the case, the two disagreed with each other on a number of issues. One of the key issues of disagreement was whether fitness landscapes are single- or multi-peaked. Wright argued that the whole problem of understanding movement of populations on a landscape boiled down to the following: landscapes are multi-peaked, and hence, populations get stuck in a local maxima. How do then populations get out of this local maxima? For Fisher, however, fitness landscapes were single-peaked structures, and selection would thus ensure that populations keep moving up on the fitness scale.

In light of out discussions on landscapes in this chapter, the following are interesting questions/thoughts to ponder over.

- Do fitness landscapes have a peak?
- Do fitness landscapes have a single peak? We have not commented on the nature of landscape. Does it have a single peak or multiple peaks? This question has important implications for evolutionary trajectories of populations. If the landscape is a single-peaked structure, then all trajectories,

starting from any place in the landscape, converge to the same peak. Thus, evolution is largely deterministic. On the other hand, if the landscape is multiple-peaked, depending on where the ancestral population lies, and which are the first mutations that occur in a population, the evolved population may result on different peaks (imagine a population on a landscape and its adaptation on a landscape with structure as depicted in Figure 6.4B [right] and Figure 6.4C).

- Can you imagine ways in which neutral mutations can influence evolutionary trajectories?
- When a beneficial mutation occurs, and the mutant corresponds to a higher fitness than the ancestral population, natural selection ensures that, as time moves forward, the progeny of the mutant replace the ancestral population. However, such a view assumes that evolutionary trajectories are deterministic. However, as we will see, evolutionary dynamics are also susceptible to noise and stochastic fluctuations. As a result, it is not necessary that the higher fitness individual will prevail in the population. More on stochastic nature of evolution in Chapter 8.

EXERCISES

1. What is the probability that an *E. coli* divides and acquires exactly three mutations in the process?
2. What is the probability that an *E. coli* divides and acquires at least two mutations in the process?
3. For a DNA sequence of length L, how many neighbors exist for a particular sequence which are at a Hamming distance equal to one?
4. For a DNA sequence of length L, how many neighbors exist for a particular sequence which are at a Hamming distance equal to two?
5. Equation (6.11) in the chapter gives the fraction of nodes in the sequence space that a node is connected to. Plot a graph of L (x-axis) versus p (y-axis). Comment on the nature of trend that you see in p as L increases.
6. What is the mode value on the fitness landscape of *E. coli*?
7. From Figure 6.4, show graphically how starting from different points on the landscape would lead a population to same peak on a smooth landscape, but can lead to a different peak on a rugged landscape.
8. On the smooth landscape shown in Figure 6.4C, if we evolve three identical genotypes independently from a starting point, sketch the trajectories of the evolving populations? Would they follow the same path?

BIBLIOGRAPHY

1. Wright S. 1932. The Roles of Mutation, Inbreeding, Crossbreeding and Selection in Evolution. *Proceedings of the Sixth International Congress of Genetics I*:356–366.

(Sewall Wright's landmark 1932 paper where he first introduced the idea of fitness landscapes.)

2. Papkou A, Garcia-Pastor L, Escudero JA, Wagner A. 2023. A rugged yet easily navigable fitness landscape. *Science* 382:eadh3860.

(A recently published fitness landscape of a sequence space size 9 for the gene *folA* in *E. coli.*)

3. Romero PA, Arnold FH. 2009. Exploring protein fitness landscapes by directed evolution. *Nat Rev Mol Cell Biol* 10:866–76.

(Fitness landscapes of full proteins or organisms remain a long way away. This is a valuable resource discussing what protein landscapes likely look like.)

7 Epistasis

7.1 INTRODUCTION

In the previous chapters, we discussed that mutations can be broadly classified into three groups:

a. Beneficial mutations are those which increase fitness,
b. Neutral mutations are those which do not change fitness,
c. Deleterious mutations are those which decrease fitness.

Based on this, we can classify a particular mutation into one of three groups.

We also saw that, based on the environmental context, the classification of the same mutation may change. For instance, we saw in Chapter 5 that the mutation G300A in the GAL2 gene in the yeast *S. cerevisiae* is a deleterious mutation in an environment where galactose is the sole source of carbon. However, the same mutation is neutral, if the environment contains glucose as the carbon source. Thus, the environment dictates the fitness effect of a mutation.

However, fitness effect of a mutation is dictated by one more factor – the genetic background or the genotype in which it occurs. This dependence of fitness effect on the genetic background is referred to as *epistasis*.

Consider the following scenario. Two strains of *S. cerevisiae* are growing in media containing glucose. The two strains are identical in their genotype except for one difference. Strain *A* does not have the gene GAL3, while strain *B* does. GAL3 is a signal transducer which processes the information that galactose is present in the media, and controls gene expression. Since the difference between the two strains lies in a gene which is responsible for utilizing galactose, they exhibit no difference in fitness in glucose.

However, when shifted to galactose, Strain *A* has considerably lower fitness f_A (0.03 h^{-1}), as compared to Strain B, f_B (0.08 h^{-1}). Next, a mutation in the promoter region of GAL3 takes place in the two strains, which stops transcription in the region of DNA upstream of GAL3. For strain *A*, since GAL3 gene was anyway absent, this mutation has no change in its fitness. Thus, the promoter mutation is a neutral one. However, in strain *B*, the promoter mutation ensures that GAL3 is no longer synthesized in the cell, thus, decreasing its fitness to 0.03 h^{-1}. Thus, the fitness effect of the promoter mutation on,

Strain *A* is zero (since its fitness remains the same),

$$\text{Strain } B \text{ is } -0.05\ (= 0.03 - 0.08)\ \text{h}^{-1}.$$

 DOI: 10.1201/9781003633662-7

The key thing to note from our perspective is that the same mutation has two different effects on fitness. This difference was only dependent on the genotype in which this mutation is introduced. This differential effect of a mutation on fitness is referred to as *epistasis*.

7.2 EPISTASIS IN AN ENZYME PATHWAY

Imagine an enzymatic cascade, where substrate *S* is acted upon by enzyme E1, resulting in P_1. Another enzyme E2 then acts on P_1 to give the final metabolite of the pathway, *P* (Figure 7.1). Let us assume that the fitness of the bacteria carrying this cascade is f_o.

Now, imagine that an individual bacterium in the population acquires a mutation (m1) in enzyme E1. The mutation changes the amino acid sequence of E1. The mutation enhances the functionality of E1, and as a result, the fitness of the mutant increases to $(f_o + \Delta f_1)$, and is, thus, greater than that of the ancestor.

Next, imagine that another individual in the population acquires a mutation (m2) in enzyme E2. This mutation enhances the functionality of E2, and as a result, this mutant has a fitness $(f_o + \Delta f_2)$, which is greater than that of the ancestor.

Based on the information above, we can say that mutations *m1* and *m2* are beneficial in nature. Both these mutations, when present individually in a bacterium, enhance fitness.

However, what can we say about the fitness of an individual which carries both *m1* and *m2*? Several possibilities exist (Figure 7.2).

7.2.1 No Epistasis

The null expectation will be that when a bacterium is carrying both *m1* and *m2*, its fitness will be simply given by the sum of the two mutations' fitness effects. That is, the fitness of the double mutant (f_{12}) will be equal to $f_o + \Delta f_1 + \Delta f_2$. If this was the case, then we say that there was no epistasis between *m1* and m2 (Figure 7.2A).

7.2.2 Positive Epistasis

Alternatively, the fitness of the double mutant can be greater than the sum of fitness effects of the two mutations. In such a scenario, the fitness of the double mutant, f_{12}, will be greater than $(f_o + \Delta f_1 + \Delta f_2)$ (Figure 7.2B).

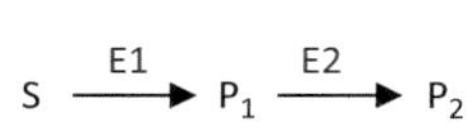

FIGURE 7.1 A hypothetical enzymatic cascade. Substrate *S* is acted upon by enzyme E1 to give the intermediate product P_1. The intermediate product P_1 is then acted upon by enzyme E2 to give the final product P.

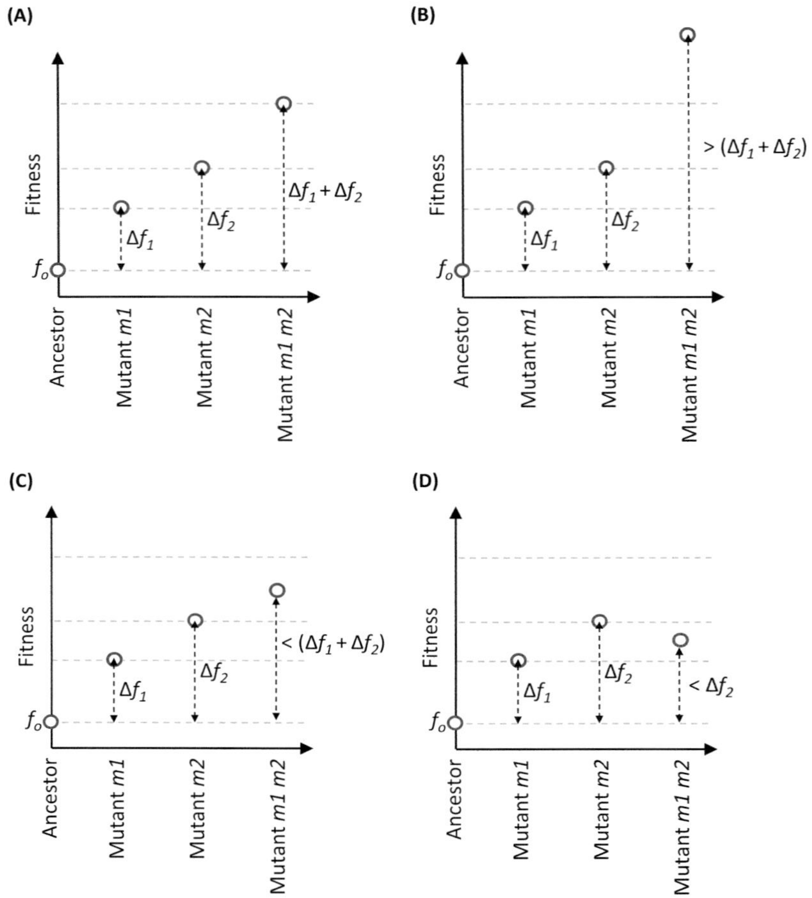

FIGURE 7.2 Epistasis between two mutations can manifest in a variety of ways. (A) No epistasis. The two mutations *m1* and *m2* individually confer a fitness benefit of Δf_1 and Δf_2, respectively. In the case of no epistasis, when present together they confer a benefit of $(\Delta f_1 + \Delta f_2)$. **(B) Positive epistasis**. When present together, the two mutations confer a benefit of $> (\Delta f_1 + \Delta f_2)$. **(C) Negative epistasis**. When present together, the two mutations confer a benefit of $< (\Delta f_1 + \Delta f_2)$, but $> \Delta f_2$. **(D) Sign epistasis**. When present together, the two mutations confer a benefit of $< \Delta f_2$. In the (D) case shown in the figure, note that mutation *m1*, when introduced in the ancestor genome, is beneficial. However, when the same mutation is introduced in the genotype with mutation *m2*, it is deleterious. Also note that the mutation *m2*, on the other hand, is beneficial when introduced in ancestor or the genotype carrying *m1*.

7.2.3 Negative Epistasis

If the double mutant fitness is greater than both the individual mutants, but is less than the sum of the effects of the two mutations (Figure 7.2C). That is,

$$f_{12} > f_o + \Delta f_1$$
$$f_{12} > f_o + \Delta f_2$$
$$f_{12} < f_o + \Delta f_1 + \Delta f_2$$

7.2.4 Sign Epistasis

Perhaps the most intriguing manifestation of epistasis takes place in sign epistasis. Epistasis between two mutations is said to be sign epistasis, when even though individually, the two mutations are beneficial, when combined the fitness of the double mutant is less than that of the single mutants. Sign epistasis, in turn, can manifest in different ways. But for our purposes, we can understand it as a scenario, where a mutation is beneficial in one background but deleterious in the other. Consider Figure 7.2D. Mutation *m1* is beneficial when introduced in the original background, and therefore, increases fitness. However, when the same mutation *m1* is introduced in a genotype which already contains *m2*, it leads to a decrease in fitness (i.e., *m1* is deleterious).

Example 7.1: Strain *A* of a bacteria has growth rate 1 h^{-1} in a particular environment. Upon acquisition of mutation *m1*, the fitness changes to 1.1 h^{-1}. However, if the ancestor were to acquire mutation *m2*, the growth rate would be 1.05 h^{-1}. A strain carrying both mutations *m1* and *m2* grows at rate 1.3 h^{-1}. Based on this information, what can we say about the nature of epistasis between *m1* and *m2*?

Solution: The fitness effect of the mutation *m1* is Δf_1, which is equal to (1.1 – 1) h^{-1}. Thus, fitness effect of *m1* is 0.1 h^{-1}. Similarly, the fitness effect of *m2*, $\Delta f2$, is 0.05 h^{-1}. The fitness effect of the double mutant, Δf_{12}, is 0.3 h^{-1}. Since $\Delta f_{12} > \Delta f_1 + \Delta f_2$, we can say that positive epistasis exists between the two mutations *m1* and *m2*. Note that since both mutations increase fitness, *m1* and *m2* are both beneficial mutations.

Example 7.2: Imagine a sequence which is *L* equals 3. Each site makes a fitness contribution depending on the identity of the nucleotide present at that particular location. These fitness contributions are as given below.

	A	T	G	C
Position 1	0.03	0.02	0.06	0.06
Position 2	0.05	0.04	0.02	0.06
Position 3	0.1	0.01	0.04	0.06

a. What is the identity of the sequence which confers the greatest fitness to an individual?
b. Suppose a population starts with a sequence AGA, map out an adaptive trajectory that a population might take to the fitness peak.
c. Is the route you have chalked out in b, unique?

Solution: The key point to note in this example is that the fitness contribution from each position is *only* dependent on the identity of the nucleotide at that position. It is *independent* of the nucleotides present elsewhere on the sequence. Thus, this is an example where epistasis is absent.

a. If we consider position 1 in the sequence, we note that maximum fitness is conferred by nucleotides G or C. Similarly, at position 2, maximum fitness is conferred by nucleotide C. Last, nucleotide C also confers the maximum fitness at position 3. Thus, the sequence that confers the maximum fitness is CCC or GCC. Convince yourself that no other sequence confers a greater fitness.
b. One possible path from AGA to CCC could be as follows:

AGA → ATA → ATG → ATC → ACC → CCC

c. It should be immediately apparent that the path in *b* is not a unique path to the peak fitness. For instance, the following path could also be taken to the peak fitness,

AGA → ATC → CAC → CCC

Moreover, in this case, two sequences confer the same maximum fitness. Hence, paths to maximum fitness can end up at two different genotypes, with identical fitness values.

7.3 IMPLICATIONS OF EPISTASIS ON EVOLUTIONARY DYNAMICS

Epistasis is ubiquitous, and manifests in biological systems. Our interest in epistasis stems from the thinking about the question of how does it influence evolutionary trajectories of populations?

7.3.1 Negative Epistasis Slows Down Evolutionary Change

From our discussion above, we should note that negative epistasis means that the effect of a beneficial mutation is greater when it occurs in the genetic background of lower fitness, as compared to when the same mutation occurs in a genetic background of higher fitness. This can be seen from Figure 7.2C, where the effect of mutation *m2* is greater in the ancestor background than in the one containing mutation *m1*.

This means, that as a population evolves toward higher fitness, the same mutation has increasingly smaller effects on fitness.

Thousands of evolutionary experiments across several environments and organisms have studied fitness trajectories. A common observation across all these experiments has been that although fitness is continuously increasing through the generations, as the number of generations increase, the rate of increase of fitness slows down. This is shown in Figure 7.3, where fitness increases rapidly at the start of the experiment. However, as the experiments move forward, the rate of increase of fitness decreases.

Thus, negative epistasis slows down adaptation, and as a result, an increase in fitness slows down as populations approach fitness peaks.

By the same token, we should also note that positive epistasis accelerates the rate of increase of fitness in a population.

7.3.2 Sign epistasis Makes the Fitness Landscape Rugged

The concept of fitness landscape, as described in the previous chapter, does not tell us about the actual structure of the landscape. A key variable which helps in

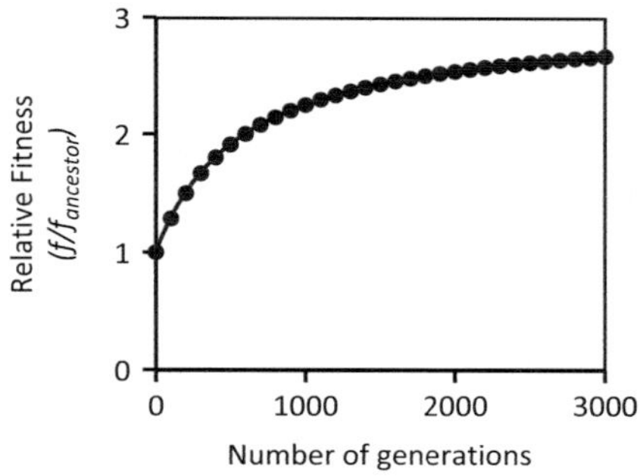

FIGURE 7.3 One of the manifestations of negative epistasis is slowing down of the rate of adaptation. In an evolution experiment, the fitness increase slows down as number of generations processed increases. Note that the fitness gain in the first 1,000 generations is greater than in the next 1,000 generations. This illustrates the fact that rate of fitness increase slows down with time. There are two possible explanations for this phenomenon. First, the high benefit mutations occur first, and after a while, all the beneficial mutations which are still available confer a small benefit. This is *not* the case. When the later occurring beneficial mutation(s) was moved to ancestral background, the benefit it confers was found to be greater than the benefit it confers in the evolved background. Second, negative epistasis – where benefit conferred by a beneficial mutation is inversely proportional to the fitness of the background in which it occurs.

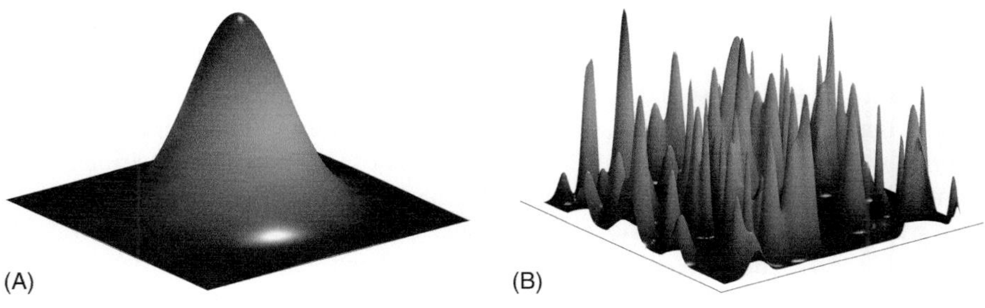

FIGURE 7.4 Sign epistasis makes the landscape more 'rugged'. A fitness landscape structure is in between the two extremes shown in the figure. In (A), we have a smooth landscape. Evolution in this case is deterministic because on this landscape, all evolving trajectories reach the same peak. However, in (B), an extremely rugged and multi-peaked structure is shown. In this case, movement of a population is strongly influenced by stochasticity – i.e., specific mutations take a population toward one peak, while another mutation takes the population toward a completely different peak. 'Ruggedness' as a phenomenon is incorporated in landscapes with the help of sign epistasis.

understanding structure of actual fitness landscapes and movement of populations on it is called 'ruggedness'.

Consider the two cases shown in the Figure 7.4. In the first case, the landscape is 'smooth', and in the second, it is 'rugged'. Being smooth or rugged has important implications on the evolutionary trajectories of populations.

Let us consider the 'smooth' landscape first (Figure 7.4A). Imagine a population starting from any point on the landscape. It increases in fitness, and, hence, moves up the fitness landscape. Eventually, the population reaches the fitness peak. Now, imagine another population starting from another point on this landscape. Note that this starting point on the landscape also ends up at the same peak. Thus, if landscapes look like the structure shown in the figure, then evolution is deterministic in the sense that all trajectories move toward the same fitness peak. Different trajectories will take different paths to the peak, but their end destination will be the same.

On the other hand, landscapes can be multiple-peaked too (Figure 7.4B). In these cases, evolutionary trajectories, depending on where we start from the sequence space and which are the first mutations that occur, a population can move toward one peak or the other. For instance, starting from any point, if the first mutation increases fitness in the direction of one peak, then the population ends up at this peak. Alternatively, if the first mutation took the population toward another peak, then the population ends up on the other peak. In this scenario, evolution is not a deterministic process. Different realizations of an evolutionary process can lead us to different fitness peaks. In addition, populations starting at different places on the landscape will end up at different peaks.

The ruggedness or smoothness of a landscape is dictated by sign epistasis on the landscape.

7.4 MODELING EPISTASIS (NK MODEL)

Efforts to model fitness landscapes were first made in the 1980s, primarily by physicists. But let us first understand what is it that we hope to achieve by modeling fitness landscapes? Very early, it was realized that fitness landscapes are large entities which are going to be difficult, if not impossible to trace experimentally. Remember that this was in a time when DNA manipulation had just become possible and was a tedious and laborious task. Thus, constructing 4^L sequences was an impossible task. Thus, given this experimental challenge, the question became, can we develop mathematical models of fitness landscapes which will tell us statistical properties of fitness landscapes? For instance, can we ask questions like,

> *with increasing sign epistasis, how rapidly does the number of peaks in the landscape increase?*

or,

> *with increasing L, how does the number of peaks change in an average landscape?*

It was with this intent that modeling frameworks to study fitness landscapes and movement on them were developed.

Our goal in this brief section of this chapter is to study one such popular class of models, called *NK* models.

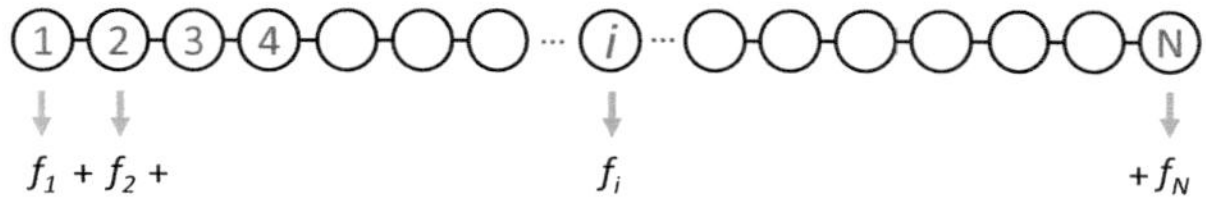

FIGURE 7.5 Fitness of an organism with N loci. In this approach, the genome of the organism is broken down into N loci. Each locus makes a fitness contribution f_i toward the organismal fitness. The total fitness of the organism is, therefore, simply the sum of the fitness contributions from the N loci.

The *NK* model is attractive because by tuning a free parameter K (which represents the extent of epistasis in the model), we can obtain landscapes with different degrees of ruggedness, and study how populations move on these structures. This feature of the *NK* model allows us to answer the questions that we raised above.

To understand how the *NK* model works, consider a genome with N loci – numbered from 1 to N (Figure 7.5). These loci can be thought of as genes, or pathways. What is important is that we have to think of these loci as parts of the genome, where each part makes a contribution to the fitness of the organism. Let us imagine that the *i*th locus makes a contribution f_i to the fitness of the organism. Thus, the fitness of the organism is simply given by,

$$F = \sum_{i=1}^{N} f_i$$

where,

f_i is the fitness contribution of the *i*th locus on the genome and is *only* dependent on what is present at the *i*th locus, and is independent of what is present at any of the other $(N - 1)$ loci on the genome. You should realize that this formulation means that we are talking of a case where there is no epistasis. This is exactly what we discussed in Example 7.2 in this chapter.

In the above scenario, the fitness contribution of a locus is only dependent on what (nucleotide, gene allele) is present at that particular locus. The fitness contribution of the *i*th locus is independent of what is present elsewhere on the chromosome. In the context of *NK* model, this is the scenario where K equals zero. That is, fitness contribution of a particular locus is dependent on zero other loci on the genome.

Thus, in the *NK* model, N represents the size of the genome (in terms of number of nucleotides, genes, loci, etc.) and K represents the number of loci (other than *i*) which dictate the fitness contribution of the *i*th locus. In the above case, since the contribution of the *i*th locus is independent of any other locus (other than *i*), K equals zero.

When K equals 1, it means that the fitness contribution of each locus is dependent on what is present at one other locus on the genome. This can be modeled by assuming that the fitness contribution of the *i*th locus, f_i, is (in addition to what is present on the *i*th locus) dependent on what is present at the $(i + 1)$th locus. For the last locus, N, the fitness contribution f_N is dependent on what is present at the first locus.

$$f_i = \text{function of } i^{\text{th}} \text{ and } i + 1^{\text{th}} \text{ loci}$$

In this scenario, the total organismal fitness is still given by the sum of N fitness contributions from the N loci, and f_i still represents the fitness contribution of the ith locus on the genome. However, the key difference between this case (K equal to one) and the one discussed above (K equals zero) is that now, f_1 is not just dependent on what is present at the locus 1, but is also dependent on what is present at locus 2. Similarly, fitness contribution of the second locus, f_2 is not just dependent on what is present at locus 2 but is also dependent on what is present at locus 3. And so on.

Similarly, we can tune the variable K and adjust the extent of epistasis in the fitness landscape. If we were to plot the fitness landscape after defining fitness landscapes in the manner above, we will note that the fitness landscape becomes increasingly rugged as K increases.

From the perspective of understanding the fundamentals of moving on a landscape, it is often assumed that, for each position, we have two options for nucleotides (0 and 1). This simplification from the reality (where there are four options for each position, A, T, G, and C) simplifies the analysis of movement on landscapes without altering the results qualitatively.

How do we define rules of epistasis? For example, imagine a landscape with K equal to 1. That is, the fitness contribution of a locus (i) is dependent on one other locus (j). Thus, the fitness contribution of allele '1' at locus i is contingent on whether there is a 0 or a 1 present at locus j. Epistasis and its rules are a subject of intense research in the last few years, and little is known about how it operates at a global scale. Hence, as a first approximation, to investigate movement of populations on a landscape, the rules of epistasis are often assumed randomly. For example, fitness contribution of allele 1 at locus i is given by f_i as,

$$\begin{aligned} f_i &= K_0 \text{ if allele at } j \text{ is } 0; \\ &= K_1 \text{ if allele at } j \text{ is } 1. \end{aligned}$$

where, K_o and K_1 are randomly chosen constants, and j is another locus on the genome. The same is done for all loci in the genome.

Note that in real cases it is not necessary (actually extremely unlikely) that every locus' contribution depends on K other loci, and this K is the same for every locus. In reality, it is very likely that some loci are of the kind whose fitness contribution is dictated by no/few loci. Whereas, there will be some loci whose fitness contribution is dictated by many, many loci.

7.5 CONCLUSION

Epistasis is a real, ubiquitous phenomenon. However, our understanding of epistasis and how it manifests is quite limited. This limited understanding seriously restricts our ability to predict evolution. As a result, intense research is currently underway toward finding the 'rules' by which epistasis manifests in cells. These efforts are best represented by four papers in *Science* that have appeared in the last decade. These references are given in the reference list for this chapter. Our research group at IIT Bombay has also made contributions in this area via computational and theoretical research, with two papers in the reference list.

In Chapter 15 of the book, we will study experimental efforts to understand empirical fitness landscapes. In particular, we will study three studies. Despite the huge amount of effort involved, these studies are only able to scratch what fitness landscapes are. This is the challenge before the field.

EXERCISES

1. In Figure 7.2, we discuss three cases of epistasis, and one case of no epistasis. Which of the four possibilities seems to you the most widely observed in biological systems? Justify your intuition.
2. An *E. coli* strain has a fitness of 1.2 h^{-1} in an environment containing glucose as the carbon source. Mutation *I* increases the fitness of the strain to 1.5 h^{-1}. The strain carrying mutation *I* then acquires another mutation (mutation II), which further increases the fitness to 1.7 h^{-1}. If we know that no epistasis exists between the two mutations, what would be the effect of mutation II in the *E. coli* strain.
3. Using the code1 shared for this chapter, simulate the fitness landscape for *N* equal to 10 and *K* equal to one to ten. What are the differences you note in the structure of the fitness landscape as *K* increases.
4. Consider the following case of no epistasis in a sequence of length three.

	A	T	G	C
Position 1	0.01	0.05	0.03	0.08
Position 2	0.02	0.04	0.01	0.03
Position 3	0.3	0.04	0.003	0.06

   a. What is the sequence that confers the maximum fitness?
   b. Starting from sequence AAA, write down two alternate paths that the evolving population could take to reach the peak fitness.

5. Consider a DNA sequence of length, *L* equal to two. Fitness contributions of each position is as per the following rules,
   Fitness contribution of position 1:

		Nucleotide at position 1			
		A	T	G	C
Nucleotide at position 2	A	0.1	0.5	0.03	0.08
	T	0.2	0.4	0.01	0.03
	G	0.3	0.4	0.003	0.06
	C	0.4	0.2	0.4	0.4

Fitness contribution of position 2:

		Nucleotide at position 1			
		A	T	G	C
Nucleotide at position 2	A	0.1	0.05	0.03	0.08
	T	0.2	0.04	0.01	0.03
	G	0.4	0.04	0.003	0.06
	C	0.3	0.2	0.4	0.4

a. What is the sequence that confers the maximum fitness?
b. Starting from sequence AAA, write down two alternate paths that the evolving population could take to reach the peak fitness.

You should realize that this problem is qualitatively more difficult to solve than the previous problem. Imagine this complexity when extended over a genome!

BIBLIOGRAPHY

1. Miko I. 2008. Epistasis: Gene interaction and phenotype effects., 1:197.
(A simple illustration of what is epistasis, and how it can manifest to control phenotypes.)
2. Johnson MS, Reddy G, Desai MM. 2023. Epistasis and evolution: recent advances and an outlook for prediction. *BMC Biol* 21:120.
(A recent excellent review of what we know and not know about how epistasis manifests in bacterial populations.)
3. Venkataraman P, Saini S. 2025. On the metabolic basis and predictability of global epistasis. *bioRxiv Cold Spring Harbor Laboratory:2025*.02.04.636564.
(Recent work from our group which attempts to explain the mechanistic origins of the patterns of epistasis we see reported in [2] above.)
4. Kauffman SA, Weinberger ED. 1989. The NK model of rugged fitness landscapes and its application to maturation of the immune response. *J Theor Biol* 141(2):211–45.
(This is a classic paper which first introduced NK models for studying shape and properties of fitness landscapes.)

8 Drift

8.1 INTRODUCTION

The late paleontologist and evolutionary biologist, Stephen Jay Gould, once asked a rhetorical question. Gould asked, what would happen if we were to go back 4.5 billion years ago to the time when Earth was formed. From there, let us imagine that evolution takes place all over again? In such a hypothetical scenario, would species like the ones we see on the planet today be around after evolution for 4.5 billion years, or would evolution take a completely different course of action? In other words, Gould is asking what are the relative roles of chance and determinism in dictating evolutionary outcomes.

If evolution is largely dictated by chance events, then we would imagine that on a re-run of evolution of life on Earth, we would see very different kinds of life forms. Alternatively, if evolution is a very deterministic process, then a repeat of Earth's history would again throw up very similar outcomes in terms of organisms we see.

Thus, we return to the question: what are the relative roles of chance and determinism in dictating evolutionary outcomes? In this chapter, we will discuss how chance events change the dynamics of evolution in a population. The role that chance events play in dictating evolution is best illustrated by an example of *marbles in a jar*, which is what we start this chapter with.

8.2 MARBLES IN A JAR

Consider a jar with 100 marbles in it (Figure 8.1). Each of the marbles is of a unique color. The marbles are identical to each other in every other way, for example, size and weight. Thus, the frequency of each color in the jar is simply the number of marbles of a particular color divided by the total number of marbles in the jar. Since, in our jar, each marble is a unique color, the frequency of each color is $\frac{1}{100}$.

> **Example 8.1:** Imagine a population with 100 people. Twenty of them write with their left hand, and 80 of them write with their right hand. What is the frequency of right-handed people in this population.
>
> **Solution:** The frequency of right-handed people in the population is simply $\frac{\text{number of right handed people}}{\text{total population}}$. In our example, thus, the frequency of right-handed people is $\frac{80}{100}$.

DOI: 10.1201/9781003633662-8

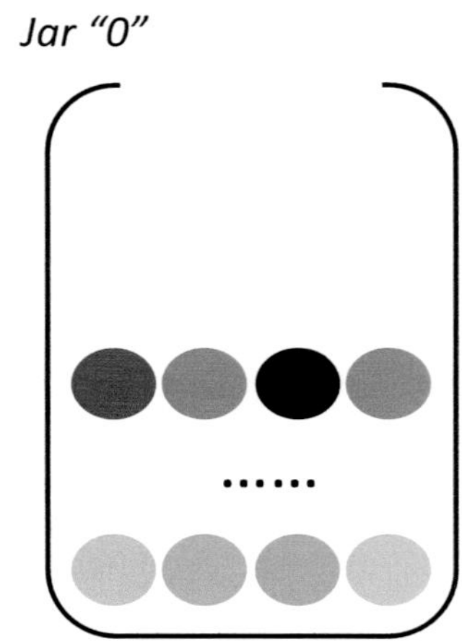

FIGURE 8.1 Marbles in a jar. A jar contains 100 marbles, each of unique color. Frequency of any color is simply equal to the number of marbles of that particular color divided by the total number of marbles in the jar. Since each marble has a unique color, frequency of each color is 1/100.

The example we discussed above is trivial, but you should note that just as we were discussing frequency of marbles in a jar, we can also discuss frequency of a particular phenotype in a population. We will be talking about these frequencies in a population quite a lot in the coming chapters.

Let us label the starting jar as Jar '0', or the starting jar. Next, we do the following.

a. Randomly pick a marble from the jar '0', and note its color (say, it is blue),
b. Put the marble drawn back in the jar '0' *and* place a marble of the same color (blue) in the next jar (Jar '1'),
c. Repeat (a) and (b) till the number of marbles in the jar '1' equals 100.

Before moving ahead,

➔ What can we say about the number of unique colors in jar '1' when its population reaches 100? Would it have reduced, or stayed the same? You should immediately note that it is impossible for the colors to increase in frequency.

What will likely happen is that because the entire process is completely randomized, some colors will be picked more than once, hence, their frequency will increase in jar '1'. However, since the total number of marbles in jar '1' is 100, some other colors may not be picked up at all. As a result, the number of unique colors in jar '1' will be lower than that of jar '0'.

For instance, if the blue-colored marble is picked twice, then, since the total number of marbles remains N, it is obvious that at least one color will not be present in jar '1'. Note that this is only possible because after drawing a marble from jar '0', we put it back in the same jar, allowing it to be picked again (see point b, above).

Let us continue the game further. Now, as per the rules $a - c$ defined above, marbles will be drawn from jar '1', and jar '2' will be populated.

The process continues from jar '*i*' to jar '$i + 1$'.

Example 8.2: Comment on what will be the final outcome of this game in terms of the number of unique colors present in the jar.

Solution: We should note that the end point of this game is when there is only one color left in the jar. Let us say that the only green marbles are left in the jar. Then we will always draw a green marble from the jar, and as a result, no other color can replace green. Hence, the next jar will contain only green marbles. The game halts at this point, because its position is static. This is the final outcome of the game.

Before moving ahead,

➔ At the start of the game, what can be say about the probability of the event that green marbles take over the jar, when the game ends?

The above question looks like a difficult question to solve, without any additional information. However, we can arrive at the answer to the above question simply using intuition and logic.

The original frequency of the green marbles is $\frac{1}{100}$ (because there is only one green marble in the jar at the start of the game).

We also know that the game ends with one of the colors taking over the jar. Since, other than their color, all marbles are identical to each other in all respects, each color has an equal probability of eventually occupying the jar. Thus, at the start of the experiment, the probability that blue marble will take over the jar is the same as the probability that green marble takes over the jar (which is the same as any other color taking over the jar). Let us call this probability p.

We also know that at the end of the game, one of the colors *does* take over the population. There is simply no other outcome of the game. Hence, the sum of these probabilities (of a color taking over the jar) equals 1.

Or,

$$p_{green} + p_{red} + .. + p_{black} = 1 \tag{8.1}$$

but,

$$p_{green} = p_{red} = .. = p_{black} = p \tag{8.2}$$

Since there are 100 colors in the jar, equation (8.2) becomes,

$$100p = 1 \quad \rightarrow \quad p = \frac{1}{100} \tag{8.3}$$

Thus, the likelihood of green marbles taking over the population is simply $\frac{1}{100}$.

The above result holds because the chance of each color taking over is *mutually exclusive*. That is, if green takes over the jar, then blue cannot. In such a scenario, the probability of one of the colors taking over the jar is simply the sum of probability of each color taking over. That is, for *mutually exclusive events*, probability of either one happening is simply given by sum of their individual probabilities.

8.3 ANALOGY BETWEEN 'MARBLES IN A JAR' AND EVOLUTIONARY PROCESSES

The 'marbles in a jar' game has a close analogy with evolutionary processes. If each jar is thought of as a generation of a population, and each marble as an individual (or an allele). Then, drawing a marble and placing the same color marble in the next jar can be thought of as equivalent to an individual giving birth to a progeny, and passing its allele to the next generation. The carrying capacity of the environment is fixed at 100, so the population size remains constant with time (100 marbles in our example).

Moreover, since each marble is equally likely to be drawn from the jar – the fitness of every individual in the population is the same.

Despite being of the same fitness – some individuals or alleles (colors) are lost from the population, while others increase in frequency. What causes this change in frequency? These changes in frequency are caused by randomness in the birth frequency. The marbles in a jar game is a simple illustration of how chance events lead to evolutionary change. Thus, natural selection is not a pre-requisite for evolutionary change.

With this toy introduction to drift or chance events in evolution, in the rest of this chapter, we will develop a basic quantitative framework to study evolution due to chance events (or drift) in microbial populations.

8.4 DRIFT IN EXPERIMENTAL EVOLUTION

Let us start with a question. Imagine a Continuous Stirred Tank Reactor (CSTR) or a chemostat (as discussed in Chapter 4) (Figure 8.2). The total carrying capacity of the chemostat is N.

This chemostat is populated by an isogenic bacterial population **A**, which has growth rate r_A. For this discussion, we will use growth rate as a proxy for fitness. Imagine that one of the individuals in the reactor acquires a beneficial mutation, and the progeny **B** has a fitness r_B.

Since the mutation that the progeny acquired is beneficial, $r_B > r_A$. Let us further imagine that the beneficial mutation confers a benefit of 2% to the progeny. Thus, $r_B = 1.02\ r_A$.

In this chapter, we seek an answer to the following question: assuming no new mutations occur in the chemostat, what is the probability that, after a sufficiently long time, progeny of **B** will entirely replace **A** from the chemostat? That is, as shown in Figure 8.3, what is the probability that starting from the image on the left, after a sufficiently long time, we will end up with the figure on the right?

From a strictly Darwinian sense, it seems that the probability of **B** (green) replacing **A** (blue) should be one. This is so because, since we are given that **B**

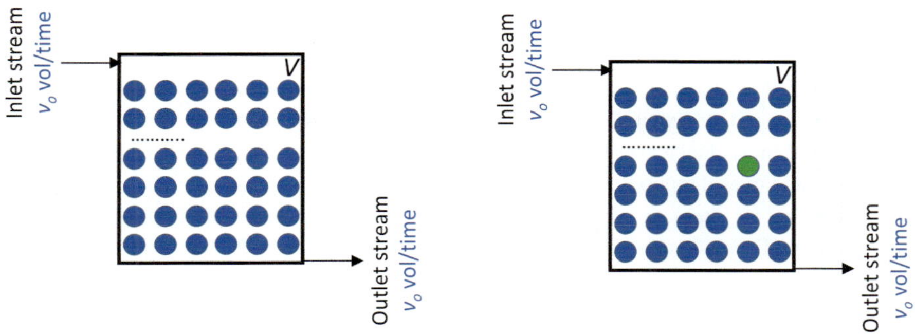

FIGURE 8.2 Evolution of a bacterial population in a CSTR/chemostat. (*Left*) A bacterial population is growing in a chemostat. All bacteria have identical DNA sequence, and in the given environment, have fitness r_A. In this operation, fresh media is continuously being added to the chemostat, and spent media is being removed at the same rate. This ensures that the volume of liquid in the chemostat does not change with time. At steady state, the number of bacteria removed from the chemostat per unit time is exactly balanced by the new births taking place in the chemostat per unit time. (*Right*) Imagine that at a certain time, one of the cell divisions leads to an individual (shown in green) which has a beneficial mutation and has a growth rate r_B ($> r_A$).

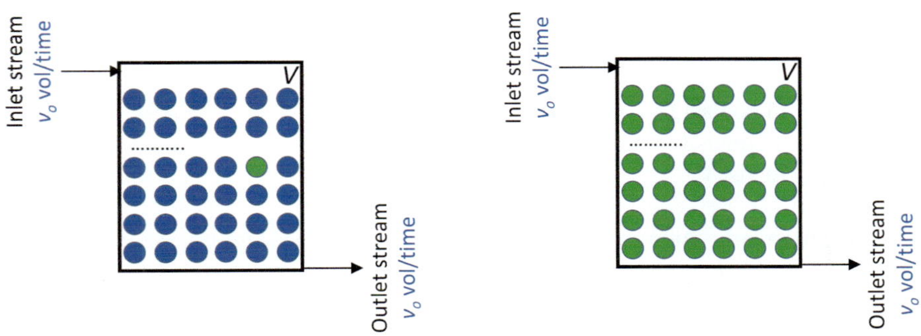

FIGURE 8.3 Imagine that the chemostat, at a given instant of time, is in position on the left. That is, it has $N - 1$ individuals (blue) with fitness r_A, and one individual (green) with fitness r_B. Given that ($r_A > r_B$), what is the probability that starting from the position on the left, the chemostat, after some time, reaches the state shown in the figure on the right. That is, what is the probability that the green individual bacteria on the left, on account of its higher fitness, is able to replace the entire blue population in the chemostat?

has a higher fitness than **A**, its progeny should replace those of **A** in every single independent run of this experiment. This is based on the fundamental principle of natural selection. However, viewing evolutionary change through the prism of only natural selection is not correct.

In the above discussion, we note that growth rate has been taken as a proxy for fitness. This is usually the case, but not necessarily universal. To see scenarios when fitness may not be best represented by growth rate, see Note I.

Example 8.3: Looking at Figure 8.3, can we imagine a scenario where B might not be able to replace A?

Solution: We can picture a scenario where the only **B** individual leaves the system through the exit stream of the chemostat even before it had a chance to replicate. Once the only **B** individual leaves the system, the only genotype left remaining is **A**. Hence, **B** cannot take over the population anymore.

Consider an alternate scenario. Imagine that the one **B** individual divided in the chemostat. Thus, the chemostat now has two **B** individuals (and $N - 2$ **A** individuals). In this scenario also, it is possible that both the **B** individuals are washed away in the exit stream of the chemostat before they divided. In such a scenario also, **B** is unable to replace **A** from the system.

The same can also happen when there are three **B** individuals in the chemostat. And so on. However, we should note that as the number of **B** individuals in the chemostat increase, it becomes increasingly unlikely for all of them to be washed away by chance.

We do not, yet, know the probability with which this might happen, but we can certainly imagine this manifestation of the chemostat. We turn to computing this probability next.

To compute the probability of **B** replacing **A** in the chemostat, let us denote the state of the system by a variable i. The variable i represents the number of **B** individuals in the chemostat. Clearly, i is a dynamic variable which keeps changing with time.

That is, when the number of **B** individuals in the chemostat is,

- One, i equals 1,
- Zero, i equals 0, and
- N, i equals N.

We are particularly interested in the probability that the system transitions from the state $i = 1$ (when there is only one **B** individual in the chemostat) to $i = N$ (when **B** has completely replaced **A** in the population in the chemostat) (Figure 8.4). Note that the transition represented in Figure 8.4 is the same as the one represented in Figure 8.3.

The state of the system, via variable i can be represented on a number line, as shown below.

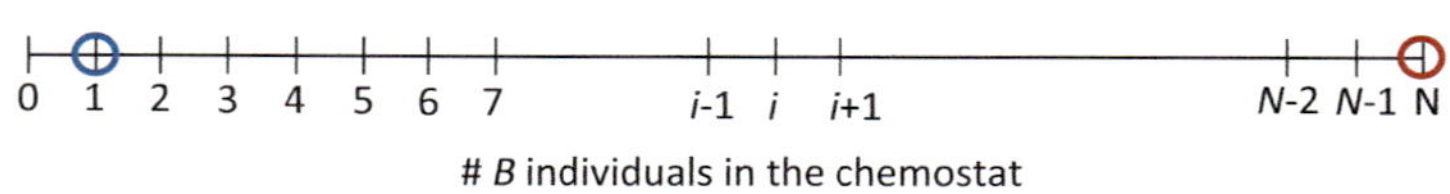

FIGURE 8.4 At any given point in time, the state of the chemostat can be represented by a number on the number line as shown above. The number line indicates the number of B individuals in the chemostat at any given point in time. Thus, as was posed in Figure 8.3, we are interested in quantifying the probability that the system is able to transition from # B individuals equal to 1 (blue open circle) to N (red open circle).

8.5 MORAN PROCESS

To model the process of bacterial growth and death in the chemostat, we first need to learn a simulation technique proposed by Moran. We mimic population growth in a Moran process by considering one single interval of time after another. In each of these intervals, exactly *one* birth and *one* death event take place. This ensures that while the population is dynamic in nature (cells are dying and born) but the population size remains constant at N (since in each time step, there is one birth and one death).

Let us imagine that the population at a given time is at a state i (number of **B** individuals in the population).

$$\#A \text{ individuals} = (N - i)$$

$$\#B \text{ individuals} = i \tag{8.4}$$

To mimic the birth process in the Moran process, we select one individual for birth. This individual is selected randomly from the population. However, this random selection is done in a way such that the individuals with greater fitness have a higher likelihood of being drawn, while those of lower fitness have a lesser chance of being drawn. Thus, the probability that an **A** individual is selected for birth is, thus, given by the fitness-weighted average of frequency,

$$P(A\text{ birth}) = \frac{\text{Fitness of } A \text{ individuals}}{\text{Fitness of total population}} = \frac{(N-i)r_A}{(N-i)r_A + ir_B} \tag{8.5}$$

If an **A** individual is selected for birth, the number of **A** individuals increases by one, from $N - i \to N - i + 1$.

Similarly, the probability that a **B** individual is selected for birth is given by,

$$P(B\text{ birth}) = \frac{\text{Fitness of } B \text{ individuals}}{\text{Fitness of toal population}} \frac{ir_B}{(N-i)r_A + ir_B} \tag{8.6}$$

If a **B** individual is selected for birth, the number of **B** individuals increases by one, from $i \to i + 1$.

From the context of the chemostat, the above probabilities are akin to the probability that an **A** or a **B** individual divides in the next cell division event. As the above equations show, the probability of division for each genotype is dependent on their number and their fitness. Note that the two probabilities in equations (8.5) and (8.6) add up to one.

Similarly, we can calculate the probability of death in the single step of the Moran process. In the chemostat, death is akin to being eliminated from the reactor via the exit stream. The exit from the stream (death) is simply dependent on the physical proximity of an individual to the exit stream, and is, thus, assumed to be independent of the fitness of an individual. Thus, the probability that an **A** individual is washed (death event) from the chemostat is simply proportional to the frequency of **A** individuals in the chemostat. Based on these,

$$P(A\ \text{death}) = \frac{(N-i)}{(N-i)+i} = \frac{(N-i)}{N}$$

and

$$P(B\ \text{death}) = \frac{i}{(N-i)+i} = \frac{i}{N} \qquad (8.7)$$

In case of death for an **A** individual, the number of individuals of **A** decreases from $N - i \rightarrow N - i - 1$. And, in case of **B** death, the number of **B** individuals decreases from $i \rightarrow i - 1$.

In the setup that we describe, in one step of the Moran process, only four transitions are possible in a single birth-death step. These transitions in a single step of the Moran process are shown in Table 8.1 and Figure 8.5.

TABLE 8.1
Transitions in One Step of the Moran Process in a Population of *A* and *B* Type Individuals

Individual Picked for Birth	Individual Picked for Death	Transition in the State of the System
A	A	$(N-i) \rightarrow (N-i)$
A	B	$(N-i) \rightarrow (N-i+1)$
B	B	$(N-i) \rightarrow (N-i)$
B	A	$(N-i) \rightarrow (N-i-1)$

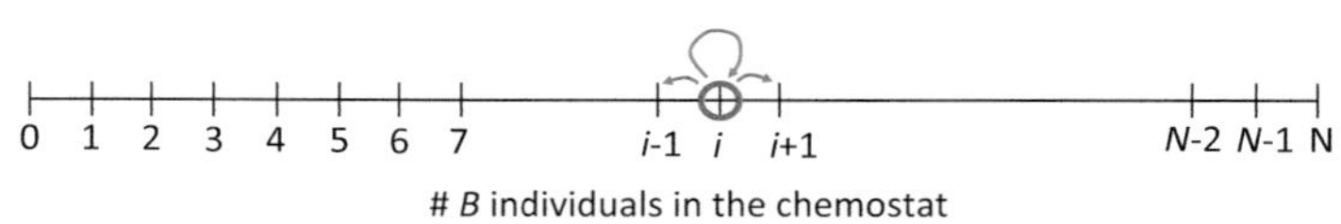

FIGURE 8.5 In one step of Moran process, three transitions are possible. From the system starting at state i (the number of B individuals in the population), the system can (i) transition to $i - 1$ (if A is picked for birth, and a B individual is picked for death), (ii) remain at i (if an A individual is picked for birth and death, OR if a B individual is picked for birth and death), or (iii) transition to $i + 1$ (if a B individual is picked for birth, and an A individual is picked for death). The probability of these three transitions is indicated by $P(i \rightarrow i - 1)$, $P(i \rightarrow i)$, and $P(i \rightarrow i + 1)$, respectively. Since the three transitions represent all possible transitions in a single Moran step, the three transitions add up to one.

8.6 A SHORT DETOUR INTO PROBABILITY

Before we go any further, we should note two crucial ideas from probability theory. These are called the *OR* and the *AND* rules of probability.

Imagine two independent events. By independent, we mean that the outcome of the first event has no bearing on what happens in the second. As an example, if we toss a coin, the outcome of the coin toss has no bearing on what number we see when we roll a dice. Thus, a coin toss and dice roll are independent events.

For independent events, we have the *AND* rule of probability. This rule says, that for two independent events, their probability is simply the product of the probability of the two events. For instance, if our first event is seeing *Heads* on the coin toss, and the second event is seeing *3* on the dice roll. Then the probability of seeing both events is given by,

$$P(Heads\ AND\ 3) = P(Heads)P(3) = \frac{1}{2}\cdot\frac{1}{6} = \frac{1}{12} \tag{8.8}$$

That is, according to the *AND* rule of probability, for independent events, probabilities multiply.

To understand the *OR* rule of probability, imagine two *mutually exclusive events*. Two events are said to be mutually exclusive if they both cannot happen together. If one happens, it is automatic that the other did not. For example, seeing the numbers 3 and 5 on a single roll of a dice are mutually exclusive events. In this case, probability that the first *OR* the second event will take place is simply the sum of the two probabilities.

$$P(3\ OR\ 5) = P(3)P(5) = \frac{1}{6} + \frac{1}{6} = \frac{1}{3} \tag{8.9}$$

Thus, according to the *OR* rule of probability, for mutually exclusive events, probabilities add.

8.7 TRANSITION PROBABILITIES

Let us now return to our discussion of transition probabilities.

Based on our discussion above, we can write mathematical expressions for the four possible transitions. These probabilities are given as,

$$P(A\ birth, A\ death) = \frac{(N-i)r_A}{(N-i)r_A + ir_B}\,\frac{(N-i)}{N} \tag{8.10}$$

In this case, the system stays at state i. Birth of an **A** individual adds one to the **A** population, but death of an **A** individual reduces the number of **A** individuals back to i. Remember we defined the state of the system as the number of **B** individuals in the population.

$$P(A\ birth, B\ death) = \frac{(N-i)r_A}{(N-i)r_A + ir_B}\,\frac{i}{N} \tag{8.11}$$

In this case, the system transitions from state i to $(i-1)$.

$$P(B\ birth, B\ death) = \frac{ir_B}{(N-i)r_A + ir_B}\frac{i}{N} \tag{8.12}$$

In this case, the system stays at state i.

$$P(B\ birth, A\ death) = \frac{ir_B}{(N-i)r_A + ir_B}\frac{(N-i)}{N} \tag{8.13}$$

Finally, in this case, the system transitions from state i to $(i+1)$.

Note again that in a single step of a Moran process, the system from a state i, can (a) transition to $(i+1)$ *or*, (b) transition to $(i-1)$ *or*, (c) remain at state i.

From the above four possibilities, we can calculate the probability of each of these transitions,

$$P(i \to i) = \frac{(N-i)r_A}{(N-i)r_A + ir_B}\frac{(N-i)}{N} + \frac{ir_B}{(N-i)r_A + ir_B}\frac{i}{N} \tag{8.14}$$

$$P(i \to i+1) = \frac{ir_B}{(N-i)r_A + ir_B}\frac{(N-i)}{N} \tag{8.15}$$

$$P(i \to i-1) = \frac{(N-i)r_A}{(N-i)r_A + ir_B}\frac{i}{N} \tag{8.16}$$

Using this framework, we note that the state of the system can be represented by a number line (between 0 and N) – which represents the number of **B** type individuals in the population (Figure 8.5). The state of the system at any given point in time can be represented by the location on this number line. We are interested in the probability of a single **B** individual in the population (location at $i = 1$ on the number line) reaching $i = N$ (as shown in Figure 8.4).

Note that, from the transition probability expressions above, we note that the likelihood of the system remaining at i, or moving to $(i+1)$ or $(i-1)$ are a function of i (the state of the system). That is, the probability of the system transitioning from i to $i+1$ is a function of i.

Before moving ahead,

➔ Go through the transition probability expressions and convince yourself that the transition probability of going from i to $i+1$ is higher when i equals $(N-1)$ as compared to when i equals 1.

Example 8.4: What do the three probabilities as indicated by equations (8.12)–(8.14) sum up to?

Solution: There are two ways to look at this question. The first is – simply sum up the three expressions. You will note that the sum of the three expressions comes out to one. I leave this exercise to the reader.

However, there is another way to look at this question. Note that according to the transitions we listed, Table 8.1 is an exhaustive list of *all* transitions. There is no other transition possible in the system. Thus, since the transitions we list are an exhaustive list of all possibilities, it must sum up to one.

To understand this better, consider a simpler example. Suppose we toss a coin. What is the sum of probabilities of seeing a Heads or a Tails? Since Heads or Tails are the only two possible outcomes of a coin toss, their probabilities must sum up to one. Alternatively, $P(Heads)$ is 0.5, and $P(Tails)$ is also 0.5. Both sum up to one.

To solve for the probability of transition from $i = 1$ to $i = N$, let us define a variable x_i.

$$x_i = P(system\ reaches\ state\ N\ starting\ from\ state\ i) \tag{8.17}$$

From our discussion above, we should note that the probability I am most interested in is x_1. That is the likelihood of starting with one **B** individual in the population, reaching a state where the population is entirely **B**.

To understand the derivation, the next step is key. Pay close attention to how this equation is framed.

Since in a single step of the Moran process, only three transitions are possible, we can write the following recursive relationship,

$$x_i = P(i \rightarrow i - 1)x_{i-1} + P(i \rightarrow i)x_i + P(i \rightarrow i + 1)x_{i+1} \tag{8.18}$$

The right side of the equation is the same probability, but after the system has taken one Moran step.

In words, the above equation represents the following. The left side of the equation is simply the probability that starting with a state of the system where there are i **B** individuals in the population, what is the probability that the system reaches a state of N **B** individuals.

However, once the system starts from state i, in one Moran step, it can reach state $(i - 1)$, remain at state i, or move to state $(i + 1)$. These three transitions are represented in the three terms on the right-hand side of equation (8.16).

The first term on the right side says that starting from i, the first step of Moran process takes the system to $(i - 1)$ with a probability $P(i \rightarrow i - 1)$. Thus, from there, if the system has to reach state N, the probability of that event is x_{i-1}. Hence, the first term on the right side of equation (8.18) says that starting from state i, the system (after one Moran step) can move to $(i - 1)$ and from there reach N.

The middle term of right side is telling us that another way for the system to reach N is to start at i, and after one Moran step, remain at i (this probability is $P(i \rightarrow i)$). From there, the probability that the system reaches N is x_i.

Finally, the last term of the right side tells us that starting from i, the system could move to $(i + 1)$ after one Moran step (this happens with probability $P(i \rightarrow i + 1)$). From there, the probability of reaching N is x_{i+1}.

Thus, while the left side gives the probability of reaching N starting at i, the right side gives the same expression but after allowing one step of the Moran process.

After having understood the equation (8.16), you should also note that the term x_i appears on both left- and right-hand side of the equation.

We can write the equation (8.16) for i equal to 1, 2, ···., $N - 1$. This gives us $N - 1$ equations.

In addition, we also know that,

$$x_o = 0 \tag{8.19}$$

Remember that x_i is the probability that the system reaches a state of all **B**, starting from state i. In this case, the starting state of the system is that there are zero **B** individuals. Hence, as there are no **B** individuals in the system, the probability that the system reaches i equal to N is zero.

And,

$$x_N = 1 \tag{8.20}$$

Since the system is already at state N, the probability it reaches N is equal to 1.

Since we know the expressions for the transition values, for a given population size, and the magnitude of the fitness advantage of the beneficial mutation, we can solve for the transition probability x_1.

For a case when the fitness of **A** is r_A, and fitness of **B** is r_B, for a large population size $(N \gg 1)$,

$$x_1 \sim \frac{r_B - r_A}{r_B} \tag{8.21}$$

Note that the probability of **B** replacing **A** is simply the selection coefficient associated with the beneficial mutation in **B**.

Before moving ahead,

➔ What are the typical selection coefficients of beneficial mutations? What does your intuition tell you?

From experimental evidence from microbial systems, we know that the beneficial mutations typically confer an advantage of $< 5\%$ (corresponds to $s = 0.05$). Mutations that confer fitness advantage greater than 5% are quite rare.

This observation leads us to a somewhat surprising result that even for a strong beneficial mutation, conferring 5% growth advantage, the likelihood that the individual carrying this beneficial mutation is able to replace the ancestral population is only about 0.05. In other words, 19 out of 20 times, the individual carrying the beneficial mutation would be lost from the system, due to the action of drift. In the chemostat example, this would be akin to the beneficial mutant being washed away from the chemostat. A beneficial mutation of this magnitude would have to take place 20 times in the chemostat for one of them to be not washed away, and replace the ancestral genotype in the chemostat.

For mutations conferring smaller fitness advantage, this probability would be even smaller than this.

Hence, most beneficial mutations are lost from the system! Thus, when the frequency of beneficial mutations is small, their fate is dictated largely by drift, and to a much lesser extent, by selection. And since beneficial mutations, when they first arise in a population, are in small frequency – drift plays a large role in dictating evolutionary outcomes.

The spread of a mutation in a population so that every individual is carrying the mutation is called *fixation*. The probability that a mutation, after having arisen in an individual in a population, reaches fixation is called the *fixation probability*.

Note that in the above discussion, x_1 is the fixation probability of a beneficial mutation.

We should consider a few points at this stage,

First, a typical trajectory of a beneficial mutation, as it spreads through the population, is often represented as below (Figure 8.6). Note that in most cases, the beneficial mutation is simply lost from the system.

Since the likelihood of being washed away from the chemostat is purely a stochastic/chance process, the system dynamics is a combined result of a deterministic force (natural selection) and a stochastic process (death) (Figure 8.7). When i (number of ***B*** type individuals) in the chemostat is small, the trajectory is largely dictated by stochasticity. However, as i increases, the chance that all individuals carrying the beneficial mutation are lost from the system (and we return to state i equals zero) are increasingly small. Hence, at higher values of i, the system is largely driven

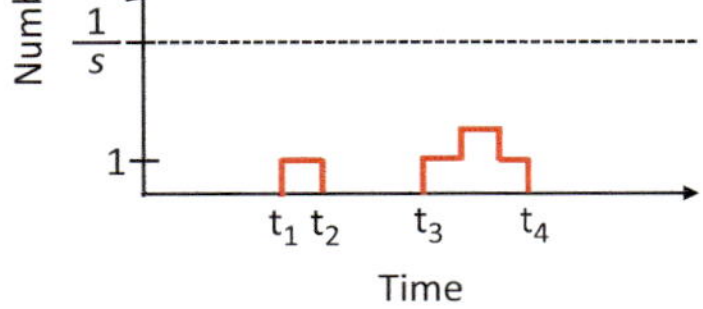

FIGURE 8.6 Most beneficial mutations are lost from a chemostat. Imagine an isogenic population in a chemostat starting at time t equal to zero. At t equal to t_1, a beneficial mutation occurs in the population (as indicated by the red line). However, before this mutant divides, it is lost from the chemostat at time t_2. As a result, the beneficial mutation is lost from the system because of the action of drift. At time t_3, another beneficial mutation occurs in the chemostat. This mutant divides, and hence, the number of individuals carrying this mutation increases to two. However, both the individuals carrying this mutation are lost from the chemostat. As a result, by time t_4, the beneficial mutation is lost from the system.

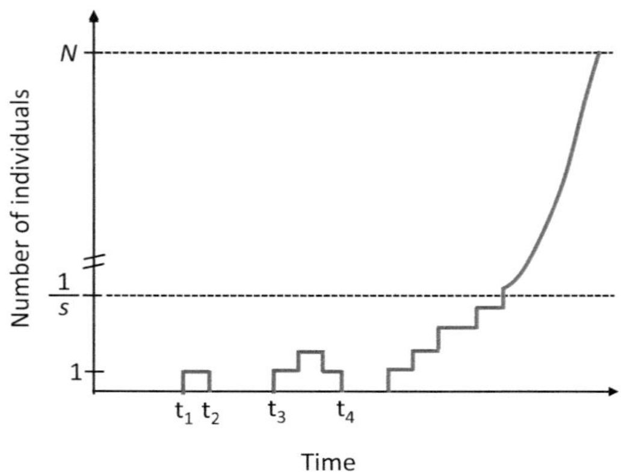

FIGURE 8.7 Beneficial mutation reaches fixation. As shown in the figure above, two beneficial mutations occur at t_1 and t_3. However, both these beneficial mutations are lost from the system. The third mutation in the system, does not get eliminated from the system. Note that, before the frequency of the beneficial mutations reaches $\frac{1}{s}$, the fate of the mutation is largely dictated by drift or chance events. Once, however, the frequency of the individuals carrying the beneficial mutation crosses this limit, the likelihood of these individuals getting lost from the system due to chance are negligible. As a result, the frequency of the individuals carrying the beneficial mutation increases exponentially thereafter. Note that the threshold of when drift or chance events become negligible in dictating the fate of a beneficial mutation is dependent on the strength of the mutation, s. If a beneficial mutation has a small s, more individuals (compared to another beneficial mutation with a higher s) carrying that mutation are needed before its fate is dictated by selection alone.

deterministically. Thus, it is important to realize that the relative significance of the stochastic and deterministic forces driving the system is a function of the state of the system.

Second, in our analysis, we have only considered a version where the mutation to have arisen is a beneficial mutation. What would happen in the system if ***B*** carried a mutation which reduced fitness? Note that natural selection would work toward eliminating such variants. However, chance would still permit the mutation to spread in the population (if the mutant escapes being ejected from the system, at least for some time). However, once the number of such ***B*** mutants enters the region where its fate is dictated largely by selection (i.e., large i), natural selection would ensure that it does not increase in frequency further. As a result, the chance that a deleterious mutation reaches fixation is negligible, and is not considered relevant as far as evolutionary change is concerned. Deleterious mutations can only spread in the population if the population underwent a large bottleneck (we will discuss this later), or if the population size was so small that stochastic forces dominated deterministic natural selection (this scenario is rarely realized in microbial populations where population sizes are extremely large).

8.8 CONCLUSION

In this chapter, we discussed an important result in evolutionary biology theory. This result emphasizes how important chance events are in dictating outcomes. More specifically, it tells us that the chance that a beneficial mutation survives in a population is extremely small. Much more likely is the fact that the beneficial mutation will be lost from the population because of a chance occurrence. Does this seem surprising?

Interestingly, the probability that a mutation reaches fixation is further reduced because of a phenomenon called *clonal interference*, which we turn to next. Thus, beneficial mutations, despite conferring an advantage to the individual they are present in, need a lot of luck to survive in a population!

NOTES

Note I

Why growth rate itself should not be used as a proxy for microorganismal fitness.

A typical microbial growth curve looks like Figure 8.8.

Upon first transferring to a flask containing certain growth nutrients, initially there is a phase when there is no growth. This phase is associated with the microorganisms synthesizing proteins which would enable it to grow on that nutrient media. For example, if *E. coli* were transferred from a media containing glucose as the carbon source to a media containing lactose as the carbon source, the cells would not be able to grow immediately upon transfer. This is because to be able to grow on lactose,

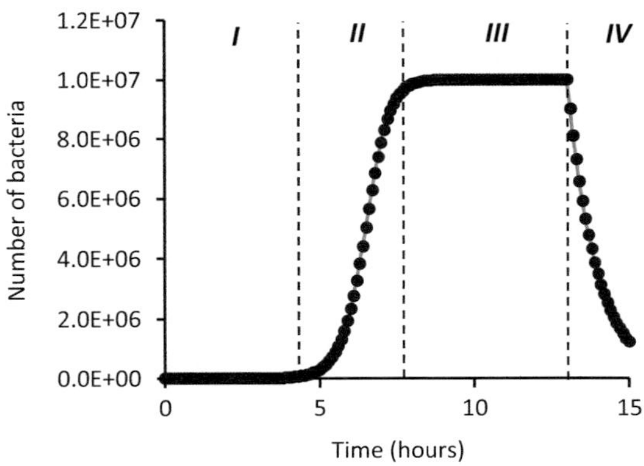

FIGURE 8.8 Typical growth curve of bacteria in a batch culture. When introduced in a media, the bacteria typically take some time before they start dividing. This phase is associated with protein production necessary for growth in that environment. This phase is referred to as the 'lag' phase and is indicated by '*I*' in the figure. In the next phase, bacteria divide exponentially with time. This phase is called the 'exponential' or 'log' phase and is indicated by '*II*' in the figure. Once all the nutrients have been exhausted from the media, there is no more growth. As a result, the number of cells does not increase with time. This phase is referred to as the 'stationary' phase, and is indicated by '*III*' in the figure. After stationary phase, the cells begin to die and the number of viable cells in the culture flask decreases with time. This phase is referred to as the 'death' phase, and is indicated by '*IV*' in the figure.

cells need several proteins, such as LacZ, LacY. The expression of these proteins is repressed in environments which contain glucose. This phase of growth when the cells do not exhibit any growth because of absence of the appropriate proteins being expressed in them is referred to as the 'lag phase'.

In the next phase of growth, the cells actively divide and grow exponentially. This phase is therefore referred to as the 'exponential phase' or also 'log phase'. Increase in cell numbers in this phase is represented by the following equation,

$$N(t) = N_o e^{rt} \tag{8.22}$$

where, N_o is the number of cells present at the start of the exponential phase, r is the growth rate, and t is the time of growth in the exponential phase. The parameter r is also referred to as the 'Malthusian parameter' and in many studies is taken as a proxy for fitness of a microbial population.

The exponential phase of growth continues as long as nutrients are present in the media. As the nutrients begin to run out, the cell growth slows down and eventually halts completely. In this phase, the number of cells remains constant. Stationary phase does not mean that the cells are metabolically completely inactive. In fact, in this phase, cell growth is supported by cell death occurring in the flask.

After the stationary phase, death events outnumber cell growth, and the total number of viable cells in the flask starts to decrease. This phase of 'growth' is referred to as the 'death phase'.

If we compete two genotypes – both in exponential phase – in a particular media, then obviously, the one with a greater growth rate is going to increase faster in this environment, compared to the other. Thus, the faster growing strain will have a higher fitness. As a result, often, growth rates of different strains are taken as proxies for fitness. While this is largely an accurate analysis, we should be aware of other possible scenarios too, where growth rate is a poor indicator of fitness.

Consider the growth curves in Figure 8.9.

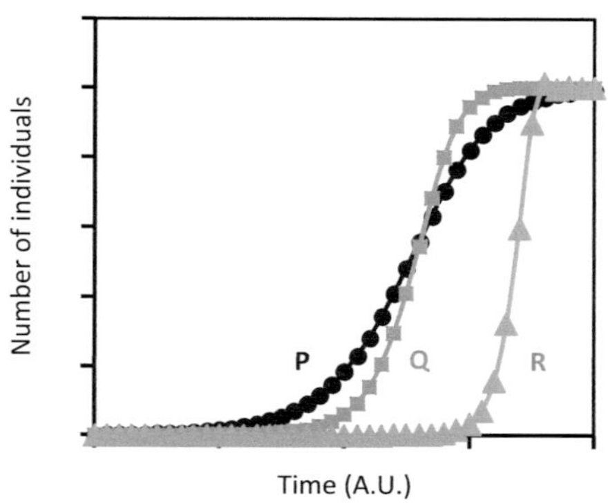

FIGURE 8.9 Growth dynamics of three different strains (P, Q, and R) in a particular growth environment. Strain P exhibits no lag phase and smallest growth rate in the exponential phase. Strain Q exhibits a finite log phase but a higher growth rate than P. Last, strain R exhibits the longest lag phase, and the highest growth rate in the exponential phase.

TABLE 8.2
Growth Characteristics of Strains *P*, *Q*, and *R*

Strain	Lag Phase Duration	Growth Rate
P	Minimum	Minimum
Q	Medium	Medium
R	Highest	Highest

Based on this, we can summarize the growth characteristics of the three strains as in Table 8.2.

Before moving ahead,

➔ Which of the three strains has a highest fitness in the given media conditions? Take a pause here, and try and reason out an answer from the data above.

If we simply take growth rate as a proxy of fitness then we would be tempted to say that the strain *R* is the fittest strain among the three and strain *P* would be the least fit strain among the three.

However, that would be wrong. Consider the following situation: what if we add to a flask with a media composition of the above growth curves, equal numbers of each of these three strains. What would be the growth dynamics then?

Take a look at the graphs again. Since the strain *P* has zero lag phase, it exhibits growth (albeit at a slower rate than other strains) right from the time of transfer. As a result, by the time the other strains even start to increase in number, strain *P* has exhibited considerable growth. As a result, the amount of nutrients that are available for strain *Q* and *R* is considerably reduced. Thus, in this initial time, strain *P* is the fittest among the three.

And after some time, strain *Q* starts to grow. This means that by the time the strain *R* enters its log phase, all the nutrients in the flask are already exhausted. As a result, when we compare the frequency of the three strains at the end of this experiment, we would find that, starting from an equal number of each genotype, strain *P* has the highest number of progeny (and hence, highest fitness), followed by *Q* and *R*, respectively.

Consider one more example, as shown in Figure 8.10.

In this case, strain *X* exhibits a high growth rate and strain *Y* exhibits a lower growth rate. Both strains exhibit an identical lag phase duration. In this case, based on the higher growth rate of *X* we would be tempted to say that *X* has a higher growth rate than *Y*. However, when we look at the total biomass (maximum cell number) of the two strains, there is a marked difference. Strain *X*, while exhibiting a higher growth rate, plateaus at a much lower cell density as compared to strain *Y*. This could be because, as it utilizes the resources in the media, it secretes a metabolic end product which halts its own further growth. Strain *Y*, on the other hand, does not get impacted by this metabolic end product, and as a result grows to much higher numbers. In this case also, if we let the growth culture run its course, we will find

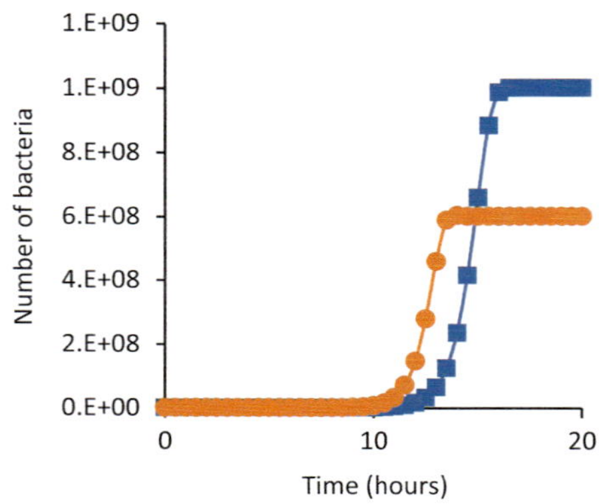

FIGURE 8.10 Growth dynamics of two strains, when grown singly, in a particular growth environment. Strain *X* (indicated by blue curve, square markers in the graph) exhibits a lower growth rate but a higher biomass at saturation. Strain Y (indicated by the orange curve, circle markers in the graph) exhibits a higher growth rate but a lower biomass levels of saturation.

that the number of progeny of *Y* is much greater than those of *X*. Hence, strain *Y* has a higher fitness as compared to *X*.

However, note that the definition of fitness also has a subjective quality associated with it. If two researchers were doing this experiment to compare the fitness of these two strains. One of them, who stopped the experiment at 10 hours, would conclude that strain *X* has a higher fitness, compared to *Y*. The other researcher, who conducted the experiment till 20 hours, would conclude that *Y* is fitter than *X*. Both are correct – because they define fitness differently!

The lesson we should learn from this is that fitness, a critical quantity in evolutionary biology, is a highly subjective, complex, and non-trivial quantity to define. This is also one of the reasons why evolutionary microbiologists simply define fitness as growth rate, as to avoid all the complications as defined above and more!

EXERCISES

1. Plot i versus x_i. Is this linear/non-linear? Before plotting it, think about the problem, and sketch a qualitative plot that agrees with your intuition. What is the reasoning behind your logic?
2. Is chance a greater force in systems with smaller N or larger N? Or, are smaller systems more susceptible to stochastic fluctuations, compared to larger systems?
3. What is the probability of fixation for green marbles in the 'marbles in a jar' game if the starting population contained four green marbles in the jar of the total of 100 marbles.
4. Remember that natural selection dictates that ***B*** should always replace ***A***, given that growth rate of *B* is greater than that of *A*. What then explains that the probability that a single mutant of ***B*** is not able to replace ***A*** individuals from a chemostat most of the times?

5. Write equation (8.16) for i equal to 1, 2, 3. Do you see the recursive nature of the equation?
6. Solve for the system of linear equations represented in equations (8.16), (8.17), and (8.18) and show that the solution of the system is equal to:

$$x_i = \frac{i}{N}$$

   In the case when **A** and **B** are neutral variants (i.e., they have identical fitness).
7. Solve for the system of linear equations represented in equations (8.16), (8.17), and (8.18) and show that the solution of the system is equal to:

$$x_i = \frac{i}{N}$$

   In the case when fitness of **A** is f_A and that of **B** is $f_A(1 + s)$ are neutral variants (i.e., they have identical fitness).

BIBLIOGRAPHY

1. Gould SJ. 1990. *Wonderful Life: The Burgess Shale and the Nature of History*. W W Norton & Co Inc. ISBN-10:039330700X.
   (Gould's book is a masterpiece and a classic. It narrates the wonderful tale of discovery of the Burgess Shale, and discusses the role of chance and determinism in dictating evolutionary fates of populations. Moreover, Gould is also a wonderful writer and we have much to learn by reading his prose.)
2. Travisano M, Mongold JA, Bennett AF, Lenski RE. 1995. Experimental Tests of the roles of adaptation, chance, and history in evolution. *Science* 267(5194):87–90.
   (This is one of my favorite papers. It uses an elegant and simple idea to decouple the contributions of adaptation, chance, and history in dictating evolution trajectories.)

9 Clonal Interference

9.1 INTRODUCTION

Consider a cellular population of size N in a chemostat. The population is isogenic, and each individual has fitness f. As time progresses, beneficial mutations will occur and individual with higher fitness will replace those with fitness f. This process of replacement can take place in one of two ways. In this chapter, we will develop an intuition and a quantitative understanding of how this takes place in microbial populations.

9.2 TWO REGIMES

First, a beneficial mutation occurs in the population. The mutant survives drift, and its progeny increase in numbers. As this happens, the frequency of the ancestral genotype decreases with time. Eventually, the mutant progeny reach fixation, and the original ancestral genotype has gone extinct. After the process of fixation, we wait for a newer beneficial mutation to occur and survive drift. The whole process then repeats itself. This process is illustrated in Figure 9.1. What is important to note here is that during the process of the beneficial mutation reaching fixation, there are only two genotypes in the chemostat – one, the ancestral genotype and two, the genotype carrying the beneficial mutation.

The above scenario can be plotted graphically in another way (Figure 9.2).

In this representation, we start with an isogenic population of size N at $t = 0$. This continues for a certain time before a beneficial mutation (indicated by red) arises. This individual carrying the beneficial mutation persists in the population for a while, before going extinct. Thereafter, another beneficial mutation arises in the population, whose numbers fluctuate with time, before this mutation, too, goes extinct from the chemostat. Finally, we have another beneficial mutation occur in the chemostat, whose frequency increases with time, and eventually, this mutation reaches fixation.

The key thing to note here is that we wait a certain time before a beneficial mutation arises and survives drift. Each beneficial mutation has two fates. First, it gets lost due to drift. In the representation in the figure, the first two beneficial mutations to arise are eliminated by drift. Second, the beneficial mutation survives drift – in which case, it increases in frequency. This is represented by the third mutation that arises in the chemostat and reaches fixation.

This process then repeats itself with the second set of beneficial mutations, indicated in green in Figure 9.2.

We should note that there are two time-constants associated with this process.

First, the time we have to wait for the first beneficial mutation that escapes drift. This is represented as τ_w in the figure. Second, the time it takes for the beneficial mutation that has escaped drift to reach fixation. This time is represented as τ_{fix}.

DOI: 10.1201/9781003633662-9

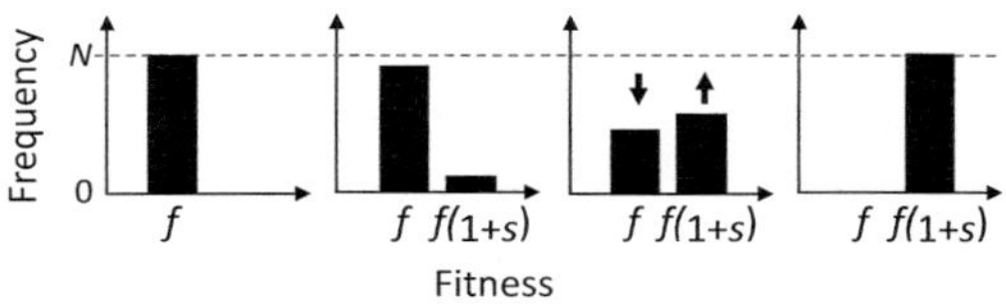

FIGURE 9.1 Imagine a population of size N in a chemostat. All individuals in the population have fitness f (left panel). After a certain time, one individual acquires a beneficial mutation and has fitness $f(1+s)$. As a result, the frequency of individuals at fitness f is $N-1$, and those at $f(1+s)$ is 1 (second panel). As shown in the third panel, the frequency of the higher fitness genotype increases, and that of the lower fitness decreases. This continues till the higher fitness genotype eliminates the original genotype from the population (rightmost panel). This process then repeats itself. Note that at any given point in time, there are only two genotypes in the population.

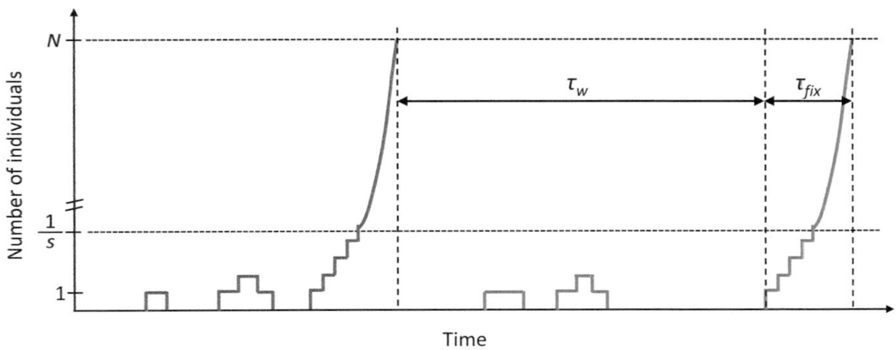

FIGURE 9.2 Starting from an isogenic population, a beneficial mutation arises in the population and reaches fixation. This is indicated by the red curve reaching fixation. In this regime, there is a time τ_w associated with waiting for the next beneficial mutation which survives drift to arise. After τ_w time, such a mutation arises and reaches fixation. The time taken for this beneficial mutation to reach fixation is indicated by τ_{fix}. In the regime shown in the figure above, $\tau_w \gg \tau_{\text{fix}}$. This ensures that at any given point in time, there is only one genotype in the population.

Note that τ_w is not the time associated with the occurrence of a beneficial mutation. This is so because, as we saw in the last chapter, a large majority of the beneficial mutations that occur are going to simply be lost due to drift. Instead, τ_w is the waiting time associated with the first beneficial mutation that escapes drift.

The two time-constants discussed above are often measured in the number of generations and not the absolute amount of time. This makes possible comparisons and analysis against populations of different generations time.

Depending on the relative magnitude of these two time-constants, evolutionary change in microbial populations can be classified into two regimes.

We will now discuss these two regimes in detail.

9.2.1 Regime I. ($\tau_w \gg \tau_{fix}$)

In this regime, the waiting time associated with the occurrence of a beneficial mutation that escapes drift is much greater than the time it takes for the mutation to reach fixation. This suggests that the system is simply waiting for a beneficial mutation to escape drift. Once that event happens, the beneficial mutation quickly reaches fixation. This is followed by a long waiting time for the next beneficial mutation to occur and escape drift. It is this regime which is represented in Figure 9.2.

The distinguishing feature of this regime is that at any given point in time, if we were to examine the individuals in the population, they would all be isogenic. It is only in a small window of time where, upon sampling, we will find that there are two genotypes coexisting in the chemostat (Figure 9.2).

Let us try and think when would a population evolve as per regime I. The mutation rate is μ per cell per generation. Of all the mutations taking place in the population, only a small fraction is going to be beneficial. Hence, let us call the mutation rate of beneficial mutations as μ_b (where, $\mu_b < \mu$). Thus, if the population size is N, the number of beneficial mutations occurring per generation is $N\mu_b$. Of these, as we saw in the last chapter, only a fraction s will survive drift. Hence, the effective number of beneficial mutations that survive drift in one generation is $N\mu_b s$. Thus, the number of generations that it will take for one beneficial mutation to survive drift is,

$$\tau_w = \frac{1}{N\mu_b s} \tag{9.1}$$

As is evident from the equation above, for τ_w to be large, we ought to be working with systems with small populations, small beneficial mutation rates, and small selection coefficients. We will discuss quantitative aspects of the dynamics between τ_w and τ_{fix} later in this chapter.

Example 9.1: Estimate τ_w in a microbial population of size 10^6, μ_b of 10^{-5} cell^{-1} generation^{-1}, and a selection coefficient s equal to 0.02.

Solution: Applying equation (9.1) to estimate τ_w, we get,

$$\tau_w = \frac{1}{10^6 10^{-5}(0.02)} = 5 \text{ generation.}$$

Thus, it takes five generations for there to be one mutation in this population which escapes drift. Note that time in this formulation is measured in the number of generations.

Example 9.2: Suppose we want to design an evolution experiment with *E. coli* (μ_b of 10^{-5} cell^{-1} generation^{-1}, and s 0.02) such that there is one beneficial mutation that escapes drift every single generation. What should be the population size that we should be working with, in this experiment?

Solution: Again, we apply equation (9.1), to estimate N, which satisfies,

$$1 = \frac{1}{N10^{-5}(0.02)}$$

$$N = 5 \times 10^6$$

Note that in this discussion, we do not take into account deleterious and neutral mutations. Deleterious mutations will be acted against by selection and hence will never increase to appreciable frequencies. The fate of neutral mutations, on the other hand, is dictated solely by drift. In large populations, the probability of their frequencies reaching appreciable numbers is small. Hence, ignoring these two types of mutations from our analysis is a reasonable assumption to make in large microbial populations.

9.2.2 Regime II. ($\tau_w \ll \tau_{fix}$)

In this regime, the exact opposite of what we discussed is true. The waiting time for beneficial mutations is much smaller as compared to the time it takes for a beneficial mutation, once it has escaped drift, to reach fixation. As a result of this, before a beneficial mutation (which has escaped drift) reaches fixation, another beneficial mutation occurs in the population and escapes drift. As a result, the two beneficial mutations compete with each other. However, in this regime, before either one of them reaches fixation, another beneficial mutation occurs and escapes drift. This regime is depicted in Figure 9.3.

As a result of this, if we were to sample a population at any given point in time, many genotypes coexist in the population. This can be represented alternatively, as shown in Figure 9.4. A beneficial mutation arises in the population (shown in red), and thereafter increases in frequency. However, before it reaches fixation, another beneficial mutation arises in the population (shown in green). Thus, at this point,

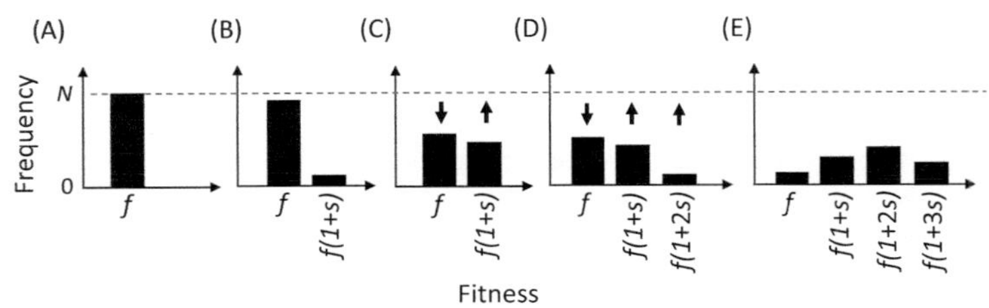

FIGURE 9.3 (A) Starting from an isogenic population, all individuals at fitness f. (B) One individual acquires a beneficial mutation. As a result, $N - 1$ individuals are at fitness f and one at $f(1 + s)$. (C) Selection dictates that the genotype at fitness f decreases in frequency, and those at $f(1 + s)$ increase in frequency. (D) As the frequency of individuals with fitness $f(1 + s)$ increases, one of the individuals acquires another beneficial mutation. This individual has a fitness $f(1 + 2s)$. (E) The same process continues, and in (E) four genotypes coexist in the chemostat.

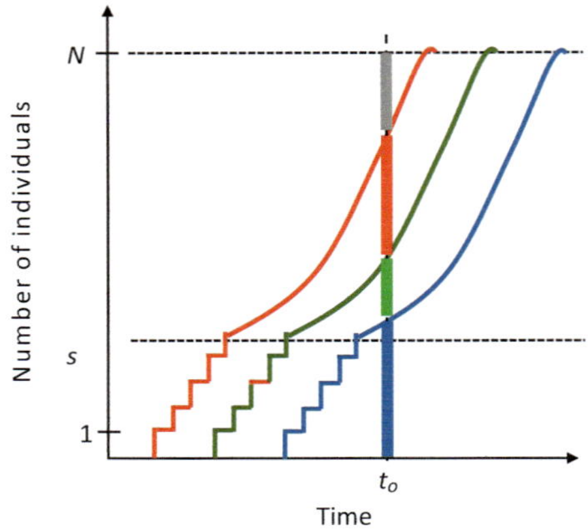

FIGURE 9.4 Starting from an isogenic population, a beneficial mutation occurs in the chemostat. The frequency of this mutation in the population is indicated by the red curve. Before this mutation reaches fixation, two more beneficial mutations (whose frequencies are indicated by the green and blue curve) occur in the population. Thus, at time t_o, the relative frequencies of the four genotypes in the population are given by the relative lengths of the four bars as shown in the figure. The gray bar represents the frequency of the ancestral genotype.

there are three genotypes in the population (ancestor, beneficial mutation indicated by red, and beneficial mutation indicated by green). Before the ancestor genotype is eliminated, or any of the two beneficial mutations reach fixation, another beneficial mutation occurs in the chemostat (indicated by the blue curve). Thus, multiple genotypes coexist in the chemostat at any given point in time.

All these genotypes, each carrying a unique beneficial mutation, are competing against each other. Eventually one of the genotypes reaches fixation, and the process continues. The process where multiple genotypes coexist and compete against each other in a population is referred to as *clonal interference*.

Before moving ahead,

➔ Before moving forward, you should pause at this point and try and reason (with the help of some back of the envelope calculations) which of the two regimes you think is more relevant for a microbial population. To estimate this, you will need some numbers (like population size in a 100 ml chemostat, *E. coli*'s mutation rate, what is a typical selection coefficient of a beneficial mutation). Look up these numbers from literature, and make assumptions to arrive at a reasonable estimate of what you think is a more appropriate regime for *E. coli* in a chemostat.

9.3 ESTIMATE OF τ_w

Let us imagine that our system is a 100 ml chemostat containing *E. coli* in LB media. The population size for this system can be assumed to be $O(10^{10})$ (although its precise value will be dictated by the rate at which dilution is taking place in the reactor). But as a first approximation, let us N as 10^{10}.

E. coli has a mutation rate, μ, of 10^{-3} cell^{-1} generation^{-1}. However, for our analysis, we are only interested in the mutation rate of beneficial mutations, μ_b. We can write the total mutation μ as,

$$\mu = \mu_b + \mu_d + \mu_n \tag{9.2}$$

where,

μ_b is the rate at which beneficial mutations take place,
μ_d is the rate at which deleterious mutations take place, and
μ_n is the rate at which neutral mutations take place.

The estimates for μ_b are not easily available. They are also dependent on the environment in which it is being quantified – for example, the Baker's yeast (*S. cerevisiae*), a common microbial model system in research labs, is extremely well adapted when the carbon source is glucose. This means that the supply of beneficial mutations in this environment is very limited. On the other hand, in an environment with galactose as the carbon source, a large number of beneficial mutations are available. As a result, it is virtually impossible to get accurate estimates of μ_b. However, we are interested only in a qualitative estimate of μ_b.

Before moving ahead,

➔ Of the three types of mutations, which do you think is the most frequent – deleterious, beneficial, or neutral? Or, what percentage of all mutations that occur are (a) deleterious, (b) beneficial, and (c) neutral? You should list numbers that agree with your intuition of biology and evolutionary processes, before we go ahead. Remember, this is a question to which we do not yet have an answer to. So, there is literally no right or wrong answer!

The common consensus is that deleterious mutations far outnumber beneficial mutation. The intuition behind this idea is that if we make a random change to a machine (enzyme/protein, in this case), chances are that we will end up making the machine worse. It will only be a very fortuitous event that a random change leads to an improvement in the machine. Hence, $\mu_d > \mu_b$. The relative frequency of μ_n is more debatable. While it is largely believed that neutral mutations outnumber beneficial mutation, the relative frequency of neutral mutations compared to deleterious mutations is not clear. However, as a first estimate, we assume,

$$\mu_b < \mu_d \sim \mu_n \tag{9.3}$$

To quantify this idea, let us assume that,

$$\mu_b = \frac{\mu}{20} = 0.05\mu \tag{9.4}$$

Although this number is a guess, remember that in these types of calculations, we are only interested in qualitative estimates. The precise value of μ_b might be 1% of μ or 5% of μ. In either case, our estimate of μ_b being 5% of μ will be off by a factor of two or so. But remember that we are interested in order of magnitude calculations for the numbers of interest here.

Lastly, we need an estimate of selection coefficient, s. Evolution experiments in lab have shown that a selection coefficient, s of 0.03–0.04 represents a strong beneficial mutation. Hence, let us for our calculations assume s to be equal to 0.03.

Substituting these numbers, we get an estimate for τ_w as,

$$\tau_w = \frac{1}{10^{10}\,(0.05)(10)^{-3}(0.03)} = 6.10^{-3} \text{ generations} \tag{9.5}$$

This suggests for a system as large as a 100 ml chemostat, the waiting time associated with a beneficial mutation to escape draft is much smaller than a generation. Or, within a single generation, the number of beneficial mutations which escape drift is significantly greater than one. Thus, beneficial mutations arise rapidly.

9.4 ESTIMATE FOR τ_{fix}

The estimate for τ_{fix} is a little more complex, and we will make a number of simplifying assumptions. Remember that in calculating τ_{fix} we are interested in calculating the time it takes for a beneficial mutation which has escaped drift to reach fixation. By a rule of thumb, a beneficial mutation is said to have escaped drift when the number of individuals carrying that mutation is $\frac{1}{s}$ or more.

That is, a beneficial mutation which is only weakly beneficial (small s), the number of individuals that need to carry this mutation before it can be said that selection dictates it fate is larger, as compared to a mutation with a relatively larger s.

When a mutation escapes drift and its fate is dictated by selection. At that stage, the mutation is said to be *established* in the population. After establishment, a mutation either reaches fixation, or is eliminated because of another beneficial mutant in the population, which confers a greater fitness advantage. Drift does not dictate this mutation's fate anymore.

Thus, when a beneficial mutation becomes established in the population, its numbers are $\frac{1}{s}$. The relative fitness advantage that the individuals carrying this mutation have over the rest of the population is s. While making this last statement, we assume that there are no other mutants present in the population. Thus, the mutant population grows in the population with an exponent of s. At time t after establishment, the number of individuals of the mutant type is thus given by $N(t)$,

$$N(t) = N_o e^{st} = \frac{1}{s} e^{st} \tag{9.6}$$

We are interested in the time it takes for this population to reach fixation – i.e., the left side of the equation to become equal to N, the carrying capacity of the chemostat. By substituting $N(t)$ by N, and solving for time, t, we get,

$$\tau_{fix} = t = \frac{1}{s} \ln(Ns) \tag{9.7}$$

Example 9.3: Using the numbers used in equation (9.5), get an estimate of τ_{fix}.

Solution: Using equation (9.7), τ_{fix} can be estimated as

$$\tau_{fix} = \frac{1}{0.03} \ln\left(10^{10}\, 0.03\right) = 200 \text{ generations} \tag{9.8}$$

From our above discussion, we note that for a chemostat of size 100 ml, we have a scenario where $\tau_{\text{fix}} \ll \tau_w$. That means that, in the given settings, we are operating in a regime where clonal interference is very relevant. Thus, any evolutionary model that we design has to take into account existence and competition between different beneficial mutations in the chemostat.

We will next examine one such model of microbial adaptation.

9.5 TRAVELING WAVE MODEL

The previous section's calculations tell us that clonal interference is a real phenomenon in microbial populations, and our understanding of microbial populations must take it into account. In fact, it is quite difficult to design experiments with microbial populations such that we are in *regime I* discussed in this chapter. Based on this, we are going to develop a model which captures evolution of a microbial population, in which multiple beneficial mutations exist together.

We will first develop this model graphically and intuitively, and then, we will develop the mathematics which describes this model.

Let us imagine that we have a population of size N in a chemostat. All individuals in the population at the start of the experiment are isogenic, and have a fitness f_o.

We will also imagine that all beneficial mutations have a fitness coefficient s_0. That is, all beneficial mutations that occur in the population confer the exact same benefit. Obviously, this is not true of real beneficial mutations. A beneficial mutation may be weakly beneficial (small s), or strongly beneficial (large s). We will discuss this in more detail in the next chapter on *Distribution of Fitness Effects* (DFE).

With these starting conditions, we will plot the population as a histogram between fitness (x-axis) and frequency (y-axis) (Figure 9.5A). As we can see in the figure, at time $t = 0$, all individuals in the population are at fitness f_o. As cell divisions take place in the population, most progeny will not have mutations, and thus they remain in the bar at fitness f_o.

- The progeny which have neutral mutations are also represented in the bar at fitness f_o.
- The individuals which have acquired deleterious mutations will be represented at fitness levels less than f_o – but these individuals will be eliminated by selection, and hence, we will ignore from the model.

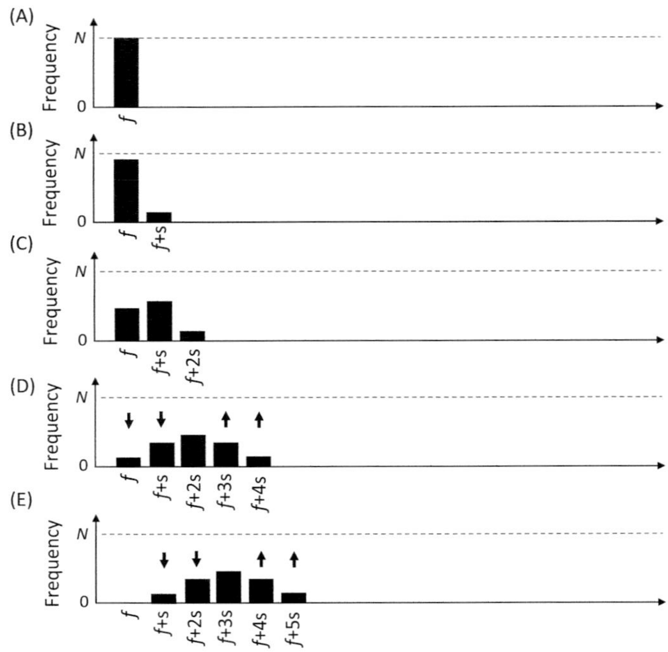

FIGURE 9.5 Starting from an isogenic population, all individuals at fitness f (A). (B) One individual acquires a beneficial mutation. As a result, $N - 1$ individuals are at fitness f and one at $f(1 + s)$. (C) Selection dictates that the genotype at fitness f decreases in frequency, and those at $f(1 + s)$ increase in frequency. While this happens, another individual acquires a beneficial mutation. Thus, there is one individual at fitness $f(1 + 2s)$. (D) At steady state, the frequency distribution of fitness levels is as shown. The up arrows indicate genotypes whose frequency increases in time, and the down arrow indicates genotypes whose frequency decreases with time. (E) As selection eliminates the genotype corresponding to fitness f, a genotype at fitness $f(1 + 5s)$ is established. This maintains the shape of the distribution as in (D), but only that the distribution moves fs units to the right.

The mutations of most interest to us are beneficial mutations. We will assume that all beneficial mutations will have a selection coefficient s. At some point, one of the progeny will acquire a beneficial mutation. The fitness of this individual will thus be $f_o(1 + s)$. This individual will then be represented as shown in Figure 9.5B.

The fate of the new mutation is then dictated by the combined forces of selection (which increases its frequency) and drift (which leads to changes randomly). If the new mutation is eliminated by drift, we are back to the original population structure, i.e., Figure 9.5A. However, if the mutation survives drift (when its frequency reaches $\frac{1}{s}$), natural selection increases its frequency. Thus, the frequency of the population at fitness f_o decreases, and that of at $f_o(1 + s)$ increases with time. This trend continues till one of the individuals at fitness $f_o(1 + s)$ acquires another beneficial mutation and we have one individual at fitness $f_o(1 + 2s)$ (Figure 9.5C). The new beneficial mutation's fate is again decided by a combination of selection and drift.

This process continues as the population adapts to its environment.
As adaptation proceeds, we note the following,

a. The population, in the graph we have described, moves to the right (to higher fitness values) with time.
b. The fittest bar (the rightmost at any given point in time) arises from the population next to it (to its left). This is so because we assume that all beneficial mutations have selection coefficient s. This rightmost population in the distribution is called the 'leading edge' of the population.
c. At any given point in time, the frequency of the population in the leftmost bar will decrease with time (as it represents the population with the least fitness at that particular time), and that of the rightmost bar will increase with time (as it represents the population with the highest fitness at that particular time).

At this point you should recall the result we derived earlier in the book on different genotypes growing together in an environment. The result told us that the genotypes whose fitness is greater than the mean fitness of the population will increase in frequency, and those whose fitness is less than the population mean fitness will decrease in frequency.

In the case we are discussing here, it is clear that the genotype represented by the leftmost bar is the least fitness genotype, and hence will decrease in frequency. And the genotype represented by the rightmost bar is the most fit in the genotype, and hence will increase in frequency.

Before moving ahead,

➔ Given the three characteristics listed above, what can we say about the frequency distribution in the graphical representation discussed above, when the shape of the population fitness distribution reaches a steady state? Take a pause at this moment before moving forward, and sketch the shape that you think this population will take.

At steady state, the population fitness distribution will take the shape as shown in Figure 9.5E. The frequency at the highest fitness levels will be small, as those genotypes (and fitness levels) have only just arrived in the population. With time, they will increase (and hence the upward arrows). The frequency at the lowest fitness levels will be small too, as these genotypes (and fitness levels) are being eliminated because of selection (and hence the downward arrows). In between, there is a mean fitness of the population, which also corresponds to the highest frequency.

Note that this population keeps moving to the right. In the next time frame of the population, the rightmost edge would have given birth to a newer fitness level on the right, and it itself would have increased in frequency. While the lowest fitness level would have gone extinct, and the level just to the right of it would have decreased in frequency. Hence, with time, the shape of the fitness distribution remains the same. This distribution simply travels to the right. Hence, this model is referred to as the *traveling wave* model of microbial adaptation.

9.6 SPEED OF ADAPTATION

What is the speed at which this wave moves to the right? In the next section, we will comment on the quantitative aspects of the traveling wave. Let us imagine that the wave moves one unit to the right in time τ. One unit move to the right means that every individual's fitness increases by exactly fs. Thus, the mean fitness of the population also increases by fs. Thus, the speed of adaptation of this microbial population is simply,

$$\text{Speed of adaptation, } v = \frac{fs}{\tau} \tag{9.9}$$

This means that if we can get estimates of τ, we can estimate the speed of adaptation of this population.

What follow is quantitatively the most challenging section of this book. If you want to skip this section, and move to the next chapter directly, there will be no loss of continuity. The important thing to keep in mind at this point is that in the regime of clonal interference, traveling wave model is one way to look at an evolving microbial population.

We assume that the population distribution in the traveling wave is symmetric around its mean. This assumption need not be exactly true in real populations, but it makes the underlying analysis simpler, and does not alter the results we will reach qualitatively. In this symmetric wave, let us assume that the leading edge is K beneficial mutations ahead of the mean fitness (which is also the most frequent fitness of the population). Thus, the fitness of the individuals in the leading edge is Ks_o fitness units higher than the population mean. Similarly, the lagging edge (to the extreme left) is K beneficial mutations behind the mean fitness of the population, and the fitness of these individuals is Ks_o fitness units lower than the population mean.

Remember that in order to compute the rate of adaptation, we need estimates of τ. We will do this by developing our analysis from two different perspectives, and then stitching the two together to solve for τ.

Analysis I. In this section, we ask, how long does it take for the leading edge to become the most frequent genotype in the population?

Note that the leading edge has an advantage of Ks fitness units over the population mean. Also, since the leading edge is established, the number of individuals in the leading edge is $\frac{1}{Ks}$. However, in τ time, the leading edge would no longer be the leading edge (as the wave would have moved to right one unit), and as a result, its fitness advantage over the population mean would be reduced to $(K-1)s$. In this τ time, the numbers in the leading edge would have grown to,

$$N(\tau) = N_o r^{rt} = \frac{1}{Ks}\, e^{Ks\tau} \tag{9.10}$$

For the next τ time, the numbers in this genotype grow with a growth rate $(K-1)s$. As a result, the number of cells after 2τ units of time would be given by,

$$N(2\tau) = \frac{1}{Ks}\, e^{Ks\tau} e^{(K-1)s\tau} \tag{9.11}$$

This analysis continues for K units of τ time. Finally, when the leading edge becomes the most frequent genotype, its numbers are given by the following expression,

$$N(K\tau) = \frac{1}{Ks}\, e^{Ks\tau} e^{(K-1)s\tau} \ldots e^{s\tau} \tag{9.12}$$

The above expression can be simplified to,

$$N(K\tau) = \frac{1}{Ks}\, e^{K(K+1)s\tau/2} \tag{9.13}$$

For large K, this can be written as,

$$N(K\tau) = \frac{1}{Ks}\, e^{K^2 s\tau/2} \tag{9.14}$$

The problem we now have is that while we have an expression for the right-hand side of the equation, we do not know what fraction of the total population is in the most frequent genome. Thus, we do not know what to place on the left-hand side of the equation above.

This is where experiments come to our rescue! We know from experimental studies that the most frequent genotype in a culture is often an order of magnitude greater than the second most frequent genotype. Thus, an overwhelmingly large fraction of the population resides in the most frequent fitness in the population. This allows us to make the following assumption: for qualitative understanding of the traveling wave, we will assume that, at an order of magnitude estimate, half the entire population is the most frequent genotype in the population. As a result, we get the following equation,

$$\frac{N}{2} = \frac{1}{Ks}\, e^{K^2 s\tau/2} \tag{9.15}$$

The above equation has two unknowns: K and τ. To solve for two unknowns, we need two equations. The first is equation (9.15). For the other equation, we will do analysis II.

Analysis II. How long does it take for the leading edge to NOT be the leading edge anymore?

The leading edge has $\frac{1}{Ks}$ number of cells, and has a Ks fitness advantage over the rest of the population. As its numbers are growing, mutations are occurring. A small fraction of these mutations are going to be beneficial in nature. However, most of these beneficial mutations, as we have seen, will be lost due to drift. We have to find an expression for the time it takes for one such mutation to become established. Once that happens, the current leading edge no longer remains the leading edge. In our framework, we know that the time taken for this to happen is τ.

To start our analysis, we note that the cells in the leading edge are growing as per the following relationship,

$$N(t) = \frac{1}{Ks}\, e^{Kst} \tag{9.16}$$

In a dt interval of time, the number of beneficial mutations occurring in this population will be given by,

$$\#\text{beneficial mutations in time dt in leading edge} = \frac{1}{Ks}\, e^{Kst}\ \mu_b dt \tag{9.17}$$

A beneficial mutation happening in leading edge only has a Ks chance of surviving drift. Therefore, of all the beneficial mutations occurring in dt time, the mutations that survive drift are,

$$\#\text{beneficial mutations in time dt in leading edge that survive drift}$$
$$= \frac{1}{Ks}\, e^{Kst}\ \mu_b dt\ (Ks) \tag{9.18}$$

This is simply equal to,

$$\#\text{beneficial mutations in time dt in leading edge that survive drift} = e^{Kst}\ \mu_b dt \tag{9.19}$$

We are interested in the time when the number on the right-hand side becomes one – i.e., when the number of beneficial mutations in the leading edge which survive drift becomes equal to one. This means that we have a new leading edge, and the existing leading edge is no longer the leading edge. Thus, we are interested in solving for time t in the following equation,

$$\tau = \int_0^t e^{Kst}\ \mu_b dt = \frac{\mu_b}{Ks}\left(e^{Kst} - 1\right) \sim \frac{\mu_b}{Ks}\, e^{Kst} \tag{9.20}$$

The above equation is our second equation between the variables K and τ. We can now solve equations (9.15) and (9.20) together to get expression for τ.

We will not get into more mathematical treatment of this subject here. For those inclined to study the underlying mathematics in greater detail, please see the references given at the end of this chapter. The important point we want to establish here is that the traveling wave model of adaptation for bacterial populations allows us to graphically and analytically study population dynamics.

9.7 CONCLUSION

In this chapter, we discovered that in an actively growing bacterial population (where growth rate is a proxy of fitness), multiple beneficial mutations exist at any given point in time. Thus, these beneficial mutations compete against each other. This phenomenon is referred to as clonal interference. Our calculations showed that clonal interference is a ubiquitous phenomenon for microbial populations. What this also means is that a newly occurred beneficial mutation in a population not only has to overcome drift, but it also has to outcompete the other beneficial mutations in the population. Thus, the chances of a particular beneficial mutation reaching fixation are smaller than what we derived in the previous chapter (where we ignored occurrence of new beneficial mutations). The task of a beneficial mutation reaching fixation got even tougher!

EXERCISES

1. What is the size of the population for which clonal interference is not relevant? That is, only one beneficial mutation exists in the population at any given instant of time.
2. Suppose μ_b increased ten-fold for a population. Would this lead to increased clonal interference, or will this lead to reduced clonal interference?
3. Given the values of s and μ_b in this chapter, at what value of N will $\tau_{\text{fix}} \sim \tau_w$. What will the sketch of Figure 9.2 look like, in this case?
4. List the assumptions of the traveling wave model of microbial adaptation? List down which assumptions you think are reasonable and which unrealistic.
5. Suppose we were to relax the assumption of the traveling wave model discussed in this chapter that all mutations have the same benefit s. How would the traveling wave sketch look in that case?
6. Solve equations (9.15) and (9.20) to estimate the speed of the traveling wave for $N = 10, 10^3, 10^4, 10^8, 10^{10}$. Plot these on a graph where N is x-axis and speed of the traveling wave is on y-axis.
7. What does the graph in question (9.6) tell you about how the speed of adaptation changes as a function of population size?

BIBLIOGRAPHY

1. Desai MM, Fisher DS. 2007. Beneficial mutation selection balance and the effect of linkage on positive selection. *Genetics* 176:1759–98.
   (The traveling wave model we have studied in this chapter. Note that the paper has more rigorous derivations than the sketch we did in the chapter.)
2. Korolev KS, Xavier JB, Gore J. 2014. Turning ecology and evolution against cancer. *Nat Rev Cancer* 14:371–80.
   (Clonal interference and how it can be exploited in the context of cancer treatment.)
3. Nguyen Ba AN, Cvijovic I, Rojas Echenique JI, Lawrence KR, Rego-Costa A, Liu X, Levy SF, Desai MM. 2019. High-resolution lineage tracking reveals travelling wave of adaptation in laboratory yeast. *Nature* 575:494–9.
   (An experimental test of the traveling wave model in yeast. Note how the assumption that all beneficial mutations confer the same benefit is violated in the experiment reported in this paper, and what it leads to.)

10 Distribution of Fitness Effects (DFE)

10.1 INTRODUCTION

One of the major assumptions of the traveling wave model that we discussed in the last chapter was that all beneficial mutations confer the same benefit. That is, the selection coefficient of every beneficial mutation is s. This assumption is clearly incorrect. When beneficial mutations occur, each would confer its own benefit, quantified by its selection coefficient.

The same also holds for deleterious mutations. Each deleterious mutation would confer a decrease in fitness by a unique amount. Thus, the selection coefficient of each deleterious mutation would be negative and unique.

In this chapter, we will discuss what does the distribution of fitness effects for beneficial and deleterious mutations look like? Since mutations provide the raw material for variation for natural selection to act on, knowing the distribution of fitness effects of mutations is key to developing a quantitative understanding of how an evolutionary trajectory would evolve.

10.2 WHAT IS DISTRIBUTION OF FITNESS EFFECTS (DFE)?

Imagine an *E. coli* genome. In a given environment, the fitness of the organism with this genome is f_o. We randomly introduce one mutation in this genome and measure the progeny's fitness. Let us call this fitness f_1. Let us only consider the case, for now, where the mutation introduced was a beneficial mutation, i.e., $f_1 > f_o$. The selection coefficient associated with this mutation is therefore,

$$s_1 = \frac{f_1 - f_o}{f_o} \tag{10.1}$$

After recording the selection coefficient of the random mutation, we go back to the original genotype and introduce another random beneficial mutation in the genome. Let us assume that this mutation changes the fitness of the organism from f_o to f_2. Thus, the selection coefficient associated with the second mutation is,

$$s_2 = \frac{f_2 - f_o}{f_o} \tag{10.2}$$

We keep doing this exercise and compute the selection coefficient of hundreds of randomly introduced beneficial mutations.

 DOI: 10.1201/9781003633662-10

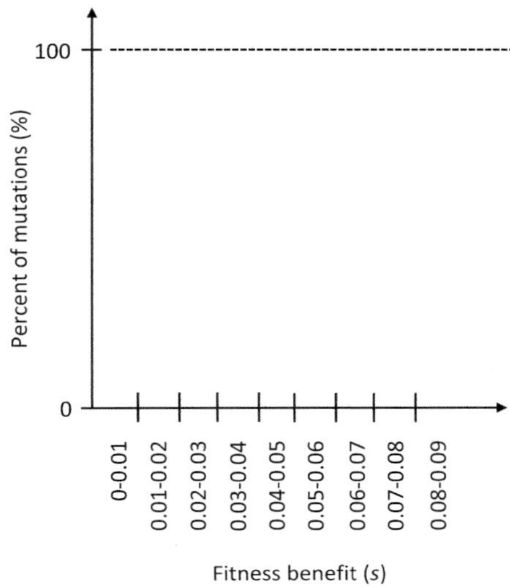

FIGURE 10.1 What does a Distribution of Fitness Effects (DFE) look like? Imagine that a large number of beneficial mutations are introduced in a genome, each conferring its selective advantage s. What is the distribution of s? Are beneficial mutations of all magnitudes equally likely? Or, are beneficial mutations with small s more likely than those with large s? Or, other possibilities?

We then plot the following graph: what percentage of the beneficial mutations have a selection coefficient between 0 and 0.01? Similarly, what percentage of all beneficial mutations confer a benefit with s between 0.01 and 0.02? And so on and so forth (Figure 10.1).

Before moving ahead,

➔ What does your intuition tell you this graph should look like? Take a pause here and fill in the graph that you think represents the distribution that we just discussed above.

Example 10.1: What does the DFE of neutral mutations look like?

Solution: By definition, neutral mutations do not effect fitness of an organism. Thus, for each neutral mutation, fitness does not change. Hence, the selection coefficient associated with each neutral mutation is simply 0. Thus, 100% of beneficial mutations confer a selective advantage of zero.

DFE is a difficult quantity to determine experimentally. Later in the book, we will discuss a technique to measure DFE in bacteria such as *E. coli*.

However, to our best estimate, the DFE of beneficial mutations in a microorganism looks like the following graph (Figure 10.2). The distribution shown in the

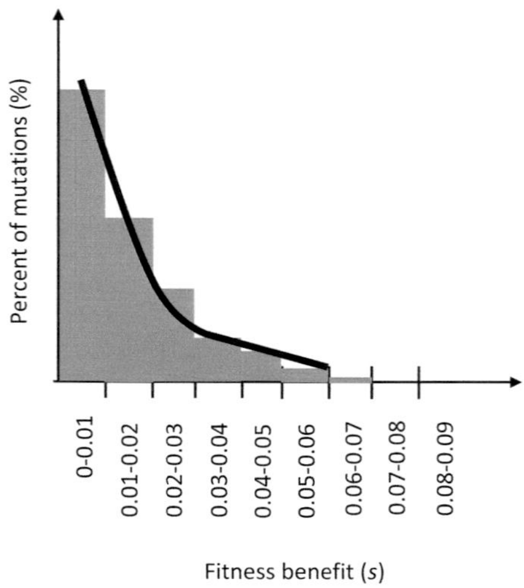

FIGURE 10.2 DFE of beneficial mutations is best represented as an exponential distribution. Mutations of small s are more frequent than mutations with a large s. Thus, there are lots of mutations available which increase fitness by only a small amount. On the other hand, there are very few mutations which increase fitness by a large amount.

Figure 10.2 is similar to what is mathematically described as an exponential distribution, which is mathematically described as,

$$P(s) = \lambda e^{-\lambda s} \tag{10.3}$$

where, λ is the parameter which describes the steepness of the distribution, and s is the selection coefficient. $P(s)$ is the probability that a beneficial mutation of selective advantage s takes place. Mathematically, we plot the above equation for a particular value of λ, say 1. We will note that the equation (10.3) represents a decreasing function, with high value of $P(s)$ for small s, and increasingly smaller values of $P(s)$, as s increases. A sketch of this distribution is shown in Figure 10.2.

What this distribution means is that, for a given genome, a large fraction of beneficial mutations are weakly beneficial (i.e., confer a small fitness advantage). There is only a very small percentage of mutations which confer a large fitness advantage.

Does this distribution agree with the DFE that you drew for Figure 10.1?

In an evolution experiment, beneficial mutations will keep on accumulating in a population. That means that beneficial mutations that are available in the DFE will get fixed and will no longer be available as a beneficial mutation thereafter.

Which mutations, the ones with low s or high s, do you think will appear and fix more frequently in an evolution experiment? Given the shape of the DFE in Figure 10.2, this could be thought of in two ways.

- The mutations with the small selection coefficients will occur at a frequency higher than the beneficial mutations with large selection coefficients. This is simply because there are so many of them, as compared to the beneficial mutations of large effects. This tells us that beneficial mutations with small *s* occur more frequently than those with large *s*.

However, we also know from the chapter on drift that each mutation which confers an advantage of *s*, only survives drift with a probability *s*. Thus, weakly beneficial mutations, although more in number, have a smaller likelihood of surviving drift and thereafter, getting established in the population. Which means that mutations with large *s* survive drift with a greater probability than those with small *s*.

Thus, two competing forces are at work here. Mutations occurring more survive less, and those which survive more, occur less.

- The beneficial mutations with large selection coefficients, on the other hand, have a relatively higher selection coefficient *s* and thus survive drift with a greater probability. However, the relative frequency, as compared to the mutations with smaller selection coefficients, is so small that they will likely not be over-represented in the mutations that we see in an actual evolution experiment.

Between these competing ideas at work here, and it is difficult to say a priori which forces are going to be dominant over the other.

To get a quantitative estimate of the distribution of fitness effects of the mutations that we see in an actual evolution experiment, we can think of this as the following flowchart in Figure 10.3.

We know that exponential distribution is represented by,

$$P(\text{occurance})\ \text{OR DFE} = P_1(s) = \lambda e^{-\lambda s} \tag{10.4}$$

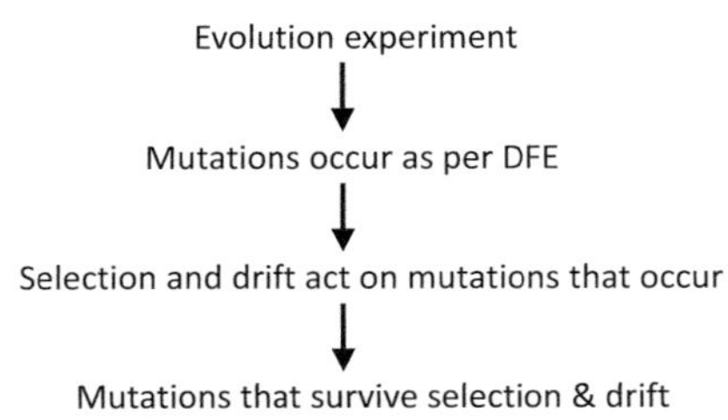

FIGURE 10.3 Starting from an isogenic population, newer mutations occur as per the DFE of the organism in the environment in which the population is evolving. The mutations that occur are then acted upon by selection and drift. What we see as an output of the evolution experiment is the subset of the mutations that occurred – i.e., the mutations that survive selection and drift. Note that because selection and drift act unequally on all mutants, the DFE of the occurrence of mutations is not the same as DFE of the mutations that we see at the outcome of the experiment.

where λ is the parameter which defines the shape of the distribution. The greater the value of λ, the steeper the distribution and the more rapid its fall with increasing s. See exercise 1 at the end of this chapter.

We also know that the probability that a beneficial mutation survives drift in a population is given by,

$$P(\text{survives drift}) = P_2(s) \sim s \tag{10.5}$$

Thus, the distribution of fitness effects that we see at the outcome of an evolutionary experiment will be the product of the two and will be given by,

$$P(s) = P_1 P_2 = \lambda s\, e^{-\lambda s} \tag{10.6}$$

We can plot the three distributions (Figure 10.4) and see that our prediction of the selection coefficients of the beneficial mutations that we will see at the output of an evolution experiment will be given by the distribution $P(s)$ as shown below. The beneficial mutations of small s are under-represented because their selection coefficient is small, and while these mutations occur most frequently, their most common fate is elimination because of drift. At the other end of the spectrum, beneficial mutations of large fitness effects are seen less in evolving populations because, although they have a higher chance of reaching fixation, they occur relatively rarely. In between the two, there is a range of selection coefficients which are over-represented at the output in an evolutionary experiment.

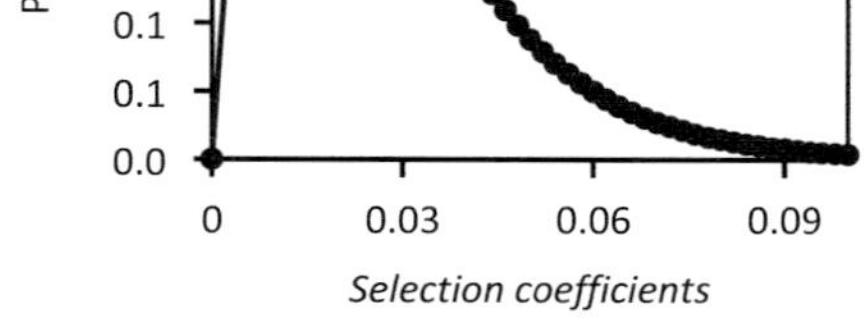

FIGURE 10.4 Probability density function of selection coefficient being observed at the outcome of an evolution experiment. Under the two assumptions (first, beneficial mutations have a DFE best represented with an exponential distribution, and second, probability that a beneficial mutation of selection coefficient s survives drift is $\sim s$), the probability distribution of a selection coefficient being seen at the output of an evolution experiment has a maxima at an intermediate selection value.

Note that in the above discussion, we are repeatedly emphasizing on two things,

- First, the mutations that are introduced have to be randomly introduced. This is so because if the mutations are a result of an evolution experiment, then only mutations that were advantageous in that particular environment would show up in an experiment. However, in our analysis, we are interested in exploring all beneficial mutations that can occur in a genome.
- Second, the mutations that we introduce randomly in the genome, have to be done in the original genome corresponding to fitness f_o. This is so because if the second beneficial mutation is introduced in the genome with fitness f_1, then epistatic interactions with the first mutation in this genome could lead to a fitness effect of this mutation which is distinct from what its effect would have been in the genome of fitness f_o.

10.3 DFE OF DELETERIOUS MUTATIONS

Just as we developed the discussion of beneficial mutations, we can also perform experiments to understand the distribution of fitness effects of deleterious mutations. In this case, starting with a genome of fitness f_o, we will introduce a mutation and measure the fitness of the resulting progeny which carries this mutation. Let the fitness of the progeny be f_1. In this case, we are only interested in the mutations which decrease fitness, i.e., $f_1 < f_o$. From these fitness values, we can calculate the selection coefficient s_1 of the deleterious mutation. We repeat this process to obtain the selection coefficient of hundreds of deleterious mutations. This data would then provide us with the information needed to plot the distribution of fitness effects of deleterious mutations.

DFE of deleterious mutations are less understood as compared to those of beneficial mutations. This is because of two reasons. One, because deleterious mutations are eliminated by selection, their role in dictating the evolutionary trajectory of a population is quite limited. Hence, determining DFE of deleterious mutations has attracted lesser interest, as compared to beneficial mutations. Second, in the few cases where attempts have been made to determine the DFE of deleterious mutations, it has been found that, unlike beneficial mutations, no simple statistical distributions mimic the trend that is exhibited by deleterious mutations. Remember that for beneficial mutations, we saw that their distribution of fitness effects is well-represented by an exponential distribution. However, no such simple distributions occur to predict the behavior of deleterious mutations.

Compared to the DFE of beneficial mutations, DFE of deleterious mutations is much less studied and understood. Since deleterious mutations are eliminated by selection, their DFE has little effect on dictating evolutionary trajectories of populations. As a result, understanding them has attracted far lesser interest than the DFE of beneficial mutations. To our best approximation, however, DFE of deleterious mutations has two major differences as compared to that of beneficial mutations.

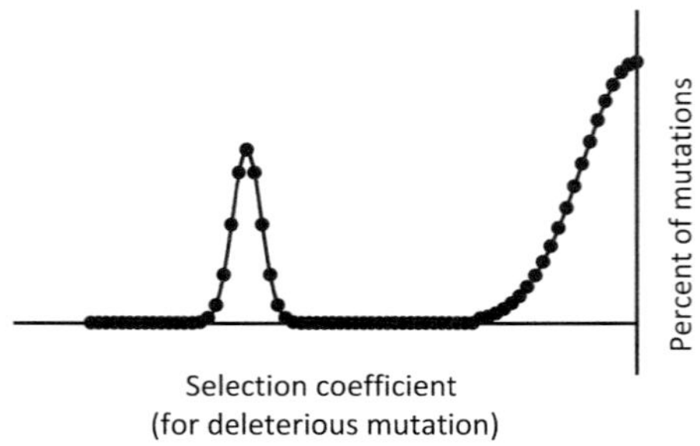

FIGURE 10.5 DFE of deleterious mutations. DFE of deleterious mutations is thought to be two-peaked. The first peak, close to neutrality, represents weakly deleterious mutations. There is another peak, which corresponds to highly deleterious or lethal mutations.

- The distribution of fitness effects of deleterious mutations is more like a normal distribution (as compared to an exponential distribution).
- For deleterious mutations, there exists a finite fraction of mutations which reduce the fitness to zero. That is, there is a finite fraction of deleterious mutations which are lethal.

Both these aspects of DFE of deleterious mutations are represented in Figure 10.5.

10.4 CONCLUSION

We studied in this chapter that not all beneficial mutations are the same. Some confer a greater advantage than others. Interestingly, the beneficial effects of randomly introduced mutations follow a predictable statistical pattern. This pattern is referred to as the Distribution of Fitness Effects (DFE). We saw that the DFE of beneficial mutations is best represented by an exponential distribution, but the DFE of deleterious mutations exhibits more complex distributions.

EXERCISES

1. Plot exponential distributions for λ equal to 1, 2, 5, and 10 on a single graph and compare these four distributions with each other.
2. What happens to the exponential distribution with increasing λ?
3. An exponential distribution is mathematically described as,

$$f(x) = \lambda e^{-\lambda x}$$

   Compute the mean of the exponential distributions for the values of λ given in question (10.1).
4. Figure 10.5 shows that the DFE of deleterious mutations is two-peaked. One peak represents mildly deleterious mutations, and another which are highly deleterious or lethal. Why do you think this DFE exhibits two peaks, while the DFE of beneficial mutations is single-peaked?

5. Imagine a genotype g, which exhibits fitness f, and DFE of beneficial mutations which is represented by an exponential distribution with the parameter λ.

   The genotype g acquires a neutral mutation to become g'. By definition, since the mutation acquired was neutral, its fitness is also f.

   Do you think g and g' exhibit identical DFEs of beneficial mutations? Why or why not?

BIBLIOGRAPHY

1. Hegreness M, Shoresh N, Hartl D, Kishony R. 2006. An equivalence principle for the incorporation of favorable mutations in asexual populations. *Science*. 311(5767):1615–7.

   (This is a very clever experiment to determine DFE of beneficial mutations from adaptive experiments. Although the authors conclude that it is quite difficult to determine DFE through their approach, the premise is really interesting.)
2. Brajesh RG, Dutta D, Saini S. 2019. Distribution of fitness effects of mutations obtained from a simple genetic regulatory network model. *Scientific Reports*. 9(1):9842.

   (Our group approached the problem of determining DFE in a novel computation approach. However, this approach can only be applied to systems which have been characterized very well. Because of this reason, this approach's general applicability is quite limited.)

11 The Idea of 'Molecular Clock' and Neutral Theory of Molecular Evolution

11.1 INTRODUCTION

Emile Zuckerkandl was a post-doctoral researcher in Linus Pauling's group in the late 1950s. A few years ago, Pauling, while visiting friends in France, had met Zuckerkandl and was impressed by the young man. Encouraged by Pauling, Zuckerkandl then moved to California Institute of Technology in the US and the two started working together.

Zuckerkandl's research got off to a rocky start in the US. Being in a Marine Research Institute, he was interested in studying crab proteins. However, Pauling, a Chemistry Nobel Prize recipient in 1954, had become more involved in his anti-war work by that time (for which he was later awarded the Nobel Peace Prize in 1962). Pauling was particularly interested in the effect of radiation on human proteins. Of particular interest to Pauling was Hemoglobin, a protein which is responsible for carrying oxygen from lungs to tissues. Thus, Pauling encouraged to drop the crab protein work, and work on Hemoglobin instead.

The early 1950s had seen the introduction of a technique which allowed researchers to study the difference in protein variants present in different individuals. For example, is the sequence of amino acids in the Hemoglobin that you and I are carrying identical? If not, what is the extent of Hemoglobin protein sequence that exists in a population. Testing this variation in a population was a challenge, up until the 1950s.

The idea behind testing this variation experimentally was quite simple. Proteins were allowed to travel under the influence of an electric field. Proteins, depending on their precise amino acid sequence, have a specific mass and carry charge. The distance they travel in gels is directly proportional to the charge, and inversely proportional to the mass. Thus, if two species (or individuals) have different amino acid sequences for a particular protein (say, Hemoglobin), they can be differentiated on a protein gel, when allowed to travel under the influence of an electric field.

When Zuckerkandl started his work, he noticed that the Hemoglobin from humans and chimpanzees were extremely close to each other, and virtually impossible to separate under the influence of an electric field on a gel. While for other pairs of species, Hemoglobin can be separated on a gel.

 DOI: 10.1201/9781003633662-11

Zuckerkandl thought that this suggested that in species which shared a common ancestor in relatively recent time, a protein-like Hemoglobin has not diverged very far from each other's sequence. While species that diverged relatively longer ago, protein sequences have diverged significantly more. Thus, the evolutionary relationship between two species can simply be determined from a protein's sequence!

When Zuckerkandl shared his results with the laboratory head, he met with more disappointment. The lab head was a creationist, and refused to allow work in his laboratory which suggested a relationship between apes and human beings.

Soon afterward, Pauling was invited to submit an article for the *Festschrift* issue for his friend and a Nobel laureate Albert Szent-Gyorgyi. Pauling shared the invitation with Zuckerkandl, and urged him to write 'something outrageous'.

Zuckerkandl's work was back on track.

In the late 1950s, DNA sequencing was not possible. However, protein sequencing was possible, and a few protein's sequences, for many species, was available. Hemoglobin was one such protein. When Zuckerkandl compared the amino acid sequence of Hemoglobin from a number of species, the differences between the sequences could be summarized via a simple relationship (Figure 11.1).

Example 11.1: Based on Figure 11.1, what can we say about evolution of the four different proteins.

Solution: It is evident that histones diverge the slowest among the four. Hence, it appears that their function is highly converged, and there is not a lot of room for natural selection to evolve this protein. On the other hand, fibrinopeptides evolve rapidly for each species. This suggests that their evolution is highly dependent on the niche and the precise physiology of the organism. Histones, on the other hand, serve something fundamentally conserved and hence, do not diverge easily. Hemoglobin and Cytochrome c are in between these two extremes.

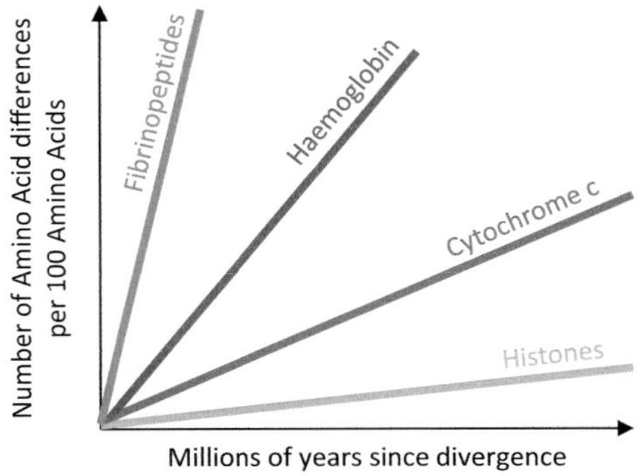

FIGURE 11.1 Protein divergence between species is linearly correlated with the time of divergence between the species. X-axis shows the time since divergence between two species, and y-axis shows the amino acid changes between two species for these proteins per 100 amino acids. As can be seen from the figure, among these four proteins, histones diverge the slowest and fibrinopeptides the fastest.

We see that the number of amino acid differences between two species' Hemoglobin sequence is linearly proportional to the time since the two species separated from their common ancestor. As a result, the difference between a chimpanzee and human Hemoglobin sequence is much closer to each other as compared to that between a human and cow Hemoglobin sequence. Mammalian Hemoglobin sequences are much closer to each other, as they shared a common ancestor in a much more recent past as compared to others.

Thus, Pauling and Zuckerkandl's results demonstrated that protein sequence tells us of evolutionary relationship between organisms! There was no need for fossils, or rocks to study these relationships. Simply studying the protein sequences from extant species would tell us these relationships.

This work was published in 1962, and Pauling and Zuckerkandl called the idea 'a molecular clock', as the data suggested that protein sequences in species were accumulating mutations at regular intervals, just like a clock!

Fifty years after the paper's publication, Zuckerkandl recalls that when the paper was published, 'Taxonomists hated it. Biochemists thought it useless'.

However, the following year, Margoliash published a study in *PNAS* which demonstrated that a similar linear relationship also holds for a mitochondrial protein, Cytochrome c.

More evidence came the following year, when in 1964, Doolittle and Blomback published a paper in *Nature*, again indicating a linear relationship between years since common ancestor and differences in amino acid sequence for fibrinopeptides in mammals.

However, note that the slopes for the linear relationship between the three proteins were different.

11.2 A PROBLEM TO SOLVE

The idea of molecular clock was not just a conundrum that warranted an explanation. It posed a serious question on how we understand evolution.

The widely held view at the time was that adaptive change is driven by beneficial mutations. Why was it that beneficial mutations in species were occurring like a 'clock' at regular intervals? This was observed despite the fact that each of the species considered had different population sizes, generation time, and mutation rate.

How do we explain this?

11.3 NEUTRAL THEORY FOR MOLECULAR EVOLUTION

An answer to the above problem was posed by Motoo Kimura in 1968, 1969. Kimura, in these papers, proposed that the above conundrum can be explained if we view the relative frequency of (a) beneficial, (b) deleterious, and (c) neutral mutations available to an organism.

The conventional thought prior to Kimura's proposal was that the fraction of all mutations available to an organism that are beneficial is reasonably high (Figure 11.2). Kimura proposed that this view is incorrect. Instead, beneficial

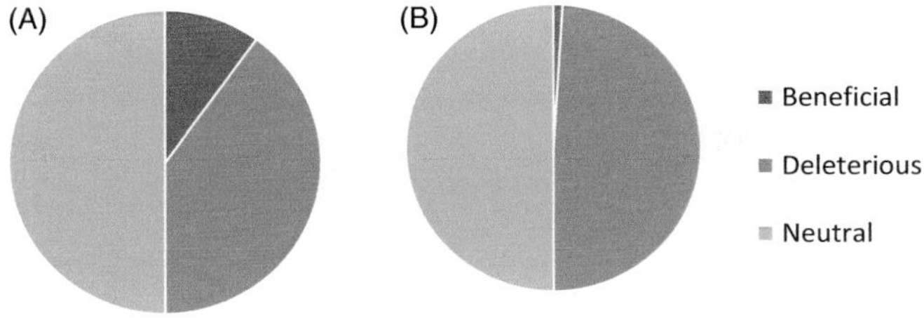

FIGURE 11.2 (A) Conventional wisdom in the middle of 20th century said the relative frequency of beneficial, deleterious, and neutral mutations would look as shown in the figure, with beneficial mutations being the least frequent, and neutral being the most frequent. (B) Kimura's proposal did not alter the relative frequency of the three types of mutations. However, Kimura proposed that the fraction of mutations that were beneficial was much smaller than thought earlier. As a result, an overwhelming majority of biological variation was neutral in nature. Beneficial mutations did take place but their occurrence was a relatively rare event.

mutations are extremely rare, and an overwhelmingly large fraction of mutations are neutral in nature, i.e., they cause no change in the fitness (Figure 11.2).

Note that both models acknowledge that deleterious and neutral mutations are most frequent among the three. However, both views agree, deleterious mutations are irrelevant as far as evolutionary change is concerned – hence, they need not be considered with respect to adaptive response of a population.

The disagreement between the two views is the relative abundance of beneficial mutations.

If we make the assumption that beneficial mutations are relatively rare – the question of variation between the protein sequences between species is largely explained by neutral variation.

In such a case, what is the rate at which species accumulate mutations? How do we explain the observation of linear divergence of protein sequences between species?

Imagine a population of size N and neutral mutation rate μ_n individual^{-1} generation^{-1}. The mutation rate associated with deleterious mutations μ_d can be ignored, since selection will reject those mutations. And, since according to Kimura's proposal, beneficial mutations are rare, mutation rate associated with beneficial mutations μ_b is ~0.

In such a scenario, the total number of neutral mutations in one generation is $N\mu_n$.

From our discussion in the chapter on drift, we know that the probability that a particular neutral mutation (in the absence of beneficial mutations) in a population of size N reaches fixation is given by the following expression,

$$P(\text{fixation of neutral mutation}) = \frac{1}{N} \tag{11.1}$$

Hence, the number of mutations that reach fixation in one generation,

$$\text{mutations fixed per generation} = \frac{1}{N}N\mu_n = \mu_n \tag{11.2}$$

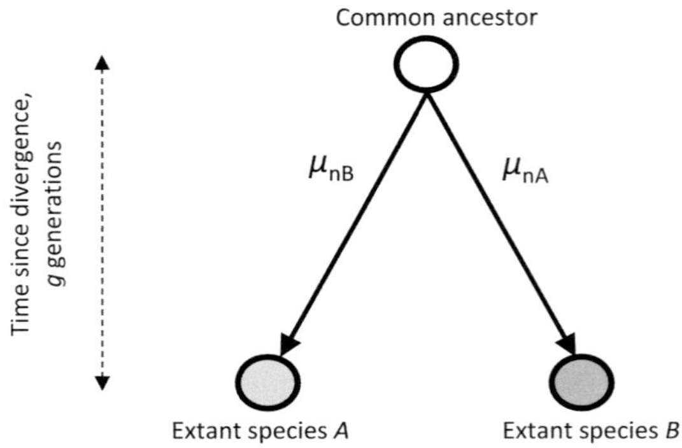

FIGURE 11.3 From a common ancestor, divergence led to two extant species A and B. The divergence took place g generations ago. As the two species diverged apart, the left arm accumulated $(g\mu_{nA})$ mutations. Similarly, the right arm accumulated $(g\mu_{nB})$ mutations. Thus, the total number of mutations between the species A and B is $[g(\mu_{\text{nA}} + \mu_{\text{nB}})]$ – i.e., a linear function of the time since divergence of the two species.

Thus, the rate at which mutations fix in a species is simply the mutation rate associated with neutral mutations. This rate is independent of the population size, and thus explains the linear relationship between the amino acid differences in a protein sequence and time of divergence for two species.

Consider two species A and B, with neutral mutation rates μ_{nA} and μ_{nB}. Species A accumulates one neutral mutation every $\frac{1}{\mu_{nA}}$ generations, where as species B will accumulate mutations at the rate of one mutation every $\frac{1}{\mu_{nB}}$ generations (Figure 11.3).

Thus, the greater the divergence time between two species, the greater the mutational distance between them. Moreover, since the rate of accumulation of mutations is independent of the population size, mutations accumulate at a constant rate for each species. Thus, Kimura's neutral theory provided a mechanistic explanation for the 'molecular clock' proposed by Pauling and Zuckerkandl in 1962.

We now turn to another important analysis using the concepts of neutral versus non-neutral mutations. We know that SNPs in the coding region of a gene can be synonymous or non-synonymous. Historically, it has been believed that since synonymous mutations do not change the sequence of the amino acids, they are neutral. And that since non-synonymous mutations change the sequence of the amino acids, they are non-neutral.

We will see next how can we use this information to gain an understanding about how sequences and proteins evolve?

11.4 WHAT IS $\frac{dN}{dS}$?

As shown in Figure 11.1, it is apparent that different proteins evolve at different rates. Why is this so? The proposal of neutral theory led to development of an idea, where, upon comparing the sequence of a gene in two species, we can comment on whether the gene has been under positive selection OR purifying selection OR is evolving under drift.

To understand this idea, consider a gene **G** in two species S1 and S2. Let the length of the gene be *L* nucleotides. With this starting point, we take the following steps.

As we take these steps, we will next work with an example of a gene, *rpoS*, from two closely related bacterial species *E. coli* and *Salmonella*. Note that *Salmonella* is a pathogen which can cause a disease, ranging from self-limiting gastroenteritis to life-threatening systemic infection.

Let the length of the gene be **L** nucleotides.

1. Count the number of changes in the DNA sequence of the gene *g* in the two species. Let this number be **T**.
2. Some of these mutations encode for a synonymous change. Let this number be **S**. Remember that a synonymous change in the DNA sequence is one where a nucleotide change does not lead to a change in the amino acid sequence.
3. The remaining mutations encode for non-synonymous mutations. Let this number be **NS**. Non-synonymous mutations are those which upon a nucleotide change, an amino acid is changed.
4. For every one of the **L** nucleotides in the gene sequence, there are three possible mutations (e.g., if the nucleotide is **A** [adenine], it could mutate to **G**, **C**, or **T**). Thus, the total number of possible mutations for the gene is **3L**.
5. Of the **3L** mutations, **K** mutations lead to a synonymous change; and **(3L-K)** mutations lead to a non-synonymous change.
6. Thus, between the two sequences, the number of non-synonymous mutations per non-synonymous site is given by the ratio,

$$dN = \frac{(NS)}{(3L - K)} \tag{11.4}$$

7. Similarly, the number of synonymous mutations per synonymous site between the two sequences is given by,

$$dS = \frac{(S)}{(K)} \tag{11.5}$$

The above two quantities provide us with a ratio $\frac{dN}{dS}$ as,

$$\frac{dN}{dS} = \frac{(NS)(K)}{(3L - K)(S)} \tag{11.6}$$

Let us consider the above using an example. We saw that in a batch culture, after a lag and an exponential/log phase, bacteria enter stationary phase. Stationary phase, when all cellular resources are gone, is all about survival. A specific set of genes is responsible for survival in stationary phase. The expression of these genes is controlled by a specific RNA Polymerase (RNAP) called RpoS. Given below is the RpoS sequence from two closely related bacteria *E. coli* and *Salmonella* – which diverged ~100 million years ago.

E. coli – rpoS gene sequence.

ATGAGTCAGAATACGCTGAAAGTTCATGATTTAAATGAAGATGCGGAATTT
GATGAGAACGGAGTTGAGGTTTTTGACGAAAAGGCCTTAGTAGAACAGGA
ACCCAGTGATAACGATTTGGCCGAAGAGGAACTGTTATCGCAGGGAGCCA
CACAGCGTGTGTTGGACGCGACTCAGCTTTACCTTGGTGAGATTGGTTATT
CACCACTGTTAACGGCCGAAGAAGAAGTTTATTTTGCGCGTCGCGCACTGC
GTGGAGATGTCGCCTCTCGCCGCCGGATGATCGAGAGTAACTTGCGTCTGG
TGGTAAAAATTGCCCGCCGTTATGGCAATCGTGGTCTGGCGTTGCTGGACC
TTATCGAAGAGGGCAACCTGGGGCTGATCCGCGCGGTAGAGAAGTTTGAC
CCGGAACGTGGTTTCCGCTTCTCAACATACGCAACCTGGTGGATTCGCCAG
ACGATTGAACGGGCGATTATGAACCAAACCCGTACTATTCGTTTGCCGATT
CACATCGTAAAGGAGCTGAACGTTTACCTGCGAACCGCACGTGAGTTGTCC
CATAAGCTGGACCATGAACCAAGTGCGGAAGAGATCGCAGAGCAACTGGA
TAAGCCAGTTGATGACGTCAGCCGTATGCTTCGTCTTAACGAGCGCATTAC
CTCGGTAGACACCCCGCTGGGTGGTGATTCCGAAAAAGCGTTGCTGGACA
TCCTGGCCGATGAAAAAGAGAACGGTCCGGAAGATACCACGCAAGATGAC
GATATGAAGCAGAGCATCGTCAAATGGCTGTTCGAGCTGAACGCCAAACA
GCGTGAAGTGCTGGCACGTCGATTCGGTTTGCTGGGGTACGAAGCGGCAA
CACTGGAAGATGTAGGTCGTGAAATTGGCCTCACCCGTGAACGTGTTCGCC
AGATTCAGGTTGAAGGCCTGCGCCGTTTGCGCGAAATCCTGCAAACGCAG
GGGCTGAATATCGAAGCGCTGTTCCGCGAGTAA

Salmonella – rpoS sequence.

TTGAGTCAGAATACGCTGAAAGTTCATGATTTAAATGAAGACGCGGAATTT
GATGAGAACGGAGTAGAGGCTTTTGACGAAAAAGCCTTGAGTGAAGAGGA
ACCCAGTGATAACGACCTGGCTGAAGAAGAGCTGTTATCGCAAGGGGCCA
CACAGCGTGTGTTGGACGCGACTCAGCTTTACCTTGGTGAGATTGGGTATT
CACCACTGTTAACAGCCGAAGAAGAAGTCTATTTTGCGCGTCGCGCACTGC
GTGGAGATGTCGCTTCTCGCCGTCGCATGATTGAGAGTAACCTGCGTCTGG
TGGTAAAAATTGCCCGCCGTTATGGCAATCGTGGACTGGCGTTGCTGGACC
TGATTGAAGAGGGCAACCTGGGGCTTATCCGTGCAGTCGAGAAGTTTGAC
CCGGAACGCGGGTTCCGCTTCTCAACATACGCAACCTGGTGGATTCGCCAG
ACAATCGAACGGGCGATCATGAACCAAACCCGTACGATTCGCTTGCCGAT
TCACATTGTTAAAGAGCTGAACGTATACCTGCGCACCGCACGTGAGTTGTC
GCATAAACTGGACCACGAACCGAGTGCGGAAGAAATTGCAGAGCAACTGG
ATAAACCGGTTGATGACGTCAGCCGTATGCTTCGTCTCAACGAGCGCATTA
CCTCGGTAGACACCCCGCTGGGCGGTGATTCCGAAAAAGCGTTGCTGGAC
ATCCTGGCCGATGAAAAAGAGAACGGTCCGGAAGACACCACGCAAGATG
ACGATATGAAACAGAGCATCGTCAAATGGTTGTTCGAACTGAACGCCAAA
CAGCGTGAAGTGCTGGCGCGCCGTTTCGGTCTGCTGGGATATGAAGCTGCG
ACACTGGAAGATGTAGGCCGTGAAATCGGTCTTACGCGTGAACGTGTTCGT
CAGATTCAGGTTGAAGGCCTGCGCCGTCTGCGCGAAATTCTGCAGACGCA
GGGGCTGAATATCGAAGCGCTGTTCCGCGAGTAA

A sequence alignment of the two genes gives us the following results. Note that the gene length for *rpoS* is 993 nucleotides. This equates to 330 amino acids (because the last three nucleotides correspond to a stop codon). Note also that the *Salmonella rpoS* does not start with the triplet ATG. In the sequence alignment, the '*' indicates the nucleotide positions where the two genes have the same nucleotide. The 'blanks' indicate the positions where the two sequences have different nucleotides.

```
E.coli     ATGAGTCAGAATACGCTGAAAGTTCATGATTTAAATGAAGATGCGGAATTTGATGAGAAC    60
Sal.       TTGAGTCAGAATACGCTGAAAGTTCATGATTTAAATGAAGACGCGGAATTTGATGAGAAC    60
           ***************************************** *****************

E. coli    GGAGTTGAGGTTTTTGACGAAAAGGCCTTAGTAGAACAGGAACCCAGTGATAACGATTTG    120
Sal.       GGAGTAGAGGCTTTTGACGAAAAAGCCTTGAGTGAAGAGGAACCCAGTGATAACGACCTG    120
           ***** **** ************ *****    *** *******************  **

E. coli    GCCGAAGAGGAACTGTTATCGCAGGGAGCCACACAGCGTGTGTTGGACGCGACTCAGCTT    180
Sal.       GCTGAAGAAGAGCTGTTATCGCAAGGGGCCACACAGCGTGTGTTGGACGCGACTCAGCTT    180
           ** ***** ** *********** ** *********************************

E. coli    TACCTTGGTGAGATTGGTTATTCACCACTGTTAACGGCCGAAGAAGAAGTTTATTTTGCG    240
Sal.       TACCTTGGTGAGATTGGGTATTCACCACTGTTAACAGCCGAAGAAGAAGTCTATTTTGCG    240
           ***************** ***************** ************** *********

E. coli    CGTCGCGCACTGCGTGGAGATGTCGCCTCTCGCCGCCGGATGATCGAGAGTAACTTGCGT    300
Sal.       CGTCGCGCACTGCGTGGAGATGTCGCTTCTCGCCGTCGCATGATTGAGAGTAACCTGCGT    300
           ************************** ******** ** ***** ********* *****

E. coli    CTGGTGGTAAAAATTGCCCGCCGTTATGGCAATCGTGGTCTGGCGTTGCTGGACCTTATC    360
Sal.       CTGGTGGTAAAAATTGCCCGCCGTTATGGCAATCGTGGACTGGCGTTGCTGGACCTGATT    360
           ************************************** ***************** **

E. coli    GAAGAGGGCAACCTGGGGCTGATCCGCGCGGTAGAGAAGTTTGACCCGGAACGTGGTTTC
                                                                           420
Sal.       GAAGAGGGCAACCTGGGGCTTATCCGTGCAGTCGAGAAGTTTGACCCGGAACGCGGGTTC    420
           ******************** ***** ** ** ******************** ** ***

E. coli    CGCTTCTCAACATACGCAACCTGGTGGATTCGCCAGACGATTGAACGGGCGATTATGAAC    480
Sal.       CGCTTCTCAACATACGCAACCTGGTGGATTCGCCAGACAATCGAACGGGCGATCATGAAC    480
           ************************************** ** *********** ******

E. coli    CAAACCCGTACTATTCGTTTGCCGATTCACATCGTAAAGGAGCTGAACGTTTACCTGCGA    540
Sal.       CAAACCCGTACGATTCGCTTGCCGATTCACATTGTTAAAGAGCTGAACGTATACCTGCGC    540
           *********** ***** ************** ** ** *********** ********

E. coli    ACCGCACGTGAGTTGTCCCATAAGCTGGACCATGAACCAAGTGCGGAAGAGATCGCAGAG    600
Sal.       ACCGCACGTGAGTTGTCGCATAAACTGGACCACGAACCGAGTGCGGAAGAAATTGCAGAG    600
           ***************** ***** ******** ***** *********** ** ******

E. coli    CAACTGGATAAGCCAGTTGATGACGTCAGCCGTATGCTTCGTCTTAACGAGCGCATTACC    660
Sal.       CAACTGGATAAACCGGTTGATGACGTCAGCCGTATGCTTCGTCTCAACGAGCGCATTACC    660
           *********** ** ***************************** ***************

E. coli    TCGGTAGACACCCCGCTGGGTGGTGATTCCGAAAAAGCGTTGCTGGACATCCTGGCCGAT    720
Sal.       TCGGTAGACACCCCGCTGGGCGGTGATTCCGAAAAAGCGTTGCTGGACATCCTGGCCGAT    720
           ******************** ***************************************

E. coli    GAAAAAGAGAACGGTCCGGAAGATACCACGCAAGATGACGATATGAAGCAGAGCATCGTC    780
Sal.       GAAAAAGAGAACGGTCCGGAAGACACCACGCAAGATGACGATATGAAACAGAGCATCGTC    780
           *********************** *********************** ************
```

```
E. coli    AAATGGCTGTTCGAGCTGAACGCCAAACAGCGTGAAGTGCTGGCACGTCGATTCGGTTTG    840
Sal.       AAATGGTTGTTCGAACTGAACGCCAAACAGCGTGAAGTGCTGGCGCGCCGTTTCGGTCTG    840
           ****** ******* ***************************** ** ** ****** **

E. coli    CTGGGGTACGAAGCGGCAACACTGGAAGATGTAGGTCGTGAAATTGGCCTCACCCGTGAA    900
Sal.       CTGGGATATGAAGCTGCGACACTGGAAGATGTAGGCCGTGAAATCGGTCTTACGCGTGAA    900
           ***** ** ***** ** ***************** ******** ** ** ** ******

E. coli    CGTGTTCGCCAGATTCAGGTTGAAGGCCTGCGCCGTTTGCGCGAAATCCTGCAAACGCAG    960
Sal.       CGTGTTCGTCAGATTCAGGTTGAAGGCCTGCGCCGTCTGCGCGAAATTCTGCAGACGCAG    960
           ******** *************************** ********** ***** ******

E. coli    GGGCTGAATATCGAAGCGCTGTTCCGCGAGTAA    993
Sal.       GGGCTGAATATCGAAGCGCTGTTCCGCGAGTAA    993
           *********************************
```

Out of 993 bases, the total number of places where the nucleotides are identical in the two sequences is 918. Thus, the number of places where the nucleotide sequence of RpoS in the two species differs is 75. Thus, **T** equals 75. A sequence alignment of the two protein sequences reveals the following.

```
ECOLI         MSQNTLKVHDLNEDAEFDENGVEVFDEKALVEQEPSDNDLAEEELLSQGATQRVLDATQL    60
SALMONELLA    MSQNTLKVHDLNEDAEFDENGVEAFDEKALSEEEPSDNDLAEEELLSQGATQRVLDATQL    60
              **********************.****** *:****************************

ECOLI         YLGEIGYSPLLTAEEEVYFARRALRGDVASRRRMIESNLRLVVKIARRYGNRGLALLDLI    120
SALMONELLA    YLGEIGYSPLLTAEEEVYFARRALRGDVASRRRMIESNLRLVVKIARRYGNRGLALLDLI    120
              ************************************************************

ECOLI         EEGNLGLIRAVEKFDPERGFRFSTYATWWIRQTIERAIMNQTRTIRLPIHIVKELNVYLR    180
SALMONELLA    EEGNLGLIRAVEKFDPERGFRFSTYATWWIRQTIERAIMNQTRTIRLPIHIVKELNVYLR    180
              ************************************************************

ECOLI         TARELSHKLDHEPSAEEIAEQLDKPVDDVSRMLRLNERITSVDTPLGGDSEKALLDILAD    240
SALMONELLA    TARELSHKLDHEPSAEEIAEQLDKPVDDVSRMLRLNERITSVDTPLGGDSEKALLDILAD    240
              ************************************************************

ECOLI         EKENGPEDTTQDDDMKQSIVKWLFELNAKQREVLARRFGLLGYEAATLEDVGREIGLTRE    300
SALMONELLA    EKENGPEDTTQDDDMKQSIVKWLFELNAKQREVLARRFGLLGYEAATLEDVGREIGLTRE    300
              ************************************************************

ECOLI         RVRQIQVEGLRRLREILQTQGLNIEALFRE    330
SALMONELLA    RVRQIQVEGLRRLREILQTQGLNIEALFRE    330
              ******************************
```

We see that of the 330 amino acids, the two sequences differ at three amino acids. At other 327 positions, the two sequences have the same amino acids. Note that despite the two nucleotide sequences being different at 75 positions at the level of DNA sequence, at the amino acid level, the two sequences differ at only three positions. Thus, **NS** equals 3, and **S** equals 72.

If we consider the nucleotide sequence of RpoS in *E. coli* and introduce all possible 2,979 (993 × 3) mutations and consider how many are synonymous and how many non-synonymous – we find that 1,445 (**K**) are synonymous and 1,534 (**3L-K**) are non-synonymous. Note that these numbers have to be calculated for each gene, as they are dependent on the sequence of the gene. For example, if a gene comprises of ATG codons only, then it cannot have any possible synonymous mutations since the amino acid Methionine is encoded by only one codon.

Substituting these numbers in equation (11.7), we get the following,

$$\frac{dN}{dS} = \frac{(NS)(K)}{(3L - K)(S)} = \frac{(3)(1445)}{(1534)(72)} = 0.04$$
$$\frac{dN}{dS} = 0.04 \quad (11.7)$$

What does this value mean in terms of gene/protein evolution?

11.5 WHAT DOES $\frac{dN}{dS}$ TELL US?

In the development of $\frac{dN}{dS}$, we will assume that synonymous mutations are neutral in nature. That is, neutral change causes no change in the organisms' fitness. This assumption is based on the fact that a synonymous mutation does not lead to a change in the amino acid sequence – and hence, the protein functionality associated with the gene sequence does not change. On the other hand, non-synonymous mutations cause a change in the amino acid sequence, and, therefore, lead to a change in the functionality of the protein. Thus, non-synonymous changes are assumed to be non-neutral (they could be beneficial or deleterious).

With these assumptions, we will discuss three regimes of the ratio $\frac{dN}{dS}$, and what does it tell us about the protein evolution.

Case I. $\frac{dN}{dS} \gg 1$ (Positive Selection)

In this regime, $dN \gg dS$, i.e., the number of non-synonymous changes (per site) is much greater as compared to synonymous changes (per site). Since synonymous changes are driven by drift (since they are neutral), and non-synonymous changes are driven by selection (selection eliminates it if the non-synonymous change is deleterious, and increases the change in frequency if the change is beneficial) – $\frac{dN}{dS} \gg 1$ tells us that beneficial (non-synonymous) mutations are being selected for at a much higher frequency, as compared to neutral (synonymous) mutations. Thus, the gene is under positive, directional selection – where, in the prevailing environment, changes which enhance the organismal fitness are being selected for, and that protein is undergoing non-neutral evolution.

Case II. $\frac{dN}{dS} \ll 1$ (Purifying Selection)

If, on the other hand, $dN \ll dS$, the number of synonymous mutations (reaching fixation under drift) per site outnumber non-synonymous mutations per site. This implies that non-synonymous mutations are largely eliminated by selection. Thus, an overwhelming majority of non-synonymous mutations are deleterious and are eliminated. This mode of selection is referred to as 'Purifying Selection' – selection works to ensure that the protein amino acid sequence is preserved.

Note that the *rpoS* example we studied above falls in this category. RpoS is essential for survival in stationary phase, and is a key protein responsible for ensuring cellular survival. Thus, the protein sequence has evolved for optimal performance. Hence, for the most part, non-synonymous mutations are not tolerated in the protein sequence.

Case III. $\frac{dN}{dS} \sim 1$ (No Selection)

In this case, $dN \sim dS$, non-synonymous mutations are being accumulated at approximately the same rate as synonymous mutations. Thus, non-synonymous mutations are also being accumulated as a result of drift. This suggests that the gene sequence of interest is not under selection, and its evolutionary trajectory is dictated by drift only.

An example of such a case would be evolution of GAL2 gene, when evolved in an environment with glucose as the carbon source. In such a scenario, GAL2 is not expressed and is not relevant for manifestations of cellular physiology. Thus, GAL2, in such an environmental context, is neither under directional selection, nor purifying selection. In fact, GAL2 is under no selection.

Thus, by comparing sequences of a gene from two distinct species, we can (a) comment on the kind of evolutionary selection pressure that the gene is under, and (b) using the ideas of molecular clock, we can comment on the time since divergence between the two species.

The above analysis assumes that synonymous mutations are neutral. However, are all synonymous mutations neutral? Are all non-synonymous mutations non-neutral? We know of several examples where this is not the case. Let us discuss the mechanistic details of how these two could be true.

11.6 SYNONYMOUS MUTATIONS MAY BE NON-NEUTRAL

Synonymous mutations can be non-neutral via a number of mechanisms.

a. *mRNA stability*. Since a synonymous mutation changes the nucleotide sequence in the mRNA, there is a chance that a nucleotide change will alter the stability of the mRNA. Suppose a synonymous mutations increase in the mRNA stability. As a result, since each mRNA lasts for longer, the amount of protein molecules from each mRNA increases, and hence, the total amount of protein in the cell increases because of the synonymous mutation. This change in the protein amount can impact a change in the cellular fitness too (Figure 11.4).
b. *Change in rate of translation*. Another mechanism via which synonymous mutations change fitness is by altering the rate at which translation takes place. mRNA molecules fold into a structure which minimizes their free energy. While synonymous mutations do not change the amino acid sequence, the change in the nucleotide sequence can lead to a change in the structure of the mRNA. This change may, consequently, lead to a change in the ease with which the ribosomes are able to translate the mRNA molecule. This change in the rate of translation leads to an altered amount of protein amounts, and consequently, a change in the organismal fitness (Figure 11.5).

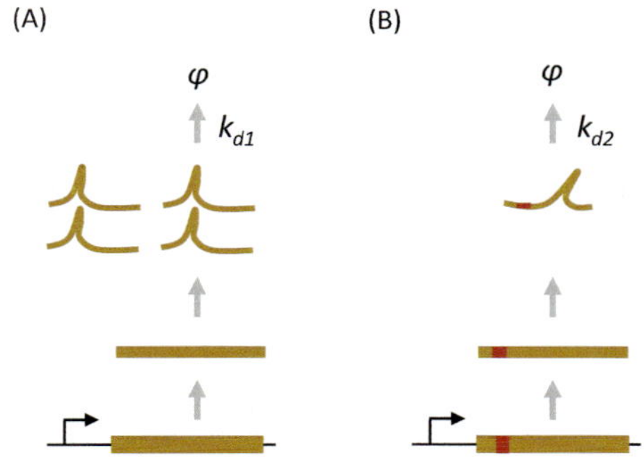

FIGURE 11.4 Synonymous mutation can lead to altered *mRNA* stability. Consider a gene sequence in (A). The *mRNA* undergoes first-order degradation with degradation constant k_{d1}. (B) The nucleotide sequence acquires a synonymous mutation (indicated in red). The altered *mRNA* sequence leads to changes in the three-dimensional structure and the stability of the *mRNA*. The degradation kinetics of the *mRNA* proceeds as per k_{d2} as the degradation constant. The change in the degradation constant leads to the two variants making different amounts of the *mRNA* in the cell, which in turn, leads to a change in the protein amounts in the cell. Hence, a synonymous mutation can have effect on fitness of the cell.

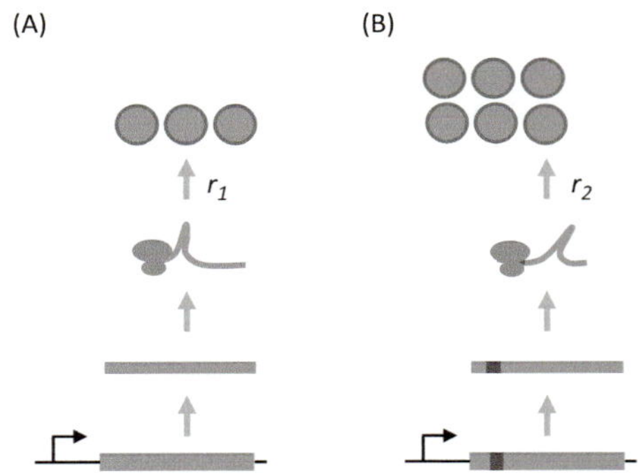

FIGURE 11.5 Synonymous mutation can lead to altered rate of translation. The altered gene sequence **(A)** and **(B)** (with synonymous mutation) leads to altered rate of translation. This altered rate of translation results because of the access that the ribosome finds toward the *mRNA*. The altered rates of translation leads to different protein amounts in the two gene sequences. The different protein amounts lead to the two variants conferring different fitness to the cell.

c. *Change in protein structure*. A synonymous mutation, by definition, does not lead to a change in amino acid sequence. However, in some cases, somewhat surprisingly, a synonymous mutation is known to lead to a change in the protein structure! This happens because of a phenomenon called 'co-translational folding'.

A protein molecule functions once it has folded in its correct three-dimensional shape. The kinetics of folding happens as the peptide chain is emerging from the ribosome. Imagine a mRNA molecule which is translated very fast. In this case, the peptide chain emerges from the ribosome quickly and the final 3-D structure that the peptide chain takes is the global energy minima.

On the other hand, imagine a scenario where the translation is slow near the middle of the mRNA molecule. In this case, half the peptide chain has come out of the ribosome, while the ribosome stalls on the mRNA. This peptide chain will, in this time, fold into its energy minima. Consequently, when the remaining mRNA molecule is translated, the peptide chain corresponding to the second half of the mRNA folds into its energy minima. The rate of translation of an mRNA molecule can thus impact the final structure of the protein. A correct structure if, of course, necessary for correct protein functionality. Hence, a synonymous mutation can have a fitness effect via change in the protein structure.

The speed at which amino acids are incorporated in the growing peptide chain is dependent on the codon being used for that particular amino acid. See the genetic code once again (Chapter 2), and note that for most amino acids, there is more than one codon. Thus, there are several codons which can be used to incorporate the same amino acid. For example, the amino acid serine can be incorporated via any of six codons. In *E. coli*, the codon `AGC` is used most frequently (25% of the times) to incorporate serine, and `TCG` is the least used codon (14% of the times). In a starker example of this bias, Leucine is encoded 47% of the times with codon `CTG`, and only 4% of the time with the codon `CTA`. Thus, there is an order of magnitude difference in the choice of codon to incorporate Leucine. This is important for the pace at which translation takes place (Figure 11.6).

Examples for each of the three cases described above are listed in 'Further Readings' at the end of this chapter.

11.6.1 Non-synonymous mutations may be neutral

In contrast with the case of synonymous mutations, non-synonymous mutations can be neutral. Proteins are large (with respect to their substrate) molecular machines. The catalytic site in a protein structure is controlled by a handful of amino acid residues, while a typical protein is a few hundred amino acids. Typically, hydrophobic amino acids are hidden deep inside the protein structure, while hydrophilic residues are on the protein structure surface. A mutation which changes an inner hydrophobic residue to a hydrophilic residue can be disastrous for the protein structure – such a change will likely cause the protein to unfold. Hence, such a change is, of course, non-neutral. However, a mutation on the surface of the protein, where a hydrophilic residue is replaced by another hydrophilic residue with similar physical properties (e.g., size), is not likely to cause change in the functioning of the protein. Hence, fitness of the organism does not change, and the mutation is neutral.

Despite the above descriptions, the assumption that synonymous mutations are neutral, and non-synonymous mutations are non-neutral is likely true to a large extent. Hence, ideas like 'molecular clock' and Neutral Theory of Molecular Evolution are still widely used in understanding sequence and evolution – at the very least as first approximation to understand evolutionary history between sequences and organisms.

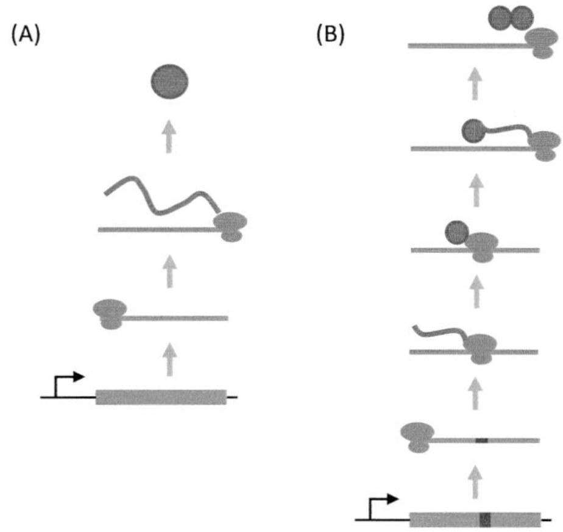

FIGURE 11.6 Synonymous mutation can lead to altered protein structure. In (A) a gene is transcribed and translated. The resulting amino acid chain folds into its minimum energy structure, giving the final protein shape and function. (B) The gene sequence acquires synonymous mutation(s) which incorporate rare codons in the middle of the gene sequence. As a result, during translation, the ribosome pauses at the site of rare codon(s). In this time of pause, the already translated chain of amino acids folds into its energy minima. Once the amino acids corresponding to the rare codons are inserted, translation resumes and the remaining amino acid chain folds into its energy minima. As a result, the three-dimensional structure of the protein in (A) and (B) are different from each other.

11.7 CONCLUSION

In this chapter, we discussed two great ideas of molecular evolution. The first one, molecular clock, was a remarkable discovery that protein sequences differ between species in a clock-like fashion. Why should it be so? While Pauling and Zuckerkandl did not answer this question, their's and other researchers' work in the 1950s paved the way for presentation of the idea of neutral theory of molecular evolution, posed by Motoo Kimura. While neutral theory has been revisited, revised, and rejected in the decades since, it is still an important null hypothesis against which observations are often stacked and measured. In my opinion, neutral theory of molecular evolution was also the last great intellectual contribution made in the field of evolutionary biology. Since the 1968 paper that Kimura wrote, and his 1983 book by the title of *Neutral Theory of Molecular Evolution*, there have been a large number of advancements in the area of evolution. However, almost all of them have been advances in technology and tools at our disposal, which have facilitated experiments and measurements that we could never make before. Intellectually, however, the field of evolutionary biology waits for the next big idea.

Having had this discussion, we now move, in the final five chapters of this book, to experimental evolution. Again, as discussed in Chapter 3, our model systems to study evolution via experiments will be bacteria. Our primary goal in these next five chapters is not to study as many experiments as we can. The number of interesting evolution experiments done is far too high to be covered in a single book, but we will only study a few experiments which, in my opinion, have either shaped how we think of evolution or have been exceptionally clever in their design.

EXERCISES

1 The genetic code has possible $9 \times 64 = 576$ possible point mutations. How many are synonymous and how many non-synonymous? Are codons corresponding to some amino acids more robust to nucleotide change compared to others?
2 See the four proteins in Figure 11.1. What are their roles in cellular physiology? Write a short note on each of them.
3 Compute $\frac{dN}{dS}$ of the following proteins in *E. coli* and *Salmonella*:
  a. *fliZ* (a regulator in flagellar synthesis)
  b. *zwf* (an important gene in glucose metabolism)
  c. *hns* (bacteria lack histones, but have 'histone-like' proteins. *hns* encodes for one such protein.
4 See reference # 10 on the next page. What is the mechanistic basis via which the synonymous mutation confers a benefit in this case?
5 In the abstract of this chapter, we saw the example of clothes. See reference # 11 for this chapter. Which gene did the researchers take to study divergence of lice on the body and on clothes? Would we get a different answer, depending on which gene we study?

BIBLIOGRAPHY

1. Margoliash E. 1963. Primary structure and evolution of cytochrome C. *Proc Natl Acad Sci U S A* 50:672–9.
2. Doolittle RF, Blombaeck B. 1964. Amino-acid sequence investigations of fibrinopeptides from various mammals: Evolutionary implications. *Nature* 202:147–52.

   (The molecular evidence of protein variation as a function of time of divergence was gathering in the years leading up to Pauling and Zuckerkandl's paper. These two papers are prime examples of that.)
3. Emile Zuckerkandl LP. 1965. *Volutionary Divergence and Convergence in Protein*. New York: Academic Press.

   (This is the classic paper by Zuckerkandl and Pauling, where they propose the idea of the molecular clock. However, note that they did not know why protein divergence should be clock-like.)
4. Kimura M. 1968. Evolutionary rate at the molecular level. *Nature* 217:624–6.

   (This is the classic paper by Motoo Kimura in 1968 where he proposes *Neutral Theory of Molecular Evolution* as a mechanistic explanation of the molecular clock. Kimura later published a book by the title of *Neutral Theory of Molecular Evolution* in 1983. The book is highly readable.)
5. King JL, Jukes TH. 1969. Non-Darwinian evolution. *Science* 164:788–98.

   (Just a year after Kimura's paper, Jukes and King published this paper in *Science* with more support for molecular clock. They somewhat playfully suggested the title, and were surprised when the paper was accepted with this title.)
6. Dickerson RE. 1972. The structure and history of an ancient protein. *Sci Am* 226:58–70 passim.

(As years went by, more evidence was coming in the form of different proteins across lineages diverging in a linear, clockwise fashion.)

7. Kreitman M. 1996. The neutral theory is dead. Long live the neutral theory. *Bioessays* 18:678–683; discussion 683.

   (An important paper by Kreitman on why, despite many criticisms, Neutral Theory is an important tool and concept at our disposal.)
8. Zuckerkandl E. 2012. Fifty-year old and still ticking··· an interview with Emile Zuckerkandl on the 50th anniversary of the molecular clock. Interview by Giacomo Bernardi. *J Mol Evol* 74:233–6.

   (An interview of Zuckerkandl on 50 years of the idea of molecular clock).
9. Bailey SF, Hinz A, Kassen R. 2014. Adaptive synonymous mutations in an experimentally evolved Pseudomonas fluorescens population. *Nat Commun* 5:4076.

   (This is one of the handful of papers where a synonymous mutation was isolated and definitively shown to be adaptive in a laboratory evolution experiment.)
10. Bailey SF, Alonso Morales LA, Kassen R. 2021. Effects of Synonymous Mutations beyond Codon Bias: The Evidence for Adaptive Synonymous Substitutions from Microbial Evolution Experiments. *Genome Biol Evol* 13.

    (A valuable review of mechanisms via which synonymous mutations can be adaptive.)
11. Toups MA, Kitchen A, Light JE, Reed DL. 2010. Origin of Clothing Lice Indicates Early Clothing Use by Anatomically Modern Humans in Africa. *Mol Bio & Evol.* 28(1):29–32.

    (This paper uses neutral theory to decipher when humans started wearing clothes.)

12 How to Do Evolution Experiments in Lab?

12.1 INTRODUCTION

This chapter marks a transition point in our study of evolution. Through the previous chapters, we have attempted to build a theoretical and a conceptual framework to study evolution. Much of what we have discussed was developed in the first half of the 20th century. Remarkably, that is before even when the structure of DNA was discovered in 1953.

Starting from this chapter, we will study, how the ideas that were developed in the 20th century are being studied in lab today. Technological advances in the last few decades allows us to perform experiments with extreme precision, and make minute measurements of aspects of microbial physiology. Moreover, with DNA sequencing becoming increasingly cheaper, we are today able to connect the physiology of the organism with the changes at the sequence level.

In this chapter, we will discuss the methodology of how we perform evolution experiments in lab, and from the next chapter onward, we will discuss how these experiments have been used in laboratories around the world to understand the principles of evolutionary dynamics we have discussed so far.

12.2 WHY USE BACTERIA TO STUDY EVOLUTION?

Darwin arrived at the theory of natural selection by observations. His journey around the world in *HMS Beagle* lead him to theorize how species arrive, and how adaptations take place. The result of his work was the publication of the *Origin of Species* in 1859. Darwin was 50, when the book was first published.

While Darwin was finishing up writing the *Origin of Species*, on continental Europe, in Brno, a Moravian priest was performing experiments to understand how traits are transmitted from one generation to the next. As we have seen in Chapter 1, the lack of explanation of how this transmission takes place was one of the weaknesses in Darwin's proposal. The Moravian priest, Gregor Mendel, was trying to solve this problem with peas as his chosen organism for experiments. Mendel's paper on genetics (the term 'genetics' was not coined till the early 20th century) was published in 1865.

The relevant time scale in evolution is the number of generations of the model organism we are able to process. In the case of Mendel, he performed experiments where one generation took one year. That is considerably faster than studying human beings, where a generation is more than two decades (the time when one generation gives birth to the next). However, evolutionary change can be slow. Hence, to be able to observe large changes which may take hundreds or thousands of generations,

 DOI: 10.1201/9781003633662-12

we need model organisms whose generation time is much slower compared to plants (~one year per generation), flies (~a few weeks per generation). Because of the long generation time of these species, studying large-scale change within a human lifespan is not likely feasible.

Are there model systems which allow us to witness large-scale changes (within a human lifespan)?

Microbes offer us that opportunity.

12.2.1 Time and Generations

As we will see in this chapter, performing evolution experiments with a bacteria like *E. coli* allows us to process ~10 generations per day. This offers a great opportunity to study evolution over thousands of generations quite easily; something that would not be possible at all working with complex sexually reproducing populations.

Compare the following.

The longest-running evolution experiment, based on duration of time the experiment has been running for, is at the University of Illinois, Urbana-Champaign, USA. This experiment, with corn plants as the model organism, was started in 1896, and in the ~125 years since, has processed exactly 125 generations.

However, the longest-running evolution experiment, based on how many generations have been processed, is currently at University of Texas, Austin. The experiment was started with *E. coli* as the model organism in 1988, and in the ~35 years since, has processed ~80,000 generations! A large part of the experiment was done at Michigan State University in Richard Lenski's laboratory. However, with Lenski retiring, the experiment was moved to Austin in the summer of 2022.

Consider the staggering number in the number of generations that we can process using the two systems. What has been done in corn in 125 years, the same number of generations can be processed in *E. coli* in two weeks! This is one of the powers of using microbial systems.

12.2.2 Control Over Selection

Microbes are grown in incubators in laboratory clean rooms. The incubators maintain constant temperature (*E. coli* experiments are often done at 37°C), constant oxygen supply (via shaking), regular supply of nutrients, and absence of any biotic (like predators) or abiotic (like pH, temperature fluctuations) stresses. If these variables are introduced in laboratory evolution experiments, they are usually introduced in a very controlled manner, with only one at a time and at a desired intensity. The idea is to make the environment the population is growing in, as precise as possible. We are then able to study the response of the population to this exact environment.

All these factors make an experimental microbial evolution set-up in the lab very removed from an ecological context. Imagine a bacterial population in soil – this population experiences temperature variation, variation in nutrient and water availability, predators, presence of other species as competitors. All these factors oscillate with time of day, season, and sometimes randomly. For example, selection pressure during a hot, sunny day is for surviving at high temperatures in the absence of water, while at night, the selection might be for survival and growth at low temperatures. Thus, selection in an ecological context is multi-dimensional. This facet of selection makes studying evolution at a molecular scale in ecology extremely difficult.

In laboratory experiments with microbes, however, by controlling the environment in which evolution is taking place, we can control selection precisely. This control helps us study cellular response to precise selection pressures with a much greater accuracy.

12.2.3 Connect Genotype with Phenotype

Evolution with a microbial population in a laboratory not just allows us to monitor the phenotypic state of the population, but also the molecular changes which enable phenotypic adaptation. This is done by allowing the population to adapt in a particular environment for a given number of generations, and then sequencing the genome of the evolved populations. The sequencing allows us to identify the molecular changes that took place in the DNA of the organism in the course of the experiment.

For example, let us say we aim to study *E. coli*'s adaptation in an environment where glucose is in limited supply and is the sole source of carbon for the population. Imagine that we perform this evolution experiment for 1,000 generations. For this, we will first sequence the genome of the bacteria we are starting with. After the evolution experiment, we will sequence the evolved populations again. Comparison of the two sequences tells us the mutations that the evolved populations acquired. Using standard molecular biology techniques, we will then study each of the mutations and decipher the role they play in the adaptation process.

12.2.4 'Frozen' Fossils

One of the challenges of evolution experiments with complex species is that we cannot directly compare the ancestor from which the experiment was started with, with the evolved organism. For example, we cannot compare the corn plant that the Illinois experiment was started with in 1896 with the evolved corn plants of today. However, this is not the case with microbial populations.

Standard and simple microbiological techniques allow us to deep freeze (at −80°C) a microbial population. These populations are metabolically completely inactive, and can be stored at that temperature for virtually any duration. And whenever we want, we can revive these stored strains by providing them conditions conducive for growth. Hence, for the evolution experiment started in 1988, we can easily grow and compare the ancestral strain from which the experiment was started with, with the evolved *E. coli* growing in the lab today. The same technique also allows us to store the intermediate population in the evolution experiment. Typically, researchers store the population every few hundred generations, each of which can be revived at any later day. This allows us to compare the evolved populations by competing against each other, which would not be possible in any complex species.

12.2.5 Sequencing

Bacteria also have smaller genomes than other laboratory model systems. Hence, sequencing genomes is cheaper. Additionally, they are haploids (i.e., carry only one copy of the genome), which makes analyzing sequencing results is simpler.

Because of all the above reasons, microbial systems have become a convenient and powerful choice to perform evolution experiments in the lab.

Through the above discussion, I hope to have communicated and convinced that bacteria and microorganisms are a powerful system to study evolution.

Somewhat surprisingly, the first evolution experiment with microbes was done a long time ago – in 1880s by William Dallinger. Curious after having read Darwin's *Origin of Species*, Dallinger asked the question if he could evolve bacteria to survive and grow at high temperatures. Starting with bacteria which grew optimally at around 20°C, Dallinger adapted these bacteria by slowly increasing the temperature over the following seven years. By the time the experiment ended in 1886 due to an explosion, Dallinger's evolved bacteria were growing at close to 70°C!

Interestingly, before the experiment's untimely end, Dallinger also demonstrated that as bacteria evolved to grow at 70°C, they were no longer growing as fast as the ancestor at 20°C. Thus, as the bacteria evolved to grow better at 70°C, their ability to grow at 20°C was compromised. Thus, making the first reported study of a trade-off in an evolution experiment.

By trade-off, we mean that as the population evolves to become specialist at growing at high temperatures, it becomes worse at growing at lower temperatures. Thus, specializing for growth at high temperatures has a cost associated with it – decreased growth at lower temperatures. This is the trade-off, advantage in one environment comes at the cost of being disadvantaged in another. A cell can be specialist in one environment (low or high temperature), but not both! Work in the last two decades has uncovered a lot about trade-offs that constrain bacterial evolution. See references for more details.

Before moving ahead,

- ➔ Why do you think trade-offs exist in bacteria? Why could the cell not evolve to become better at growing at higher temperatures without compromising its ability to grow at lower temperatures?

Next, we will study what are the different ways in which we can perform evolution experiments with microorganisms in lab. As we will see, there are three distinct ways to perform evolution experiments in lab. Each method has its benefits and disadvantages. In addition, some methods are more apt for a certain type of question that we want to answer, as compared to the others. We will now discuss these three methods.

12.3 SERIAL SUB-CULTURE

The most common way of performing an evolution experiment is by serially sub-culturing the cells in the media of interest. Suppose we are interested in studying the evolutionary trajectory of *E. coli* in a particular environment, where carbon is present only in the form of galactose. To study this, we will inoculate *E. coli* in a flask containing growth media with a defined chemical composition.

In this defined growth media, carbon will be supplied in the form of galactose, and other nutrients like sources of nitrogen, phosphorus, etc., will be provided. Since we are interested in studying the population's response to galactose limitation, galactose will be the limiting agent of growth. This means that if we increase the concentration of galactose in the media, the growth rate of the bacteria increases. If, however, we increase any other constituent of the media (like the nitrogen source), the growth rate does not increase. Thus, carbon (in the form of galactose) is the growth-limiting agent in the media.

As cells grow in this media, they utilize and eventually run out of galactose. At this point, growth halts, and cells enter the stationary phase. If we continue to keep the cells in this environment longer, we are testing the cells for their ability to survive in the stationary phase. Whereas the goal of our experiment was to test the adaptation of a population in galactose limiting environment. Hence, we must supply the population with more nutrients to allow growth.

To do this, we take a fraction of the cells in the flask (e.g., 1:100 volume) and sub-culture them in the fresh media with the exact same composition as the one we started with. The cells, having found more nutrients, grow in the second flask and then reach stationary phase. We then sub-culture in the next flask with the identical media composition.

This process is continued for as long as we want to study the adaptive response of the population.

Let us look closely at how this experiment works (Figure 12.1). As cells are growing in one flask, mutations occur. The deleterious mutants that come up grow slower than the ancestral genotype, so their numbers remain small. Neutral mutants grow at the same rate as the ancestor. While beneficial mutants arise and grow faster than the ancestor. The three types of variants keep growing till the carrying capacity of the flask is reached.

Remember that the frequency of each type of variants (beneficial, deleterious, and neutral) is dictated by when the mutation arises. Mutations that arise early will

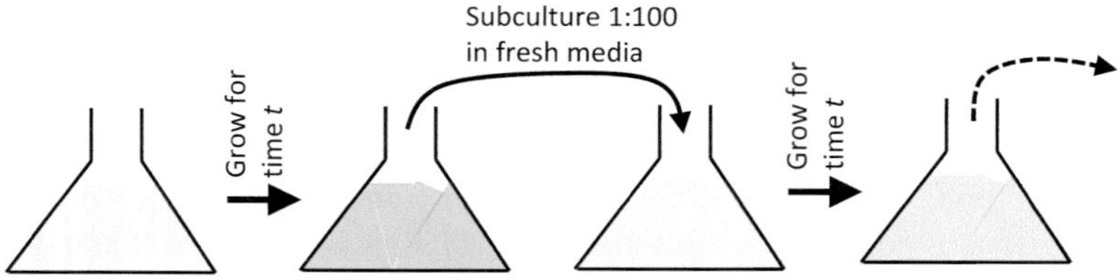

FIGURE 12.1 An evolution experiment is started when a defined culture media is inoculated with a bacterial strain. The flask is then allowed to grow for time *t* at a given temperature. After growth for time *t*, 1/100 of the culture media is propagated to a fresh flask containing the defined media. The culture is then allowed to grow again for time *t*. The process is repeated over and over again for any number of generations. A dilution of 1:100 in every flask corresponds to ~6.67 generations.

increase to higher frequencies, while those that arise late will remain at very small frequencies.

Once the carrying capacity is reached, we transfer 1:100 of the total volume (and hence, the cells in the flask) to a new flask containing fresh growth media. Since only 1:100 of the total volume is transferred to the next flask – some of the individuals carrying beneficial mutations might get left behind in the original flask. Imagine a beneficial mutation which is present in only two individuals in the flask. If none of these two individuals is transferred to the next flask, then these mutations are lost from the experiment.

Note that in such a context, it is chance events which lead to loss of these mutations. These mutations are, therefore, lost due to drift.

On the other hand, beneficial mutations that get transferred to the next flask increase in frequency in the next phase of growth. As the experiment proceeds forward, some beneficial mutations will reach fixation. And hence, evolutionary change proceeds.

A sub-culture of 1:100 corresponds to ~6.67 generations per transfer. Imagine that of the N_o cells in the first flask, $\frac{N_o}{100}$ cells are transferred to the next flask. After one generation of growth, the number of cells in this flask doubles to $\frac{2N_o}{100}$. In another generation, the number of cells increases to $\frac{4N_o}{100}$. Thus, after k generations, the number of cells in the flask equals $\frac{2^k N_o}{100}$. However, we know that, as the cells enter stationary phase, the number of cells equals N_o. Thus, the number of generations k in which the number of cells increases to N_o is therefore found from the following equation,

$$N_o = \frac{2^k N_o}{100} \tag{12.1}$$

Solving for k, the number of generations, we get from the above equation that k equals ~6.67. Thus, every 1:100 sub-culture in an experiment corresponds to ~6.67 generations. This is the sub-culture fraction that is used in the *E. coli* evolution experiment that has been going on for >75,000 generations. The sub-culture takes place every 24 hours.

Example 12.1: Suppose in an evolution experiment, we sub-culture 1:1000 every 24 hours. In the 24 hours, five generations of growth takes place. What is the evolutionary change that takes place in this experiment?

Solution: There are two important numbers to note in this experiment. First, a dilution of 1:1000 translates to ten generations ($2^{10} \sim 1000$). Second, growth of five generations means that population expands by a factor of 2^5 (~32). Thus, the population contracts by a factor of 1,000 when we shift from one flask to another, and it expands by a factor of 32 in the growth phase of the bacteria. Thus, dilution is much more than contraction in the population size.

In this context, if population size in a flask is N, after a 1,000-fold dilution, the number of bacteria transferred to the next flask is $\frac{N}{1000}$. These bacteria then grow for five generations, taking the number of bacteria to $\frac{2^5 N}{1000}$ or $\frac{32N}{1000}$. But at this point, we transfer 1:1000 to the next flask. Thus, the number of bacteria transferred to the next flask is $\frac{32N}{1000^2}$.

You should see a pattern here. The starting number of bacteria in each successive flask is becoming smaller. This is because, with each flask, the number of bacteria is being reduced by a factor of 1,000 (due to dilution), and increased by a factor of 32 (due to growth). Thus, overall, the number of bacteria is reducing. Hence, as we keep processing dilution every day, the population numbers keep getting smaller, eventually reaching extinction.

The important point to keep in mind here is that while designing evolution experiments by serial sub-culture, the dilution factor we apply to the population as we move from one flask to the next should be less than or equal to the factor by which population grows in a flask. Otherwise, the population will simply go extinct.

Example 12.2: Let us look at another aspect of evolution via serial sub-culture. In this instance, let us imagine that we start an evolution experiment with a population size 10^6. We allow a 1,000-fold increase in the population size in a flask, when it reaches its carrying capacity. Hence, population increases to 10^9. We sub-culture this population 1:100 in a new flask. What happens in an experiment when the size of expansion allowed by growth (1,000-fold in this case) exceeds the dilution that we are applying in every transfer (100-fold in this case)?

Solution: Flask #1 is seeded with 10^6 cells, and the population increases to 10^9. A 1:100 dilution means that 10^7 cells are then transferred to flask #2. Note that after this transfer, the population size in flask #2 will not be 10^{10} (a 1,000-fold expansion), but will still be 10^9. This is because the carrying capacity of the flask is 10^9. Hence, in the second flask, starting with 10^7 cells, the population reaches a size of 10^9. Thereafter, a 100-fold dilution means that 10^7 cells go to flask #3 followed by a 100-fold expansion. And so on. Hence, in the case when the factor of expansion or growth is greater than the factor of dilution, an equilibrium between the two is reached and the population size is maintained at a constant number.

In 1988, the paleontologist Stephen Jay Gould asked a rhetorical question. Gould asked us to imagine that if the entire 4.5-billion-year-old history of our planet were repeated in an independent experiment, would the evolution of life forms take the same trajectory as has happened on Earth? As a result, would species like us be the dominant species again? Or, would stochasticity in evolutionary processes mean that the trajectory on this planet would be completely different from what has happened on Earth? In essence, we are asking what are the relative roles of chance and determinism in dictating evolutionary trajectories. This is a major research theme in evolutionary biology even today.

While Gould's question was rhetorical, using microbes to do an evolution experiment in lab, we can attempt to provide an answer.

One of the main advantages of performing evolution experiments by serial sub-culture is that these experiments can be performed quite easily in independent repeats. Evolution is inherently a stochastic process. Imagine that the experiment described above is performed with the same ancestor in two independent parallel experiments. Will the evolutionary trajectory of the two lines in terms of (a) fitness of the population and (b) mutations they acquire be the same or different?

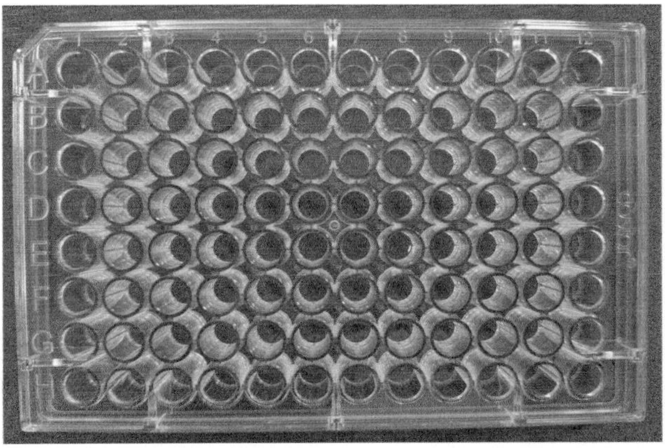

FIGURE 12.2 A 96-well plate allows 96 independent repeats of an evolution experiment. A 96-well plate carries 12 × 8 independent wells, each with a volume capacity of 250 μl. Growth can be started from a common ancestor in each of these wells, and then independently propagated from one plate to another. This number of repeats of the same experiment allows us to seek an answer to the question of necessity and chance in an evolutionary process.

Before moving ahead,

➔ For the two independent lines in our hypothetical experiment, plot the following, how does fitness change over the 2,000 generations that the experiment was done for? Take a pause and sketch the fitness trajectory of this experiment before going forward.

A typical representation of a serial sub-culture evolution experiment is in a 96-well plate (Figure 12.2), where 96 wells (8 rows × 12 columns) in the plate each correspond to an independent line, started from the same ancestor. When cells reach stationary phase in the wells, a fraction of them (1:100, for example) is transferred to a fresh plate containing media with identical composition. Thus, the logistics of handling 96 (or more) independent repeats of the experiment are trivial in a sub-culturing experiment.

12.3.1 Drawback

Evolution by serial sub-culture has one serious drawback. In our experiment, where *E. coli* is being evolved in low galactose environment, at the start of the culture, the bacteria are in an environment where galactose concentration is low, say 0.1% (a typical experimental value). However, as the experiment proceeds, the concentration of galactose decreases, eventually reducing to near zero as cells enter stationary phase. This means that the selection pressure on the cells is constantly changing with time. At the beginning of the experiment, selection acts to identify individuals which have the highest fitness when the sugar concentration is 0.1%. However, as time progresses, selection acts to select individuals for a continuously changing environment.

Thus, while at the beginning of this discussion, we mentioned that laboratory evolution experiments allow us to ensure that selection is unidimensional, this is not precisely true for evolution via serial sub-cultures.

Despite this drawback, >99% of all evolution experiments with microorganisms are performed using this technique. As we will see, the alternate techniques of performing evolution experiment in lab offer greater limitations. Moreover, the flexibility that serial sub-culture technique offers far outweighs the drawbacks.

12.4 CHEMOSTAT

The disadvantage of the changing selection pressure with time in a serial sub-culture evolution experiment can be circumvented by performing the evolution experiment in a chemostat (Figure 12.3).

Remember that in a chemostat we have a reactor of volume V. There is an inlet stream which supplies fresh media at rate v per time, and an exit stream which removes spent media (along with the cells growing in the reactor) at the same rate v per time.

When a chemostat is inoculated with an ancestor, the nutrients in the reactor provide the environment for growth. The steady rate of supply of fresh media and removal of spent media ensures that there is a constant supply of nutrients for growth. After growth for a certain amount of time, the system reaches steady state – i.e., the composition of the chemostat and the number of bacteria in the chemostat stay constant with time.

At this time, for each of the nutrients, the rate of supply (from the incoming stream) is exactly balanced by the rate of consumption (by the growing bacterial population). In addition, the number of bacteria being washed away from the reactor per unit time is exactly balanced by the increase in the population due to cell division in the same amount of time.

We evolve the population in this state. As beneficial mutations occur in the chemostat, some survive drift. These mutants will divide faster than the ancestral

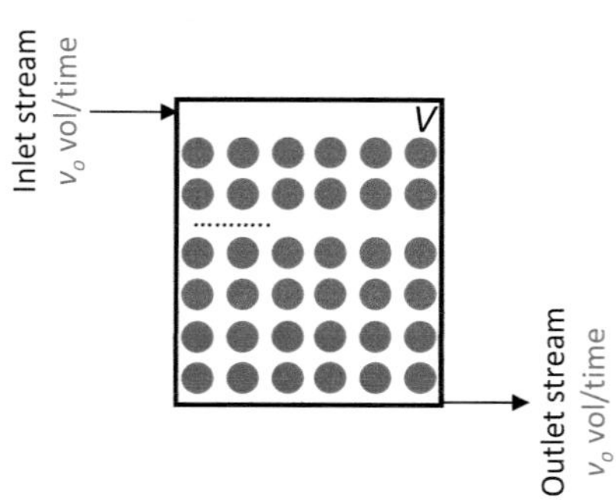

FIGURE 12.3 A chemostat allows for constant conditions of growth for any amount of time. Newer mutations keep occurring in the chemostat. These mutations may be rejected by selection (for deleterious mutations), or their fate dictated by drift (for neutral mutations), or their fate dictated by a combined action of selection and drift (for beneficial mutations).

population. This change would result in the rate of bacterial birth (which has increased because of the beneficial mutation) increase. As a result, the density in the chemostat would increase. This results in a greater number of bacteria being washed away from the reactor per time. This dynamic leads to an establishment of a new equilibrium in the chemostat.

This process continues as we move forward in time. At any point in the course of the evolution experiment, we sample and store the population being washed away from the reactor (as it is representative of the population in the chemostat at that particular time).

Evolution in a chemostat ensures that selection pressure does not change with time, since the chemical composition in the chemostat does not change with time. Hence, the population is evolving in a constant environment through the course of the experiment.

However, despite this advantage, a chemostat is rarely used in experimental evolution. The major reasons for this are (a) maintaining the sterility of a chemostat equipment for long durations is a big challenge and (b) the difficulty in running several lines in parallel.

12.5 MUTATION ACCUMULATION (MA) EXPERIMENTS

We know that mutations provide the fodder for evolutionary change. For calculations in Chapter 6 we used *E. coli*'s mutation rate, μ as 10^{-3} cell^{-1} generation^{-1}. But what we did not answer in Chapter 6 is how do we estimate the mutation rate of an organism?

A typical experimental technique to estimate mutation rates is via Mutation Accumulation (MA) experiments.

Why can we not estimate mutation rates using the above two techniques? We could simply evolve a population for a given number of generations and then sequence the evolved genome. The number of mutations accumulated in this time divided by the number of generations would provide us with an estimate of mutation rate μ.

Before moving ahead,

➔ Take a pause here, and think of a reason why this way of estimating the mutation rate is incorrect.

Mutation rates cannot be estimated using the above two techniques.

This is so because in the above two experimental designs, deleterious mutations are eliminated by drift, neutral mutations' fate is dictated by drift, and beneficial mutations are under selection and drift. Thus, an overwhelming majority of all mutations that we note in these experiments are beneficial in nature. The deleterious and neutral mutations are simply lost from the system.

Thus, these experiments only provide an estimate of the rate at which beneficial mutations fix in evolution experiments. Whereas, what we are interested in is the rate at which mutations (of any kind – beneficial, deleterious, and neutral) are occurring in the population.

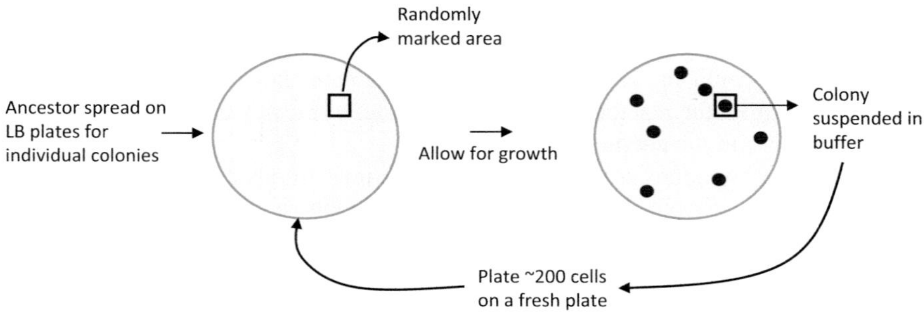

FIGURE 12.4 Mutation accumulation (MA) experiment with a microbial population. An area is marked on a fresh plate, and a culture spread to as to lead to ~200 colonies (starting from ~200 cells). The colony growing in the area marked is selected, and the rest are rejected from the experiment. This randomizes the colony picked for propagation in the experiment. The cells from the selected colony are suspended in buffer, and a volume equivalent to ~200 cells is taken and spread on a fresh plate. The choice of these 200 cells is also completely randomized. As a result, the choice of which cell is propagated in the experiment is completely randomized. Thus, the role of selection is completely eliminated in this experiment. This process is repeated for a number of transfers. The mutations thus picked up in this fashion are completely due to drift. Many lines (typically ~100) are evolved like this in parallel, and the mutation rate is estimated from each. The average of these estimates of mutation rate is considered a quantitative estimate of mutation rate.

Hence, we need experimental designs where the effect of selection is eliminated or reduced to the extent possible. This goal is accomplished by MA experiments.

Before discussing them in detail, let us first describe an MA experiment for a bacteria like *E. coli* (Figure 12.4).

An ancestral population, with ~100 individuals, is spread on a solid media. Since individual bacteria are too small to be seen with a naked eye, when we spread, we do not know where each of these 100 bacteria is on the plate. At this time, we mark a randomly selected area on the plate. Next, the plate is kept in an incubator at 37°C (*E. coli*'s preferred temperature for growth) overnight. When we observe the plate the following morning, the 100 bacterial would have replicated several times, and each would have grown into a small lump of cells (called a 'colony').

Next, we identify the colony closest to the mark on the plate and suspend the colony in buffer. A colony contains $O(10^8)$ cells. Of these, we take ~100 and spread on a fresh plate and repeat the process (typically ~100 times).

Note that in the steps described above, we have randomized (a) the colony which gets propagated to the next plate, and (b) the 100 individuals from the selected colony which get propagated further.

Thus, the identity of the individual which gets propagated in the experiment is completely randomized. Thus, the evolutionary fate of the population is dictated purely by chance, and selection has no role in the process.

At the end of the experiment, one colony is selected and sequenced. The genome sequence of the evolved colony is compared with that of the ancestor. Since each colony originated from a single colony, we can easily calculate the number of generations in each colony. The number of mutations in the sequenced genome divided by the total number of generations provides us with an estimate of the mutation rate.

To minimize the role of stochasticity in dictating the mutation rate estimates, several independent MA lines are started in experiments. The number of lines is typically O (few dozens) – each providing an estimate of the mutation rate. The average from all the lines is used as an estimate of mutation rate of the species. Of course, the longer the MA experiment (measured as number of transfers) and higher the number of independent lines – the more accurate is the estimate of the mutation rate.

Using MA experiments, mutation rates have been measured for a number of species (see Table 12.1).

Example 12.3: A typical *E. coli* colony on a plate contains around 10^8 cells. This colony, obviously, started with a single cell. How many generations transpired in this time in this colony?

Solution: We go back to the formula that starting with a single cell, after n generations, we have 2^n cells. In this case, the total number of cells after n generations is 10^8. Therefore, we solve for n from the following equation,

$$10^8 = 2^n$$

Solving for n, we get,

$$n \sim 26 \tag{12.2}$$

Thus, in a single colony of *E. coli*, more than 25 generations pass.

TABLE 12.1
Mutation Rates Estimated from MA Experiments

Organism	Mutation Rate Estimate (per Site per Generation)
E. coli	10^{-10}
Chlamydomonas reinhardtii	3.2×10^{-10}
Saccharomyces cerevisiae (haploid)	3.3×10^{-10}
Drosophila melanogaster	3.5×10^{-9}
C57BL/6 mice	5.4×10^{-9}
Caenorhabditis elegans	2.1×10^{-9}
Schizosaccharomyces pombe (haploid)	2.00×10^{-10}

Example 12.4: How many mutations take place in the colony we discuss in Example 12.3?

Solution: We often think of a colony as an isogenic entity. But through this example, we will see that that's hardly the case. In transitioning from one to 10^8 cells, $(10^8 - 1)$ cell divisions take place. This is ~10^8. We know that the mutation rate in *E. coli* is 10^{-3} per cell per generation. Thus, the total number of mutations that take place in the colony is 10^5 $(10^8.10^{-3})$.

12.6 CONCLUSION

In this chapter, we discuss three techniques of performing evolution experiments in a laboratory setting. These three are critical techniques, and depending on the research question we ask, we design an appropriate experiment, by choosing a technique apt for what we want to understand. Having gone through these methods, we will now turn to actual evolution experiments performed in laboratory conditions and see how these experiments have enhanced our understanding of how evolution and evolutionary change proceed in real time.

EXERCISES

1. Solve Equation (12.1) to show that a dilution of 1:100 equates to 6.67 generations.
2. Suppose we sub-culture 1:1000 (and not 1:100) in the evolution experiment. How many generations does this correspond to every transfer?
3. The long-term evolution experiment with *E. coli* has processed 75,000 generations to date. A sub-culture is done every 24 hours and is equivalent to 6.67 generations. How many transfers have been done in this experiment since its start?
4. Imagine an evolution experiment where ten generations are processed in two different designs. The two designs are run in identical environments. In the first, the population is grown to a size 10^7, and then sub-cultured 1:1000 in fresh flask. In the second, the population is grown to a size 10^{10}, and then sub-cultured 1:1000 in fresh flask. Thus, every transfer processes ~10 generations in each design. The only difference between the two designs is the population size that cells are grown.

   After evolution for 1,000 generations, in which design,

   a. would drift be stronger?
   b. would adaptation be faster?
   c. will the population have greater fitness?
   d. would a greater number of mutations fixed?

   Sketch the adaptive trajectories (fitness versus number of generations) for the two designs on the same graph.
5. How does your answer compare with the quantitative answer obtained for these population sizes if we were to use the analysis in Chapter 9 to estimate adaptation rates?

BIBLIOGRAPHY

1. Daniel L, Halligan PDK. 2009. Spontaneous Mutation Accumulation Studies in Evolutionary Genetics. *Annu. Rev. Ecol. Evol. Syst.* 40:151–72.
   (An excellent, comprehensive summary of mutation accumulation experiments and lessons from them.)
2. Katju V, Bergthorsson U. 2019. Old Trade, New Tricks: Insights into the Spontaneous Mutation Process from the Partnering of Classical Mutation Accumulation Experiments with High-Throughput Genomic Approaches. *Genome Biol Evol* 11:136–165.
   (An interesting article combining mutation accumulation with genomics.)
3. Mahilkar A, Raj N, Kemkar S, Saini S. 2022. Selection in a growing colony biases results of mutation accumulation experiments. *Sci Rep* 12:15470.
4. Wahl LM, Agashe D. 2022. Selection bias in mutation accumulation. *Evolution* 76:528–540.
   (The above two papers show that mutation accumulation experiments with microbes are not without the effect of selection. The two papers quantify how much selection biases results in an MA experiment via theory and experiments.)

13 Lessons from Evolution Experiments
The Long-Term Evolution Experiment (LTEE)

13.1 INTRODUCTION

In 1988, the celebrated paleontologist Stephen Jay Gould asked a rhetorical question: if the history of our planet Earth were repeated from its birth ~4.5 billion years ago, would the trajectory of life on Earth be the same as what we see around us? That is, would biped species like us be the dominant species on the planet, or would life's trajectory on the planet take a completely alternate path? In this second scenario, what kind of organism would be on the planet?

What Gould meant to ask through this question is to what extent is evolution a process which is driven by only selection (in which case evolutionary outcomes may be to a large extent deterministic) and to what extent is this process driven by chance events (in which case evolutionary trajectories can be very different in separate independent runs of an experiment). For example, 65 million years ago as asteroid collided with Earth. This collision led to extinction of dinosaurs on the planet. If the asteroid had not collided with the planet, would the evolutionary trajectory of the planet have been the same?

The question regarding the relative roles of chance and determinism in evolution has been a major debating point since Gould formulated his rhetorical question.

The same year, a microbiologist, Richard Lenski, started the following experiment in California. Lenski was interested in studying adaptation of *E. coli* in environments with limited carbon (supplied in the form of glucose). Hence, he grew *E. coli* in a flask containing salts, glucose, and (a lot of) citrate. *E. coli* in presence of oxygen cannot utilize citrate for growth (*E. coli* can utilize citrate in anaerobic conditions). In fact, this phenotype is a clinical identifier of *E. coli* as a species (see Note I for details of why Lenski added citrate to the recipe of the liquid media to start the experiment). To study *E. coli*'s adaptation in this environment, Lenski used the serial sub-culture method for propagating generations.

However, Lenski made one interesting addition to this experimental design. Instead of starting only one culture flask, he started 12 flasks (each identical in the media composition) and each seeded with an isogenic bacterial population.

The 12 flasks can be thought of as 12 independent Earths that Gould was referring to, and studying the convergence or lack of convergence in the evolutionary path of

DOI: 10.1201/9781003633662-13

the 12 flasks can provide insights into the relative roles of chance and determinism in evolutionary processes.

The experiment that Lenski started continues till date. Lenski retired from Michigan State University (where he moved to in the early 1990s) and after his retirement, the experiment moved to University of Texas in the summer of 2022.

Overall, the experiment has processed ~80000 generations, and is referred to as the 'long-term evolutionary experiment' (LTEE). Because of the length of the experiment, the LTEE has become an invaluable source in understanding evolutionary processes. In this chapter, we will discuss the experiment and some major results and insights that have been drawn from this work. LTEE has led to a more than 100 research publications, and we will, in this chapter, only scrape the surface. I share some of the more interesting outcomes from the LTEE in the section 'Further Readings' in this chapter.

13.2 LTEE'S EXPERIMENTAL DESIGN

The LTEE was designed in the following manner. *E. coli* ancestor was introduced in 12 flasks, each containing identical media composition (Figure 13.1). The characteristic of the media composition is that carbon is supplied in the form of glucose and is limiting in nature. Moreover, the flasks have citrate in the media. The cells are allowed to grow overnight, under vigorous shaking (to maintain supply of oxygen) at a temperature of 37°C. After growth for 24 hours, 1/100 of the volume is taken from the flask, and transferred to a new flask containing unspent media. A 1:100 dilution every 24 hours corresponds to 6.67 $[= \ln(100)]$ generations per day. Thus, a 75,000 generation experiment means that the cultures in the 12 flasks have been transferred >11000 times in the last 36 years.

In this chapter, we will discuss the major lessons from such a long-term evolutionary experiment and how they have enhanced our understanding of evolution as a process.

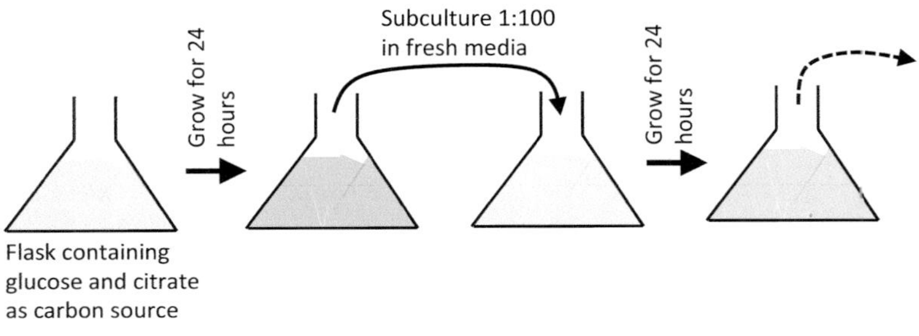

FIGURE 13.1 LTEE design. Each flask contains 25 mg/l glucose as the sole carbon source for *E. coli*, and grown in aerobic conditions at 37°C for 24 hours before being transferred to a fresh flask. In addition, each flask also contains citrate. However, *E. coli* does not utilize citrate in aerobic conditions.

13.3 PHENOMENOLOGY OF ADAPTATION IN LTEE

13.3.1 Rate of Adaptation Slows Down

One of the first results from the LTEE was that the rate of adaptation (the rate at which fitness increases) slows down with increasing generations. In the initial phase of adaptation, fitness increase can be modeled as more or less a linear increase with the number of generations. However, the slope of this curve decreases as more generations are processed (Figure 13.2). This phenomenon has been observed in many evolution experiments performed with a range of organisms in a variety of experimental contexts.

Before moving ahead,

➔ Does this agree with your intuition of how fitness should change with number of generations?

Before moving ahead,

➔ Why should the rate of adaptation decrease? Do beneficial mutations 'dry up', or do beneficial mutations confer a higher fitness advantage in an individual with lower fitness as compared to the benefit conferred by the same mutation in an individual with higher fitness?

13.3.2 Do Fitness Landscapes Have a Single Peak or Are They Multi-peaked Structures?

Imagine a fitness landscape with a single peak (Figure 13.3A). From the same starting point (12 identical flasks), it is likely that each flask will take an independent path to the landscape peak. Moreover, each trajectory will be associated with its unique speed and path at which it moves along the landscape. This is because the

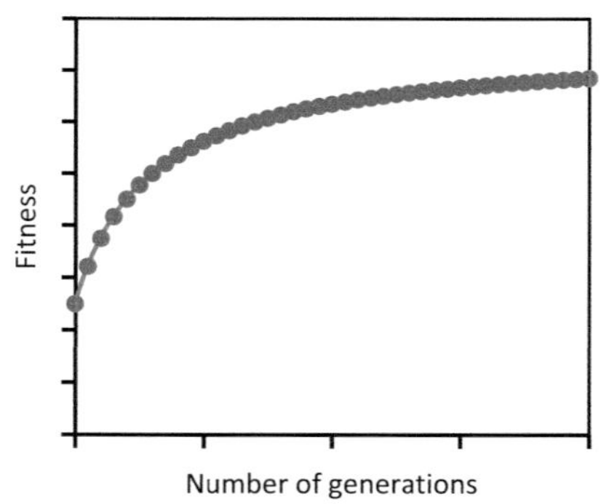

FIGURE 13.2 Rate of increase of fitness in an adaptive experiment decreases with the number of generations. Upon the start of the experiment, the fitness increases at a certain pace, as can be calculated from the slope of the curve in the figure. However, as the number of generations increase, the rate of adaptation decreases with time.

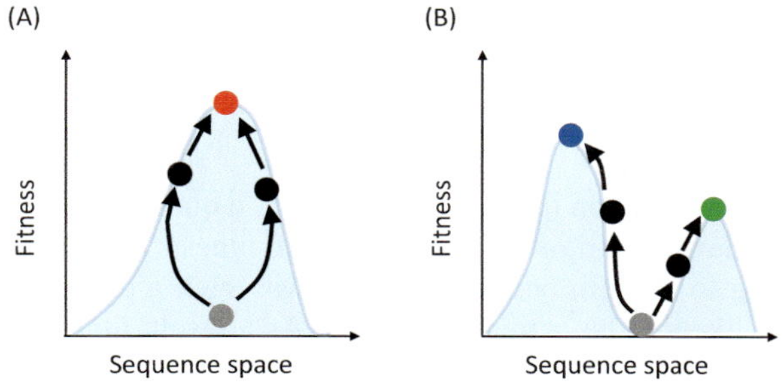

FIGURE 13.3 The structure of the fitness landscape dictates evolutionary trajectories. (A) If the landscape is a single-peaked structure, then every evolutionary trajectory starting from the same point (gray circle) on the sequence space moves toward the same peak (red circle). (B) If the landscape is a multiple-peaked structure, then different trajectories starting from the same point (gray circle) on the sequence space can lead to different peaks on the landscape (blue, or green). In this scenario, the first mutation from the starting point dictates which of the two peaks the trajectory moves toward. Note that in (A) both trajectories move toward the red peak. Hence, as all independent trajectories move toward the red peak, the variance of the fitness of the lines goes to zero. On the other hand, in (B), half the trajectories move to the blue peak, and the other half move toward the green peak. Hence, at steady state, the variance of fitness of all lines is non-zero.

waiting time associated with a beneficial mutation reaching fixation in each flask will be a stochastic process. Also, the fitness benefit conferred by beneficial mutations in each flask will, in general, be unique. As a result, the speed at and path via which any trajectory moves up the fitness landscape will be unique. However, in this view of evolution, all trajectories will eventually move toward the same peak.

How would we observe this in an experiment?

Note that as the 12 populations start from the same point on the fitness landscape, their starting fitness is identical. Hence, the variance in the fitness in the population is zero. As they evolve toward the peak via their respective paths, at a given point in time, their fitness varies, and variance increases to a non-zero number. However, given more time, the trajectories all converge toward the peak, and the fitness of the 12 lines approaches the same value. As a result, the variance between the fitness values of each trajectory will decrease with time.

Thus, this model predicts that if the 12 trajectories move on a single-peaked landscape, the variance in the fitness values of the 12 lines will first increase with time. However, as time moves forward, the variance between the lines' fitness will decrease.

On the other hand, if a fitness landscape has a structure with multiple peaks, each of different height (Figure 13.3B), an alternate scenario plays out. In this case, different trajectories may move toward different peaks. And once a trajectory reaches a peak, it remains there.

Hence, this model predicts that as the 12 lines are allowed to evolve, the variance in their fitness levels will increase with time, as they start from identical fitness. As the lines reach fitness peaks, the variance stabilizes to a constant value.

Before moving ahead,

➔ Take a pause here and think about which of the two predictions (or is there a third way?) agrees more with your intuition of how populations move on a fitness landscape.

Historically, movement on fitness landscapes was a question of a great intellectual debate between Sewall Wright (the proposer of fitness landscapes) and Ronald Fisher. According to Wright, because epistasis was such a pervasive phenomenon, landscapes were likely to be extremely rugged. As a result, fitness landscapes were likely to be multi-peaked structures. In fact, for Wright, the whole question of explaining evolutionary processes was equivalent to explaining how populations move from one peak to another. In other words, for Wright, the question of adaptation of a population boiled down to the following: a population evolves to reach a fitness peak. From there, selection does not permit the population to move down, and hence, while there may be higher fitness peaks available on the landscape, they are not accessible to the population stuck in a local maxima. How does a population stuck in a local maxima get out of it? Thus, as far as Wright was concerned, of the two predictions above, the second one makes more sense.

Fisher, on the other hand, argued that while it is true that epistasis was a pervasive phenomenon, it was also true that real fitness landscapes have a dimensionality of thousands (unlike three-dimensional structures represented on this piece of paper). This meant that for a point in the sequence space to be a peak, it would have to be a fitness maximum among its immediate neighbors in all 1,000 dimensions. According to Fisher, the probability of this event was quite unlikely. He imagined that given any point, there must be at least one dimension in which the population could move and increase in fitness. Hence, natural selection alone would ensure that the population keeps increasing in fitness and reaches the global fitness peak. There was no need to invoke any other evolutionary force to explain evolution. Fisher, in our debate, would argue that all 12 lines would move to the same fitness peak.

Before moving ahead,

➔ Do the arguments by Fisher and Wright change your intuitive answer above?

13.3.3 Do Fitness Landscapes Have a Peak?

The *E. coli* genome is ~5×10^6 bases long. This means that there are $4^{(5 \times 10^{\wedge}6)}$ unique sequences of this length possible. Since each of these sequences can be attributed a fitness number, one (or more) of the sequences must exhibit the highest fitness level. Hence, a fitness landscape must have a fitness peak. And hence, a population must be able to reach this fitness peak. Hence, populations evolving on a landscape must stop adaptation as they reach the peak.

Can this phenomenon be observed in experimental populations? The LTEE sought to answer this question.

As discussed in **I** above, the rate of adaptation slows down with the number of generations. This trend was observed after evolution for a few thousand generations in the LTEE. After 20,000 generations, however, the authors fit the fitness data with two distinct mathematical functions. In the first one,

$$\text{fitness after } g \text{ generations, } F(g) = \frac{a.g}{b+g} \tag{13.1}$$

where a and b are constants and g is the number of generations. The authors then determined a and b, which best fit the experimental data. The agreement between the experimental data and the model was found to be excellent.

Note that in this model, fitness can never exceed a, no matter how long the evolution experiment proceeds. Thus, agreement with the above equation suggests that landscapes do indeed have a fitness peak, and adaptation, eventually, would halt. The model also suggests that fitness will never be equal to a. That is, it will keep getting increasingly closer to a, but never actually be equal to a.

Lenski and his team, however, fit another model to test adaptive speed with the number of generations. In this formulation, they proposed the following equation relating fitness to the number of generations,

$$\text{fitness after } g \text{ generations, } F(g) = (1 + a.g)^b \tag{13.2}$$

Here too, a and b are constants, and g is the number of generations. The values of the constants were determined so that the model is best able to explain the experimental data. This model's agreement with the experimental data was also found to be excellent.

Note, however, that the second model is fundamentally different from the first model above. While the first model has a horizontal asymptote (i.e., fitness can never exceed a), the second model has no such maxima. For all positive values of parameters a and b, fitness continues to increase indefinitely.

Since both the models agreed with the experimental data for the first 20,000 generations equally well, the performance of the two models could not be differentiated. How, then, can the two models be compared to ask the question if fitness landscapes have a peak or not?

The authors used the two models to predict the evolutionary trajectory for the next 20,000 generations (i.e., from generation 20,001 to 40,000). Remember that the models were constructed with the fitness data from generations 0 to 20000. The predictions for generations 20001–40000 from the two models were then compared with the actual experimental data for evolved strains from the generations 20001 to 40000. And this comparison would tell us which of the two models better *predicts* the evolutionary trajectory of the population.

Before moving ahead,

➔ which of the two models do you think predicted the evolutionary trajectory from generations 20,001 to 40,000 better?

When Lenski and his team compared the experimental data for the next 20,000 generations with the predictions from the two models, they found that the second model (in Equation 13.2) was a better predictor of the evolutionary trajectory, as compared to the first one.

This is perhaps surprising. That the second model predicts that there does not exist a fitness maxima for an evolving population. This seems an unrealistic (or even unbelievable!) feature of the model. How do we reconcile the fact that the second model was a better predictor with the intuition that landscapes must have fitness peaks?

We should first note that, in the second model, even if the fitness trajectory does not have a maxima in the second model, the rate of increase of fitness decreases continuously. The slowdown in the speed of adaptation is to an extent that the second model predicts that after evolution in the carbon-limiting media for 2.5 billion generations (!), the evolved strain will divide every ~6 minutes or so.

To get a better intuition of this prediction, the model predicts that this fitness level is achieved if the evolution experiment were to be continued for another 350 million years! While it is impossible to think about or predict evolution experiments of that length of time, it certainly does not appear inconceivable to me that 350 million years of evolution would lead to such fitness values. Thus, model in Equation (13.2) seems acceptable for not only short durations of evolution (a few thousand generations), but also for a much longer duration of hundreds of millions of years.

Would it play out in a fashion represented by Equation (13.2) or not is anyone's guess. In fact, one of the challenges of evolutionary biology is development of models which connect microevolution (short-term) with the longer-term macroevolution patterns.

In a shorter time frame, the two models differ in the sense that the first model predicts a slower rate of adaptation, when compared to the second one. The lesson for us here is the evolution finds a way! When cells are posed with a challenge in their environment – some mutations facilitate adaptation which enables cells to overcome the challenge and increase fitness.

13.3.4 Role of History, Selection, and Chance in Dictating Evolution

Evolutionary trajectories are dictated by selection, drift, and also on the evolutionary history of the population. How do we decouple the relative roles of these three variables? In 1995, in a paper published in *Science*, a simple, elegant experiment was reported which enabled this decoupling.

Imagine a population with a certain trait value (e.g., division time in glucose) adapt to another carbon environment, say galactose. After adaptation to galactose for g generations, the growth rate in a galactose environment increases. However, what if instead of one line, we started off a dozen independent lines to adapt to galactose, all starting with the identical isogenic ancestor? Would we expect that all 12 lines exhibit identical growth rates, after g generations in galactose?

As shown in the Figure 13.4, several possibilities exist. In the first, after the period of adaptation, all 12 lines exhibit identical growth rates in galactose. In such a scenario, the evolutionary fate of the populations is completely dictated by selection and randomness (or drift) does not play any role in the evolutionary process.

Alternatively, all 12 lines could exhibit an increase in the growth rate in galactose, but this increased growth rate was non-identical. Some of the 12 lines exhibited a higher growth rate, as compared to the other. In other words, selection played a role

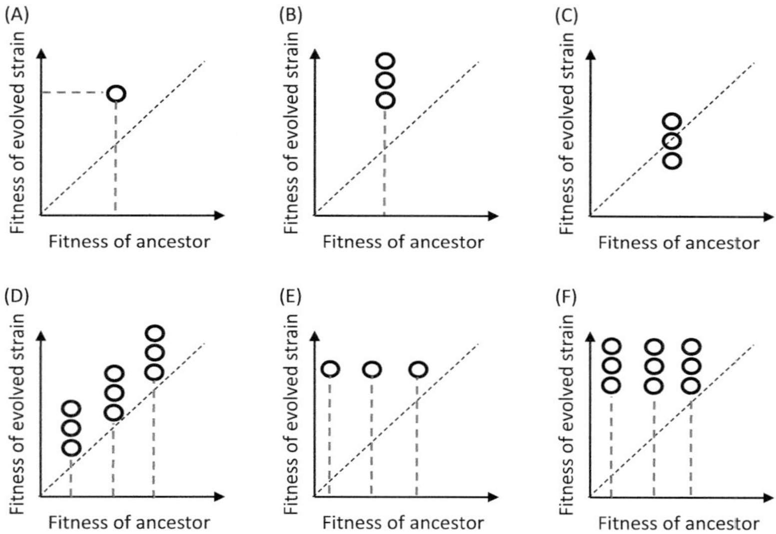

FIGURE 13.4 Decoupling the role of selection, chance, and history in an evolutionary process. (A–C) Imagine three lines of isogenic *E. coli* evolved in glucose for *g* generations. After the period of adaptation, the fitness of the three lines on another carbon source (galactose) is measured. This fitness is compared with the fitness of ancestor in galactose. (A) The fitness of all three lines in galactose is identical and higher than that of the ancestor in glucose. In such a case, selection has shaped the evolutionary process. (B) In comparison with (A), the fitness of the three evolved lines is higher than that of the ancestor, but not equal to each other. In this case, the increase is due to selection. However, the difference in fitness between lines is because of chance. (C) In this case, the fitness of the evolved lines is centered at the same value as the ancestor. Randomness (chance) leads to deviations of fitness around the ancestral fitness levels. Thus, in this case, selection plays no role. (D–F) To decouple the role of history on adaptation, the evolution experiment for *g* generations is started from three different starting genotypes, each with different fitness in galactose. After adaptation for *g* generations, the fitness of evolved lines (3 × 3) is measured in galactose. (D) Selection, chance, and history dictate adaptation in galactose. This is so since strains with higher initial fitness in galactose lead to higher galactose fitness after *g* generations. (E) Only selection plays a role in evolution. (F) Selection and chance play a role in evolution.

which led to an overall increase in the growth rate of the 12 lines. However, along with selection, drift or randomness in the evolutionary process meant that the response of the 12 lines was not identical. Thus, evolutionary fate was decided as a result of both, selection and drift. By comparing the increase in fitness in galactose of the 12 lines (evolutionary response due to selection) with the variance in the fitness values of the 12 lines (evolutionary response due to drift), we can decouple the roles of selection and drift in dictating evolutionary processes.

To understand the role of history in dictating evolution, a slightly different approach has to be undertaken. We first need to create populations which have undergone different evolutionary histories. To understand this, imagine three populations of *E. coli*, all starting from the same ancestor, which are evolved in glucose for g, $2g$, and $3g$ number of generations, respectively. After the period of adaptation, the fitness of the three populations in glucose is quantified, and represented as shown in the figure below. Consistent with our intuition, the population which evolved in glucose for the longest time ($3g$ number of generations) has the highest fitness in glucose. These three populations form our three ancestor populations which have undergone three distinct historical evolutionary paths. Starting from each of the three ancestors, we start 12 lines to evolve in galactose for g number of generations. In such a scenario, two outcomes are possible.

In the first, the qualitative spread of the fitness of the 12 lines from each of the three ancestors is similar to each other. In such a case, the differences in the evolutionary history of the three ancestors played no part in dictating the evolutionary fate of the populations in galactose. However, alternatively, we might note that the fitness in galactose is dependent on the fitness of the starting ancestor (see Figure 13.4). In this scenario, the adaptive response of the population to galactose is closely linked with the fitness (or evolutionary history) of the ancestor population. Thus, evolutionary response is closely linked with the history of the adapting population.

13.4 GENETIC BASIS OF ADAPTATION

One of the key phenotypic observations from the LTEE was that there was a striking resemblance in the fitness trajectory of the 12 lines. After evolution for g generations, cells from any two lines exhibit remarkable convergence as far as their fitness levels are concerned. This leads us to the question of whether this phenotypic convergence is a result of genetic convergence in the 12 independent lines. In other words, are the fitness changes in the 12 lines occurring because of mutations in the same genes? Or, how similar or dissimilar are the mutations facilitating adaptation in the 12 lines? These questions can be summarized in the following two,

a. Does phenotypic parallelism between the 12 lines of the LTEE extend to genetic parallelism? If so, to what level does the parallelism extend – pathway, gene, or nucleotide?
b. Is most of the change occurring neutral or adaptive?

The first step toward answering this question is to sequence the genome of the ancestral *E. coli*. This sequence provides us with a reference to compare the genome of the evolved lines from the LTEE. In early work that was published in this direction, in 2009, the LTEE team of researchers published the list of mutations that had occurred in the first 20,000 generations of the experiment.

Before moving ahead,

➔ What is your intuition about the number of mutations that occur in a serial transfer experiment, such as LTEE, in 20,000 generations? (handful of mutations/few dozen/hundreds).

What was found was that after 20,000 generations, one of the lines had 29 point mutations (where a single nucleotide had changed), 15 insertions-deletions (indels),

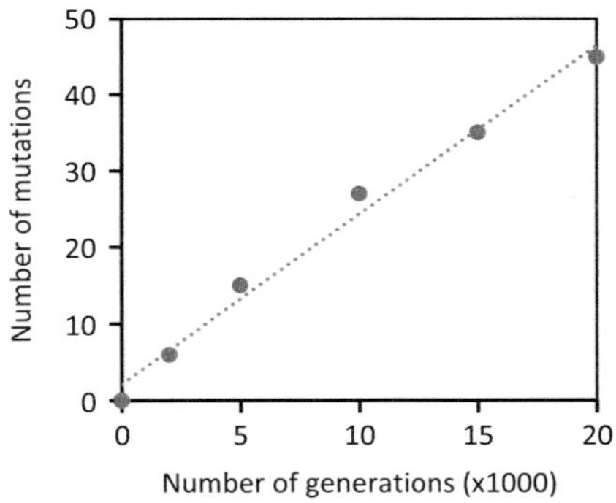

FIGURE 13.5 Number of mutations in the LTEE as a function of number of generations. Data from Reference 8.

and one inversion of the region of the chromosome. In all, after 20,000 generations, this strain had 45 mutations accumulated in its genome.

One of the striking features of this adaptive trajectory is how constant the rate of genomic evolution is. The number of mutations versus the number of generations is shown in Figure 13.5. We learned in the chapter on Neutral Theory that a constant rate of accumulation of mutations is a signature of neutral evolution, or drift. This is usually not the expectation from Darwinian adaptation. However, we also know that the fitness of these strains was increasing with the number of generations (see Figure 13.2). So, we know that at least some of these mutations are adaptive in nature.

Of the 45 changes that had occurred in the genome of the bacteria, there were 22 mutations which occurred in the coding sequence of genes. Sequencing revealed that all 22 changes were non-synonymous in nature. That is, all 22 changed lead to a change in an amino acid in the protein sequence. We learned in the chapter on neutral theory that non-synonymous changes are highly likely to be adaptive, while synonymous mutations are more likely to be neutral. The fact that none of the changes were synonymous is a strong indicator that the mutations that occurred were adaptive in nature.

Another strong indication that the mutations occurring were adaptive in nature came from the following. When 14 genes which had acquired mutations in one line were sequenced in the remaining 11 lines, the following was observed,

a. Three genes had mutations in all other 11 lines,
b. Nine genes had mutations in *at least* two more lines,
c. Only two genes had mutations in only the one line.

If mutations were occurring because of drift only, we would not expect such remarkable convergence in where these mutations occurred.

After 30,000 generations, one of the 12 lines evolved the ability to utilize citrate. As we mentioned, citrate was added to the culture media at the start of the experiment. However, *E. coli* under oxic conditions cannot utilize citrate as a carbon source. This change was readily noticed in the LTEE – because the line utilizing citrate had access to much more carbon than the others, which were growing on glucose only. As a result, this line grew to much higher density as compared to the others.

Interestingly, even though the cells in the population had the ability to utilize citrate, they did not drive to extinction the cells that could not utilize citrate.

Before moving ahead,

➔ Why should this be so?

The fact that the two genotypes (citrate utilizers and the non-citrate utilizers) coexist should tell us that the ability to utilize citrate must have come at a cost of compromised ability to utilize glucose. As a result, while the evolving strain grew to become better at utilizing glucose, the citrate utilizing mutation must have severely compromised the ability of the bacterium to utilize glucose. As a result, the two genotypes coexist in the population. The citrate utilizer primarily growing on citrate, and the ancestor evolving strain growing on glucose.

When tested, the LTEE team found that this coexistence comes from the fact that when the citrate utilizing strain was shifted to glucose, the transition time (lag phase) of switching from citrate to glucose was extremely long. As a result, in this time, the ancestral evolving individuals, which did not have this novel trait, grew on glucose – leading to coexistence of the two strains.

13.5 EVOLUTION OF NOVELTY IN LTEE

At about 30,000 generations into the experiment, one of the 12 lines evolved a striking feature. Remember that the growth media for *E. coli* in this experiment contained glucose as well as some citrate. One of the diagnostic features of *E. coli* is that it cannot utilize citrate in the presence of oxygen. Hence, in all 12 lines, *E. coli* was unable to utilize citrate for growth. Until about 30,000 generations, when one of the 12 lines started using citrate (in addition to glucose) for growth and energy.

This was discovered because after every 24 hours of growth, at the time of subculture, the research team is accustomed to a certain density of the culture media. This density corresponded to growth on glucose. However, when this one line started using citrate, it grew to a much higher density. This difference in density was easily seen by the naked eye. Clearly something weird was going on in that flask.

The usual suspect in cases like this is that there must have been some contamination in the flask because of which an external bacteria sneaked in, and was growing alongside the *E. coli* that was added to the flask. However, as the research team tested this possibility, they found out that the sole occupant of the flask was the bacteria that they added to the media.

How then did the bacteria in this flask evolve to utilize citrate? More intriguingly, how is it that this ability only evolved in one flask, and in none of the other 11. Interestingly, even after another 50,000 generations of evolution, bacteria in none of the other flasks have evolved the ability to utilize citrate. What is going on?

To explain this, the researchers tested two competing hypotheses.

Hypothesis I. Maybe it was an extremely rare mutation to have happened which facilitated this transition from lack of citrate utilizing capacity to being able to utilize citrate. This extremely rare mutation could be an inversion of a very specific region of DNA, for instance.

In such a case if all lines were evolved again, then any of these lines could get the lucky mutation and, hence, evolve ability to use citrate.

Or,

Hypothesis II. Alternatively, this particular line acquired a series of mutations leading up to 30,000 generations, such that it was primed to utilize citrate via one more mutation. And when this final mutation was acquired, citrate utilization started. And since the identity of mutations in all lines is different, no other line was able to utilize citrate.

In such a case, if all lines were evolved again, from say 27,000 generations, only this line would evolve the ability to utilize citrate. This is referred to as historical contingency in evolution.

Before moving ahead,

➔ Which of the two hypotheses do you think successfully explained the phenotype of citrate utilization?

So, all 12 lines were evolved from generation 20,000 again (remember this is easy to do, since the cells are stored in a deep freezer). After testing about 40 trillion cell divisions, the team found that none of the other 11 lines evolved to utilize citrate. On the other hand, in the line where citrate evolution did take place, the same phenotype evolved 19 times independently.

This clearly established that it was Hypothesis II which was driving the evolution of citrate utilization in *E. coli* in oxic conditions.

Sequencing results then demonstrated that the mutations responsible for this phenotype were a rare duplication of a specific part of the genome followed by point mutations. And hence, this ability has evolved only once in the LTEE to date.

13.6 CONCLUSION

Since its inception, LTEE has gone through several phases. Lenski describes that seeking funding to run the experiment was not easy in the initial years. Then, there was a phase when he was seriously thinking of abandoning the experiment since nothing 'exciting' was happening in it. But that all changed with the evolution of citrate utilization, and that too, in only one line. This goes to show that while adaptation is parallel and the improvement in fitness is nearly identical in all lines, evolution also has surprises in store for us. Today, LTEE has become an institution in itself. Post-Lenski's retirement, the experiment has moved to Jeffrey Barrick's laboratory in Texas, US. It is not quite clear what all surprises LTEE will keep throwing at us in the years, decades to come.

NOTES

NOTE I

A large number of practices in microbiology are a result of accidents. Lenski adding citrate to the starting media is one example of this phenomenon. In the earlier days of microbiology, the supply of clean water to make culture media was a big challenge. The variability of nutrients, salts, and impurities in the water supply would make the growth dynamics of bacterial growth vary from one batch of growth media to another. As a result, the analysis of results was difficult. A potential solution to reduce variation between different batches of growth was adding citrate to the media. Citrate, being a good chelating agent, binds to ions (like, Fe^{2+}) and makes supply more uniform. Today, with exquisite control of the water supply in research labs, repeatability of growth kinetics is no longer a concern. However, when Lenski started this experiment, this issue was very relevant. As we will see in the chapter, addition of citrate lead to one of the most surprising results of the evolution experiment.

EXERCISES

1. Give reasons why the experiment done to determine whether fitness landscapes were single or multi-peaked was not an inappropriate experiment to answer that particular question.
2. As LTEE is progressed, cells have evolved to grow faster. What do you think has happened to the cell size during this process? Are the evolved faster-growing cells larger, smaller, or the same size as the ancestor the experiment was started with? Why should this change (if any) take place?
3. Some of the lines of LTEE have evolved to increase their mutation rate, μ, by several fold. Can an increase in mutation rate be an adaptive strategy? If so, how?
4. How would you check if there has been a contamination in the evolution experiment you are performing? List all methods, techniques you would use to confirm this.

BIBLIOGRAPHY

LTEE is a long-standing experiment and has many facets to it. The number of publications arising from the experiment exceeds 100. Covering the papers from the experiment would be several books! Below, I list seven papers which are insightful, interesting, and give us thoughts about evolution to wonder about.

1. Arjan JA, Visser M, Zeyl CW, Gerrish PJ, Blanchard JL, Lenski RE. 1999. Diminishing returns from mutation supply rate in asexual populations. *Science* 283:404–6.
2. Blount ZD, Borland CZ, Lenski RE. 2008. Historical contingency and the evolution of a key innovation in an experimental population of Escherichia coli. *Proc Natl Acad Sci U S A* 105:7899–906.
3. Lenski RE, Travisano M. 1994. Dynamics of adaptation and diversification: a 10,000-generation experiment with bacterial populations. *Proc Natl Acad Sci U S A* 91:6808–14.
4. Maddamsetti R, Hatcher PJ, Green AG, Williams BL, Marks DS, Lenski RE. 2017. Core Genes Evolve Rapidly in the Long-Term Evolution Experiment with Escherichia coli. *Genome Biol Evol* 9:1072–83.

5. Sniegowski PD, Gerrish PJ, Lenski RE. 1997. Evolution of high mutation rates in experimental populations of E. *coli. Nature* 387:703–5.
6. Stanek MT, Cooper TF, Lenski RE. 2009. Identification and dynamics of a beneficial mutation in a long-term evolution experiment with Escherichia coli. *BMC Evol Biol* 9:302.
7. Travisano M, Mongold JA, Bennett AF, Lenski RE. 1995. Experimental tests of the roles of adaptation, chance, and history in evolution. *Science* 267:87–90.
8. Wiser MJ, Ribeck N, Lenski RE. 2013. Long-Term Dynamics of Adaptation in Asexual Populations. *Science* 342:1364–7.

   (See this paper for declining rate of adaptation for the first 50,000 generations of the experiment.)
9. Barrick JE, Yu DS, Yoon SH, Jeong H, Oh TK, Schneider D, Lenski RE, Kim JF. 2009. Genome evolution and adaptation in a long-term experiment with Escherichia coli. *Nature* 416: 1243–47.

   (Data for Figure 13.5 is from this paper.)
10. Blount ZD, Borland CZ, Lenski RE. 2008. Historical contingency and the evolution of a key innovation in an experimental population of Escherichia coli. *Proc Natl Acad Sci USA* 105(23):7899–906.
11. Blount ZD, Barrick JE, Davidson CJ, Lenski RE. 2012. Genomic analysis of a key innovation in an experimental Escherichia coli population. *Nature* 489(7417):513–518.

   (The above two references give details of the citrate utilization evolution in *E. coli*. The 2008 paper describes the phenotypic observation, and the 2012 paper describes the molecular details driving this phenotype.)

14 Lessons from Evolution Experiments

14.1 INTRODUCTION

In this chapter, we will discuss a few experimental evolution studies of interest. Experimental evolution in controlled laboratory studies has a rich tradition of more than a hundred years. In the last two chapters, we have seen the longest-running (in terms of number of generations) evolution experiment with *E. coli*. We saw that while the experiment is extremely simple (growing and sub-culturing *E. coli* in glucose-limited environments), the experiment during its run in the last ~35 years has led to several interesting results, and has enhanced our understanding of evolutionary processes significantly.

However, in one sense, LTEE is also a very simple and very limited experiment. The researchers started growing *E. coli* on low-glucose media, and recording its adaptive response. It's a simple question with a broad goal of 'lets see what happens'. This is also true for most evolution experiments. *Researchers evolve a population under a specific environment and report what happened under such conditions.* A large fraction of experimental evolution literature belongs to this category.

However, there is another type of experiment in evolutionary biology literature. These experiments are simple, clever, and designed with the broad aim of selecting for a particular phenotype. These experiments can be classified as asking the following: *what should be the evolution experiment if we want a particular trait to evolve in the population?* For example, in the first example we study in this chapter, the researchers ask the following question: yeast is unicellular. Under what environment should we evolve it so that it becomes multicellular?

Before moving ahead,

➔ How would you select for multicellularity, starting from a unicellular population?

What would you do? It's worth taking a pause here, and thinking about this question. What would be your experimental design that leads to evolution of multicellularity? To answer this question, we have to think of an experiment, where a property which is associated with multicellularity is selected, and is absent in unicellular organisms, is selected for. What would be that property? And once we identify this property, how would we design an evolution experiment to select for it? These are all key questions when it comes to design of lab evolution experiments.

It is quite impossible to do justice to the volume and diversity of these experimental studies. Our goal in this chapter is to discuss a few experiments that have been, in my opinion, creative and yet simple in their design, and have led to results

 DOI: 10.1201/9781003633662-14

which are of broad significance toward enhancing our understanding of how evolution proceeds.

Let us start with the first one.

14.2 EVOLUTION OF MULTICELLULARITY

Life evolved with single-celled prokaryotes – bacteria and archaea. This form of life continued for around two billion years, when the first eukaryote cell came into existence. The transition to eukaryotes was fundamental in how life forms evolved thereafter – eukaryotic cells could evolve to form multicellular entities.

If we think about it – there is a curious fact about the differences in how prokaryote and eukaryote cells have evolved. Prokaryotes have existed on the planet for nearly four billion years, almost twice as long as eukaryotes have existed for. However, prokaryotes never evolved to form multicellular organisms. Why would this be so? It appears there was a fundamental necessity for eukaryotic cells to evolve, before multicellular organisms could evolve.

Thus, while in terms of their biochemical capacities, prokaryotes are much more complex and diverse than eukaryotes; in terms of their morphological complexity, prokaryotes did not diversify like eukaryotes. For example, why did prokaryotic cells do not evolve to form multicellular organisms such as us? (Figure 14.1).

Multicellularity offers several advantages. It offers protection from predators because of increased size, allows compartmentalization (and hence cellular specialization), and offers faster settling in liquid pools. The origins of multicellularity are quite well understood, and it is known that multicellularity evolved more than two dozen times, independently.

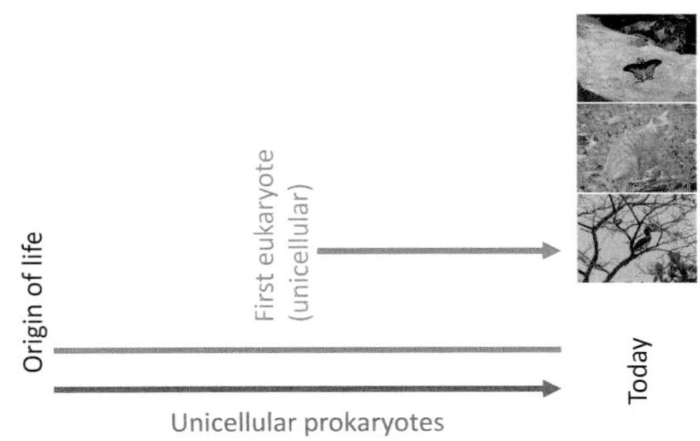

FIGURE 14.1 Evolution of multicellularity. Life evolved on earth around four billion years ago. This origin of life lead to bacteria and archaea occupying Earth's niches. Bacteria and archaea have existed for this time, but multicellularity did not evolve in these organisms. On the other hand, once eukaryotic cells evolved around two billion years ago, multicellularity evolved more than two dozen times independently in eukaryotic cells, and led to divergence of life into all the complex life forms we see around us. Why did eukaryotic cells need to evolve for evolution of multicellularity?

From the context of fitness, multicellular life meant a change in the objective function of what it meant to be of higher fitness. Remember that fitness is quantified as how many and how fast do I leave progeny for the next generation.

For single-celled organism, fitness equates to the ability to divide quickly. In a given environmental context, a variant which divides faster will outcompete its competition. Hence, faster growth rate equates to higher fitness.

However, fitness for complex multicellular organisms such as us means a completely different thing. If my cells divided as fast they could – it would likely result in me having cancer. In such a scenario, I will likely not survive to have kids – an opportunity to pass my genes to the next generation. Hence, fast-dividing cells mean that my fitness equals zero. The fitness of a complex multicellular organism is enhanced best when the constituent cells learn to cooperate, hold off untimely cell division, and give the organism the best possible chance of passing genes to the next generation.

Hence, multicellularity was a big transition in life forms on the planet.

Can we design an evolution experiment in lab, where we can observe a transition from single-cellular organism to a multicellular organism?

Such an experiment was conducted ~15 years ago. In this experiment, a yeast strain (a single-celled multicellular organism, also used in baking) was allowed to grow, while shaking in a flask containing glucose as the carbon environment. After a period of growth, the culture media was kept on a bench and the cells allowed to settle under gravity for a specified amount of time. After this period, only cells from the bottom of the flask were propagated to the next flask, for the process to be repeated over and over again.

Let us think carefully about what we expect to happen in this experiment. Only the cells which settle fast have a chance to be propagated to the next flask. Any cell which does not settle, or settles slowly, will be rejected from the experiment.

Before moving ahead,

➔ Thus, the question is what makes a cell settle faster? What do you think?

Yeast has two strategies available to settle faster. The first is flocculation. Several yeast strains produce cellular adhesins which allow cells to stick to each other. Cells sticking to each other will allow for faster settling of the cell aggregates. However, single cells sticking with each other do not equate to evolution of multicellularity.

Alternatively, what was actually observed in the experiment was that a single mutation lead to evolution of multicellularity in the culture media. As a result, the cells did not separate at the time of division. The lack of separation lead to larger cell aggregates which settle faster.

The single mutation that facilitated the transition from uni to multicellularity was found to be in a transcription factor, ACE2. The mutation leads to the cells not making ACE2 protein, which is responsible for controlling the expression of proteins which are responsible for the separation between mother and daughter cells, at the time of cell division. In cells which do not produce ACE2, the proteins necessary for mother-daughter cell separation are not produced, and as a result, multicellular aggregates are produced.

The multicellularity evolution experiment has now continued for more than 10,000 generations, and has led to several observations and insights of great importance. The most exciting among them is that as this experiment is propagated further and multicellular clusters continue to evolve, within a single cluster, we begin to see division of labor. That is, some cells in a cluster specialize to do one particular job, and others specialize to do another. For instance, cells near the center of the cluster have a gene expression profile which gives them greater rigidity and strength (as it helps them hold the cluster together), while those near the edges specialize in transporting nutrients from the surrounding media to inside the cluster (this is important because it is these cells which have the most access to the nutrients).

The progress made in understanding of evolution of multicellularity is reported in a recent book by William Ratcliff.

14.3 EVOLUTION OF BET-HEDGING

There is a famous problem in economics. Imagine you have Rs. 100/- to invest. You could invest money in a scheme which gives you a lower return, but is safe. Alternatively, you could also invest money in another scheme which offers higher return, but is risky in nature. By risk, we mean that there is a finite chance that all money invested in that scheme is lost.

Now, we have a choice to invest a fraction of money in the safe and low-returns scheme. Let us call the fraction of money invested in this scheme p. Then, it automatically means that we invest the remaining money in the high-returns but risky investment. This fraction will be $(1 - p)$ (see Figure 14.2).

The question we have at this point is: how should we divide the money between the two schemes so that our *long-term* returns are maximized?

It is obvious to see that if we invest all our money in the low-return and safe scheme, we will consistently get returns on all our money, but the return will be quite

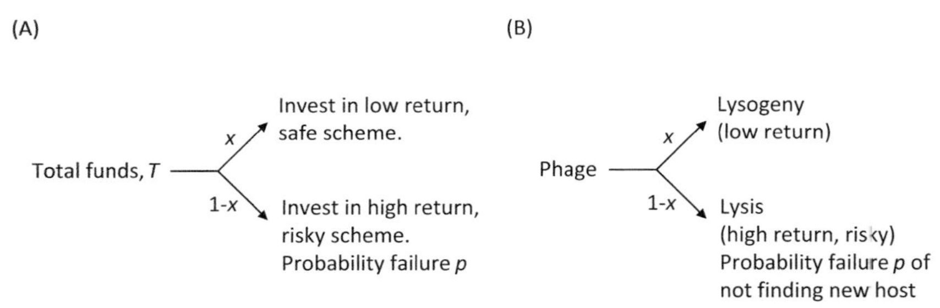

FIGURE 14.2 Bet-hedging in economics and biology have parallels. (A) Funds can be invested in two schemes. What fraction x should be invested in a safe and low return scheme and the remaining $(1 - x)$ in a risky and high return scheme that maximizes the long-term return? (B) A parallel exists in biological systems. Imagine a population of phage and *E. coli*. What should be the phage's strategy in terms of investing x toward lysogeny (safe, low return strategy) and $(1 - x)$ toward lysis (risky, high return strategy), which maximizes the phage numbers long term.

low. Alternatively, if we invest all the money in the high-risk scheme, the returns will be higher, but there is a chance that all the money we invest in that scheme will be lost. The optimal investment strategy is somewhere in between.

The optimal strategy takes into account 'bet-hedging' – that we split our investment of resources into two different strategies because each offers something desirable and something undesirable. The optimal strategy depends on p and also on the rates of return that we get from the two schemes.

Biological systems, too, exhibit bet-hedging.

Phage are viruses that infect bacteria. A phage called λ infects *E. coli*. Post-infection, the virus can follow one of two life cycles. The biological objective of the phage is to produce as many copies of its genetic material as possible.

The first is called 'lysogeny'. In this, the phage attaches its genome to the bacteria's and every time the bacteria divides, the phage DNA divides too. This is equivalent to the 'safe strategy' in the economics example. The bacteria provide a safe environment to the phage, and the phage's growth rate (or of its DNA) is at a slower pace (as the bacteria divides).

The second strategy (high return but risky) is called 'lysis'. In this, upon infection, the phage makes several dozen copies of itself inside the bacterium. The assembled phage particles are then released into the environment, while the host bacteria are killed in the process. Lysis is high return since each bacterium produces several dozen phage particles (called 'burst size') in a short time. This strategy is risky since if the newly released phage particles degrade in the environment, in case they may be unable to find a new host.

From the virus' perspective, what fraction of the phage particles should undergo lysis and what fraction undergo lysogeny for the maximization of the phage particles in the long run? Analysis has shown that several similarities exist between the economics/investment problem and the λ-phage *E. coli* problem! Viruses also hedge their bets and commit a fraction of their population to lysogeny and another to lysis.

More importantly, such bet-hedging behavior can be seen in a wide variety of contexts in microbial populations. It is important to note that the differential behavior (phenotype) is exhibited by an isogenic population. Lysis and lysogeny are exhibited by virus particles with identical genotypes. Think of bet-hedging as a strategy which a population employs to exhibit different phenotypes, despite not having genotypic diversity.

Imagine if all virus particles were lytic. Then, the progeny so produced have to find a new host in a relatively short amount of time. In a scenario where the bacterial population goes extinct because of lysis, the newly formed virus particles will degrade in the environment, and the virus population go extinct. Thus, committing fully to lysis is not a smart strategy. Conversely, if the entire population commits to lysogeny, then growth of virus particles is contingent on bacterial growth, which is slow. Hence, it would make sense to commit some fraction of the population to lysis to speed up the growth of the virus particles.

From the context of design of laboratory evolution experiments, we are interested in learning whether bet-hedging can be evolved in a population? This was a question asked in a beautiful paper published in *Nature* in 2009. For this evolution experiment, the authors chose the bacterium *Pseudomonas*.

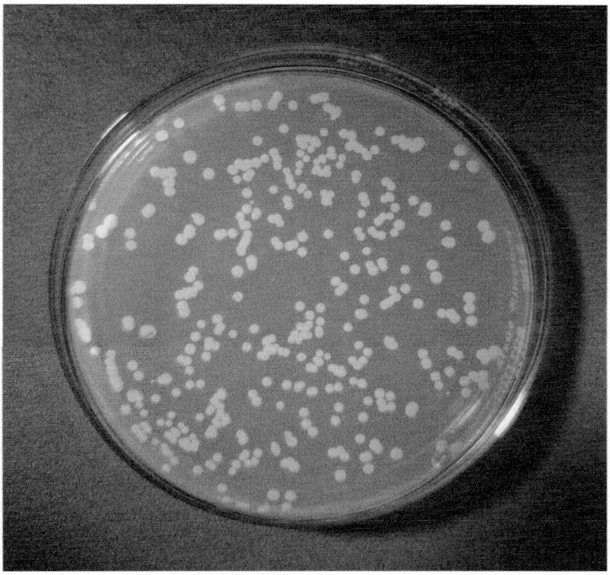

FIGURE 14.3 Colonies on a plate. The figure shows colony (each circle) of yeast *Saccharomyces cerevisiae* after growth at 30°C on rich YPD media for 48 hours. Note that each colony arose from a single cell which was spread on the plate. At the time of spreading, we did not know where each cell was being placed and hence, we cannot know the location of where a colony is going to come up.

In a common microbiology technique, ~100 bacteria are spread on an agar plate. After spreading, this plate is then kept in an incubator to allow for bacteria to divide. Typically, after overnight growth, the cells have divided to an extent that the collective mass is visible as a little mound. In microbiology, this mound is referred to as a 'colony'. Thus, a plate which had 100 bacteria spread will have 100 colonies the following morning. A typical plate is as shown in Figure 14.3.

Before moving ahead,

➔ How would you go about designing an experiment where bet-hedging evolves in a population?

The idea behind the experiment is that given a population's phenotype, we are looking for a characteristic that a part of the population exhibits another manifestation of the phenotype. What should the phenotype be? In the experiment, the research team chooses a simple phenotype: appearance of a colony on the plate.

In the experiment, the authors spread 100 or so bacteria on a plate and allowed colonies to form. Since all bacteria were isogenic, the colonies should all contain bacteria with identical DNA. However, individuals with isogenic DNA can also exhibit different phenotypic states (like, some members of λ phage exhibiting lysogeny, and others exhibiting lysis). From the hundred colonies on the plate, the

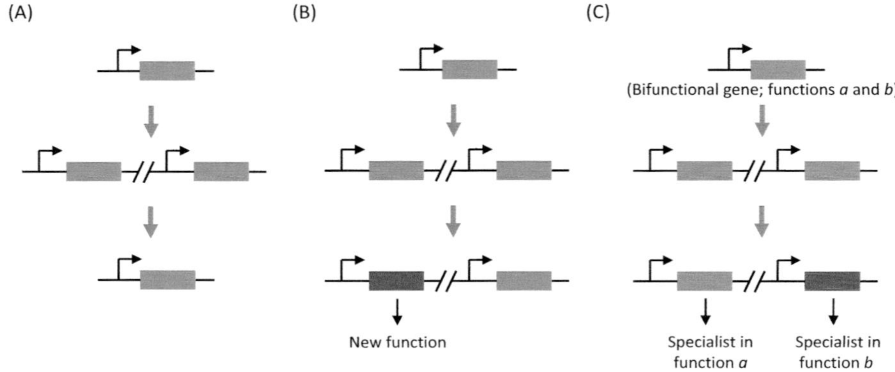

FIGURE 14.4 Possible fates of gene duplication. (A) Gene duplication results in two copies of the same gene. Redundancy in gene copies means that the additional copy serves no additional purpose in the genome. Thus, the additional copy of the gene is lost. This is the most common fate of gene duplicates. (B) In another fate, one of the copies of the gene acquires mutation. These mutations lead to the copy of the gene acquiring a novel function, which provides an adaptive benefit to the cell. This process of acquisition of a new function is referred to as 'neofunctionalization'. (C) If the ancestral protein was bifunctional – i.e., served two functions *a* and *b*, a single copy cannot evolve to be specialist in both the functions. After duplication, the two copies acquire mutations such that each copy becomes a gene specialist in one of the two functions. This process is referred to as 'sub-functionalization'.

authors select one colony to get propagated, and eliminate the other 99 from the experiment. Hundred or so cells from the selected colony are again plated on a fresh plate. So, what should be the selection criteria for one among the hundred colonies to get selected?

In their study, the authors chose the most 'different' looking colony for propagation in the experiment. The difference that they looked for could be in color, texture, or size of the colony.

One hundred of the cells from the chosen colony were then spread on the next plate, and allowed to form colonies. Again, the most 'different' colony was chosen for propagation from the second to the third plate, and so on.

Within a few dozen transfers, it was seen that bet-hedging evolved in the bacterial population, where two different phenotypes emerged from a single genotype.

From an experimental context, it is quite remarkable that a behavior as complex as bet-hedging evolves in a short space of time, in a cleverly designed experiment. Bet-hedging, or phenotypic variability among an isogenic population, has been characterized in a number of systems, and some well-studied examples of this phenomenon are listed in references.

In the two experiments discussed above, we should again note that these were not experiments where the researchers exposed a population to an environment, and asked, *how does the population respond to a particular stress, when evolved for a certain number of generations*? Instead, the experiments ask, *what should be the experiment so that a particular manifestation is seen*? The manifestation in the first experiment is unicellular to multicellular transition. And in the second case, it is the evolution of bet-hedging in a population, which does not exhibit variability with respect to a trait at the start of the experiment.

14.4 PHENOTYPIC DIVERSIFICATION

Darwin envisioned evolution to be a very slow process, to the point that it would be impossible to witness them in one human lifetime. However, in our recent past, we have witnessed several examples of rapid evolution (e.g., SARS CoV-2; HIV; Antibiotic Resistance in bacteria). We now know that evolution can bring about rapid change also.

Darwin viewed the evolution of biological diversity as a process where an ancestral population diversifies into different groups, each occupying a separate niche in a given environment. However, how fast or slow are these processes? Is it possible to view this process of adaptation and diversification in real time?

Toward this end, in a famous, now classic paper in 1998, the authors started a culture of an isogenic population of the bacterium *Pseudomonas* (the same species as we discussed in the previous example). In this experiment, the bacterial population was allowed to grow and adapt to the culture tube kept static.

Before moving ahead,

➔ In a static tube containing liquid nutrient media, how many niches are there?

If we consider carefully, a culture-tube kept static, offers three distinct niches.

1. air-media interface,
2. glass tube surface, and
3. bulk liquid.

Keeping a tube creates niches by creating gradients of entities. For example, oxygen will be available at the liquid-air interface, but almost absent near the bottom of the tube. Similarly, cells will settle down near the bottom of the tube, and hence, there would be greater density of cells near the bottom and fewer near the interface. Thus, depending on the location of an individual cell in a tube, the local environment it encounters is also varied.

Note that these niches are not available when the tube is shaking. The continuous mixing of liquid (and hence cells) would ensure that the contents of the tube are well-mixed, and that all gradients discussed above are destroyed. Hence, all cells 'see' an identical environment in the well-mixed tube.

In a handful of transfers, it was observed that the starting isogenic population had diversified into three distinct genotypes – each specialized to occupy the three niches available in the tube. Thus, microbial populations diversify rapidly to occupy all niches available to them. Perhaps this is the reason that bacteria colonize almost all niches available to them in the ecosystem.

Before moving ahead,

Read the paper, and expand on the following issues,

- ➔ What does the rapidity with which this diversification (this process is also called adaptive radiation) takes place tell us about the radiative potential of a population?
- ➔ Do all genotypes (organisms) have the capacity to exhibit rapid adaptive radiation? Or, were the authors fortunate in the choice of the organism?
- ➔ What characteristic would you expect a genome to have so that it has the capacity to exhibit rapid radiation?

14.5 GENE DUPLICATION AND ADAPTIVE DIVERGENCE

While most of mutational events that we have discussed are single nucleotide changes (SNPs), mutations of other kinds are also quite frequent. Among the list of the nature of mutations that can take place is duplication. In this mutational event, while the DNA Polymerase is copying the DNA of the organism, a part of the genome is erroneously copied twice. As a result, this region of the DNA (and all genes present in this region) is present in two copies in the progeny's DNA.

What is the fate of these duplicate genes? More often than not, the two copies serve the same function in the cell, hence, the loss of one of the two copies is not deleterious to the cell. In fact, losing one of the copies results in the cell not having to invest in the DNA synthesis of the duplicate copy. As a result, the most common fate of duplicate genes is that one of the two copies is lost from the cell (Figure 14.5A).

Alternatively, the two copies can diverge via acquisition of mutations. This can happen via one of two ways.

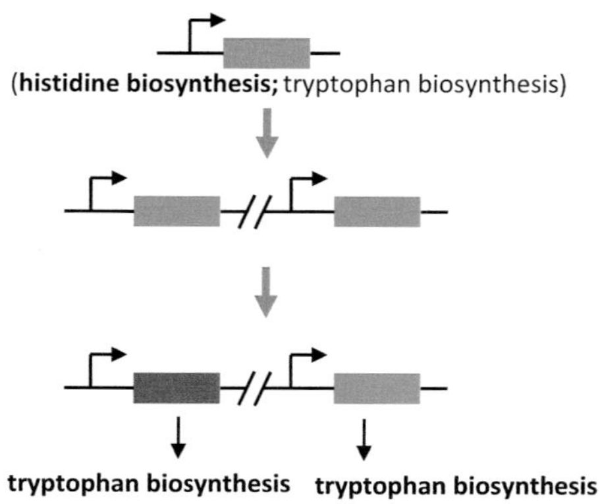

FIGURE 14.5 Real-time evolution of gene duplication and diversification. In bacteria *Salmonella*, an ancestral strain was started with a gene which is a good catalyst for histidine biosynthesis (in bold) and a poor catalyst for tryptophan biosynthesis. After evolution in media lacking both histidine and tryptophan, gene duplication leads to two copies of the ancestral gene. Thereafter, one of the copies acquires mutations that make biosynthesis of tryptophan much more efficient. Thus, exhibiting an example of duplication and diversification.

In one such scenario, one of the copies of the gene can acquire mutations and, as a result, acquire novel functionality. Thus, the two copies diverge, where one of the copies is retained intact, and the duplicate copy mutates to serve another function. Thus, the evolved individual acquires the capacity to perform a novel function that its ancestor was not able to. This phenomenon of gene duplication and subsequent diversification is referred to as 'neofunctionalization' (Figure 14.5B).

In the second scenario, imagine that the original gene encoded for a protein which was bifunctional (that is, served two functions in the cell, shown as functions *a* and *b* in Figure 14.5C). Imagine the functions as catalysis of two distinct reactions. The functional constraints on a single protein serving two functions were such that the protein could not become very good at either of the two functions. Such trade-offs limit protein evolution, and as a result, the single copy of the gene performs the two functions mediocrely. This can constrain the evolution of the organism's fitness. In this case, should a gene duplication result in two copies of the gene, the two copies can then diverge from each other to become specialists at the two functions. One copy becomes a specialist at performing function *a* and the other a specialist at performing function *b*. Such a phenomenon is called 'Subfunctionalization' (Figure 14.5C).

In both *neofunctionalization* and *subfunctionalization*, gene duplication takes place first. Thereafter, the two copies of the genes diverge and acquire different functions. Collectively, the two are referred to as 'duplicate and diverge'.

We know of many examples of gene duplication and divergence. One of the more dramatic manifestations of duplication is in the yeast *Saccharomyces cerevisiae*, which underwent a whole genome duplication (WGD) event. In this event, the entire genome of the organism was duplicated. Thus, all 3,000 genes of the organism were copied. Thereafter, about 2,500 of the gene duplicates were lost from the organism's genome. Today, *S. cerevisiae*'s genome contains around 550 duplicate and diverged genes in its genome. Among the most well-studied pairs of these duplicate genes are GAL1–GAL3 (involved in galactose utilization) and ADH1–ADH2 (responsible for production and utilization of ethanol).

However, for our discussion, we are interested in studying how laboratory experiments can be designed to study duplication and divergence in real time. This was first demonstrated in a paper in *Science* in 2013 (Figure 14.5).

Using a common gram-negative bacterium and a food-borne pathogen *Salmonella typhimurium*, the authors created a strain which carried a single gene for biosynthesis of two amino acids – tryptophan and histidine. The gene encoded for a protein which catalyzed the biosynthesis reaction for histidine efficiently, but was a poor catalyst for tryptophan biosynthesis.

This strain was grown in media which lacked both, tryptophan and histidine. Hence, growth was contingent on the gene catalyzing biosynthesis of the two amino acids. Thus, any mutation which made the cell more efficient for production of tryptophan would be a big beneficial mutation.

This strain was evolved in the media lacking the two amino acids. After evolution for a few hundred generations, it was observed that the evolved strain was synthesizing both, histidine and tryptophan, at high efficiency. Genome sequencing and analysis revealed that this increase in biosynthesis ability was obtained by the gene first duplicating into two copies. Thereafter, one of the copies diverged to become a better catalyst of tryptophan biosynthesis.

Since the ancestral gene had the capacity to biosynthesize both the amino acids – the example we discussed above represents the case of 'subfunctionalization'.

To date, this study remains the only example of real-time demonstration of duplication and divergence. Much remains to be understood of how this process develops in real time, and for this, more model systems are needed. However, there is unanimity about the significance of gene duplications and divergence in dictating the evolutionary trajectories of species.

14.6 MEGAPLATE RESISTANCE EVOLUTION

When antibiotics were first discovered in the first few decades of the 20th century, there was a wide belief that microbiology and the behavior of microorganisms was well understood. This was particularly thought to be true for pathogens, against whom such effective agents like antibiotics had been discovered. However, soon afterward, it was discovered that resistance to antibiotics started emerging in the microbial populations. Today, we know of the serious challenge that antibiotic resistance offers to human health.

However, how fast does antibiotic resistance (can) evolve?

This question was answered in a study published in 2010 in the journal *Cell*. To understand what the authors did, we first have to understand a term associated with antibiotic use – Minimum Inhibitory Concentration (MIC).

Suppose we grow the bacteria *E. coli* in a nutrient-rich environment which contains no antibiotic. In such an environment, the bacteria will grow at a certain rate. What is our expectation will happen to the growth rate, if we add an antibiotic (say, ampicillin) at a very small concentration?

What is observed is that the growth rate of the bacteria slows down, because of the small quantity of the antibiotic added. If we keep increasing the antibiotic concentration in the media, the growth rate of the bacterial population keeps decreasing. At a certain concentration of the antibiotic, the bacterial population is no longer able to grow. This concentration is referred to as the Minimum Inhibitory Concentration (MIC) of that particular antibiotic (Ampicillin, in this case) for the bacterial species in question (*E. coli* in this case) in that particular environment (nutrient-rich in this case).

Now that we understand what is meant by MIC, let us go back to the experiment we wish to discuss. A typical agar plate on which bacteria are grown in research labs is ~ five centimeters in diameter. For the purpose of their study, the team developed an agar plate which was four feet by two feet in size.

Along its length, the plate was divided into five sections of equal width. The leftmost section contained no antibiotic. The next section contained antibiotic at MIC. This was followed by three sections which contained the antibiotic at 10×, 100×, and 1000× MIC.

On a normal agar plate, the bacteria form little mounds, called 'colonies'. The agar concentration in these plates is usually ~1.5%. This makes the plate media hard enough for bacteria not to be able to swim through the media. However, in media conditions where the agar concentration is low (~0.3% or lower), the media is soft and dilute enough, that bacteria can swim in the media. Hence, when grown in agar concentrations so low, bacteria first consume resources in their neighborhood, and then swim to other parts of the plate to find and consume resources. The swimming in liquid media is accomplished via long surface appendages called flagella.

With this setup, the experiment was started by introducing *E. coli* on the left edge of the plate.

Before moving ahead,

- ➔ What do you think will happen as the experiment proceeds?

Starting from the left edge, the first section contains no antibiotic, and because the agar concentration is low to enable bacteria to swim – the bacterial population expands to occupy the entire leftmost section of the plate. This trend continues till the bacteria encounter the boundary between the leftmost section (without antibiotic) and the next section (antibiotic at MIC). Since the starting bacterial population cannot grow at MIC, growth pauses at the boundary.

However, after some time, one (or more) individual at the boundary between the two regions will acquire a mutation which enables growth at MIC. The bacterial population expands in the second region from the point where the mutant(s) arises. Thus, the region of the plate containing the MIC comes to be occupied.

Next, when the bacterial population comes to the boundary of the region which contains 10× MIC, the population pauses. There is a waiting time for another mutant to arise in the population which can grow and expand at 10× MIC.

This process repeats itself at the boundaries of 100× and 1000× MIC. The experiment ends when the entire plate comes to be occupied by the bacterial population. Genome sequencing of the bacteria isolated from different parts of (1) the plate then reveals the mutations which facilitate growth in regions of the plate containing antibiotics. The video of the experiment is available at: https://www.youtube.com/watch?v=plVk4NVIUh8, and the paper is reference (6) in the list given at the end of the chapter.

Before moving ahead,

- ➔ How many mutations (order of magnitude) do you think are needed for a susceptible bacteria to become resistant at 1000× MIC?
- ➔ How long do you think it takes for the bacterial population to expand to occupy the entire plate, and in the process evolve resistance to 1000× MIC? Do you think the time is in weeks, days, hours, or minutes?
- ➔ Why could this experiment not have been done using a plate of regular size (a few inches)? What would have been the difference in that case?

Thus, in a matter of days, a bacterial population is able to evolve and increase its MIC by a factor of 1,000. Thus, a 1,000-fold greater antibiotic concentration was needed to stop growth of the evolved bacteria, as compared to what the researchers started with in the experiment. As far as antibiotic usage, and implications of evolution of resistance are concerned, this is a frightening experiment. How are bacterial supposed to be controlled if not via antibiotics? This is the reason why an enormous effort is on to not only find newer antibiotics (which is an exceptionally difficult task) but also to judiciously use the existing antibiotics. As we saw, indiscriminate use of antibiotics leads to rapid evolution of resistance, thus, rendering the antibiotic ineffective.

14.7 DIRECTED EVOLUTION

One major class of evolution experiments is performed not with organisms but with proteins. Suppose we have an enzyme E, which catalyzes a reaction from substrate S to product P (Figure 14.6).

However, enzyme E may be a poor catalyst, and the reaction proceeds at a very slow speed. How would we increase the speed of the reaction? Ideally, we would like to engineer the enzyme E by introducing mutations in it so that it conducts the reaction faster. But which mutation do we introduce in the enzyme? This question is very hard to answer, and for most enzymes, we have little idea.

We turn to evolution to solve this problem. This approach is called *directed evolution*.

In this approach, we create thousands (or as many as we can) variants of the gene sequence corresponding to enzyme E. This is done by randomly introducing mutations in the gene sequence. Remember that there is no rhyme or reason to the mutations. We just introduce mutations randomly and create as many variants as we can.

Then, we quantify the performance of each variant, and choose the best one among all the variants created. As shown in the Figure 14.7, let the best variant be E'.

$$\mathrm{S} \xrightarrow{E} \mathrm{P}$$

FIGURE 14.6 Enzyme catalysis. Enzyme E catalyzes reaction of substrate S going to product P.

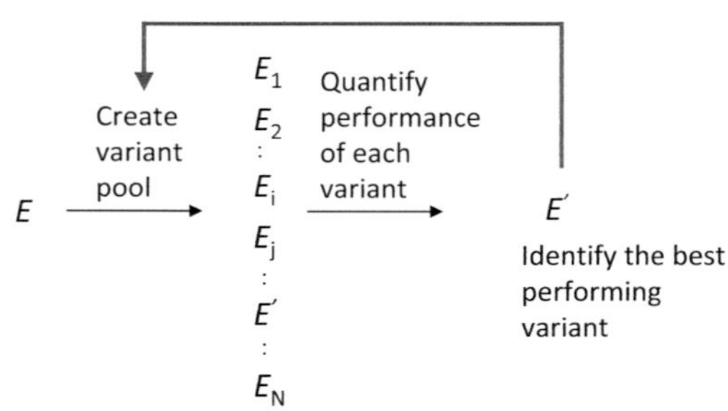

FIGURE 14.7 Design of a directed evolution experiment. Variants of enzyme sequence E are generated. The performance of each variant is quantified in terms of the ease with which it catalyzes the reaction. The best performing variant E' is taken ahead, and the process is repeated.

The entire process of introducing errors and quantifying the variants is then repeated with E'. This process is continued till we either attain the desired enzyme activity, or as long as enzyme performance shows an improvement.

Two things should be apparent here. First, this process is akin to natural selection, where the activity of the enzyme is a proxy for fitness. High activity variants are taken ahead, and the others are rejected. Second, this approach has a lot of significance in a commercial sense, where biotechnology companies are interested in making better catalyst enzymes.

The power of Directed Evolution led to the award of the Nobel Prize in 2018. The Nobel Committee called the approach, 'revolution based on evolution'.

14.8 CONCLUSION

In this chapter, we studied a handful of examples of laboratory evolution which I find creative, novel. These experiments also suggest that we are only limited by our imagination and creativity in finding the right experiments to evolve organisms, genes of novel function – for either intellectual curiosity or commercial value.

EXERCISES

1. What would happen to the evolution of multicellularity experiment if the tubes were allowed to stand stationary and cells settle for 24 hours, before sub-culturing them?
2. In the multicellularity experiment, are we also selecting for high growth?
3. In question (1), instead of 24 hours, what if we allowed cells to select for 24 seconds? Would multicellularity evolve then?
4. In the megaplate experiment, suppose there was a sudden jump from no antibiotic to 1000× MIC. What would be the fate of the experiment then?
5. Why did the bet-hedging experiment work? Can you think of alternate designs where bet-hedging could evolve?
6. Look up papers by Francis Arnold from the 1990s. Identify three enzymes on which the approach of directed evolution was applied. Give details of the reactions these enzymes catalyze.
7. Adaptive diversification was seen in the *Pseudomonas* population when allowed to evolve in a stationary tube. This is a scenario when different niches were present in the tube. Think of contexts in which diversification can take place within a single niche.

BIBLIOGRAPHY

1. Matthew D. Herron PLC, Ratcliff WC. 2022. *The Evolution of Multicellularity*. CRC Press.
2. Ratcliff WC, Denison RF, Borrello M, Travisano M. 2012. Experimental evolution of multicellularity. *Proc Natl Acad Sci U S A* 109:1595–600.

   (The above two references discuss the evolution of multicellularity and the subsequent developments in the 10,000 generations of evolution of the multicellular cluster.)

3. Beaumont HJ, Gallie J, Kost C, Ferguson GC, Rainey PB. 2009. Experimental evolution of bet hedging. *Nature* 462:90–3.

(Paper on evolution of bet-hedging.)

4. Rainey PB, Travisano M. 1998. Adaptive radiation in a heterogeneous environment. *Nature* 394:69–72.

(Adaptive radiation of *Pseudomonas* in a static test tube. Here's an interview by one of the authors on 25 years of publication of this work: https://reflectionsonpaperspast.wordpress.com/2021/02/28/revisiting-rainey-travisano-1998/.)

5. Nasvall J, Sun L, Roth JR, Andersson DI. 2012. Real-time evolution of new genes by innovation, amplification, and divergence. *Science* 338:384–7.

(In recent years, duplication rates have been found to be very high. Despite that, evolution experiments where duplications and diversification happen are difficult to design. This study remains the only one which explicitly demonstrates this in a laboratory evolution. It makes one wonder, if duplication and diversification are difficult to observe in a lab experiment, or is it just that people haven't tried it much.)

6. Baym M, Lieberman TD, Kelsic ED, Chait R, Gross R, Yelin I, Kishony R. 2016. Spatiotemporal microbial evolution on antibiotic landscapes. *Science* 353:1147–51.

(Megaplate evolution experiment – real-time evolution of resistance. The YouTube video of the duration of the experiment is available at: https://www.youtube.com/watch?v=plVk4NVIUh8.)

15 Empirical Fitness Landscapes

15.1 INTRODUCTION

In this chapter, we will consider three cases of empirical fitness landscape. The first case is from an experiment in 2006, when an allele which confers antibiotic resistance to *E. coli* was analyzed against the parent allele. The Hamming distance between the two alleles was five.

In the second case, we again look at two strains which are separated by a Hamming distance of five. But in this case, the mutations are in different parts of the genome, in five distinct genes. These five mutations were the first five mutations to have fixed in one of the lines of long-term evolution experiment (LTEE).

In the third case, we discuss an extensive fitness landscape of a gene *folA* in *E. coli*. The landscape comprises of more than 250,000 experimental sequences, and is one of the most extensive efforts to build a fitness landscape till date.

15.2 CASE I: β-LACTAMASE AND ANTIBIOTIC RESISTANCE IN *E. COLI*

β-lactamases are enzymes which confer resistance to bacteria against β-lactam antibiotics. Interestingly, there are two distinct alleles of a β-lactam gene in *E. coli*. One group carries allele 1 and the other group carries allele 2. The two alleles differentially impact the ability of the bacteria to grow in presence of antibiotic. This ability is quantified with respect to Minimum Inhibitory Concentration (MIC), which is the minimum antibiotic concentration of an antibiotic which stops bacterial growth.

Allele 2 confers an MIC which is 1,000 × higher than the MIC conferred by allele 1. Thus, in the presence of antibiotic, a strain carrying allele 2 will grow much faster as compared to allele 1. In fact, in a concentration higher than MIC of allele 1 (and below that of allele 2), only the strain carrying allele 2 will grow.

When we compare the sequences of the two alleles, we find that the Hamming distance between the two sequences is five. Four mutations are in the coding region of the gene β-lactamase, and the fifth one is in the promoter region of the gene.

The question that the authors asked in this study was, how does the transition from the sequence of allele 1 to sequence of allele 2 take place? How does MIC change as mutations are acquired? Does each mutation progressively increase MIC?

Let us denote the sequence of allele 1 as '-----', where each '-' indicates lack of the mutation. Sequence of allele 2 is, therefore, '*abcde*', where each letter indicates one mutation in the sequence. How does the MIC change as we move from allele 1 sequence to that of allele 2?

DOI: 10.1201/9781003633662-15

This is important because the mutations that increase MIC would have taken place one at a time. Thus, as allele 1 evolved to allele 2, did the five mutations need to happen in a sequence such that MIC continuously increased, or could any sequence of the five mutations lead to increase in MIC?

You will note here that there are many ways to transition from '-----' to '*abcde*'. For example, two such possible transition paths are shown below.

----- ➔ *a*---- ➔ *ab*--- ➔ *abc*-- ➔ *abcd*- ➔ *abcde*

or,

----- ➔ ----*e* ➔ ---*de* ➔ --*cde* ➔ -*bcde* ➔ *abcde*

Example 15.1: How many ways are there to transition from '-----' to '*abcde*'?

Solution: The simplest way to solve this question is to see that as we transition from '-----' to '*abcde*', the first mutation that can take place can be any of the five. The next one can be any of the remaining four. The third one, any of the remaining three and so on. Thus, the total number of 'paths' to transition from '-----' to '*abcde*' is 120 ($= 5 \times 4 \times 3 \times 2 \times 1$).

The question then becomes, how many of the 120 paths are *adaptive*. By *adaptive*, we mean paths where every successive acquisition of a mutation increases MIC. For example, consider the two scenarios in Figure 15.1.

In the first (Figure 15.1A), the path that the population takes from zero to five mutations is (----- ➔ *a*---- ➔ *ab*--- ➔ *abc*-- ➔ *abcd*- ➔ *abcde*). In this path, every successive mutation increases MIC. Thus, the MIC curve is a monotonically increasing one. Hence, in a Darwinian sense, these paths are said to be permissible, as far as natural selection is concerned.

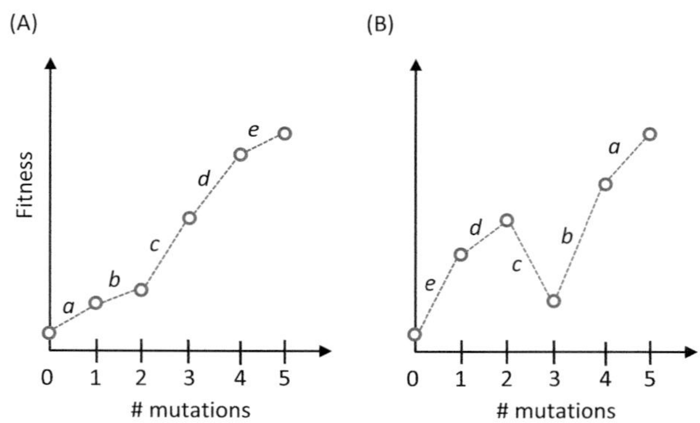

FIGURE 15.1 An adaptive and a non-adaptive path. (A) A path is said to be adaptive or Darwinian or permissible, if while traversing on it, fitness is continuously increasing. There is no step in the path where the fitness remains the same or decreases. (B) A non-adaptive is one where fitness decreases or remains the same in at least one of the steps. In the figure, the mutation *c*, when acquired in the background of mutations *de*, is non-adaptive.

However, consider the path and the corresponding MIC as shown in Figure 15.1B. In this path, the order of mutations is (----- ➔ ----*e* ➔ ---*de* ➔ --*cde* ➔ -*bcde* ➔ *abcde*). Note that, in this path, the MIC increases in the first two steps but then decreases after mutation *c* is acquired in the background ---*de*. Hence, the path shown in Figure 15.1B is not strictly increasing, and hence, not permissible in a Darwinian sense.

The question then becomes how many paths are permissible (strictly Darwinian) and how many non-permissible?

Example 15.2: Why do we say that paths with strictly increasing MIC are permissible in a Darwinian sense and the others not?

Solution: We have made an implicit assumption in the analysis above. That assumption is that we are treating MIC as a proxy for fitness. Under such an assumption, strains which have greater MIC are fitter and those with lower MIC are less fit.

So, if we treat MIC as a proxy for fitness, strictly increasing paths imply a continuously increasing fitness, as mutations are acquired. Thus, starting from the original sequence ('-----'), mutations are acquired, and fitness increases. Natural selection thus dictates that these paths continue to increase in fitness and end up at sequence '*abcde*'.

On the other hand, paths which are not strictly increasing will have a peak in between. For example, in Figure 15.1B, the genotype '--*cde*' has a greater MIC than both its neighbors ('---*de*' and '-*bcde*'). This starting from the ancestor sequence, natural selection will favor movement of the population to the sequence '--*cde*'. But thereafter, mutation in either direction decreases MIC (and hence fitness). As a result, natural selection will not permit this, and the population remains at the sequence '--*cde*'. As a result, the population does not end up at the fitness peak.

Note that a greater MIC only confers an advantage when the environment contains the antibiotic. If the environment does not contain an antibiotic, then MIC is irrelevant.

So, we return to the original question. How many of the 120 possible paths can be called permissible in a Darwinian sense?

Before moving ahead,

➔ What does your intuition say about the number of paths which are strictly Darwinian?

To answer this question, the scientists in the study tested all paths, and classified them as either permissible or non-permissible in a Darwinian sense. Somewhat surprisingly, they noted that 102 paths out of 120 were non-permissible, and fitness (MIC) increased strictly in only 18 paths.

Thus, only 15% of the paths were permissible. This makes the process of evolution a bit more predictable. Note that if all 120 paths were permissible, then our uncertainty about which path natural selection takes is big. However, because most paths are non-permissible, natural selection *has* to take one of the permissible paths.

Why are there intermediate peaks?

Note the two paths in Figure 15.1 again. In the first, when mutation *c* occurs in the background '*ab*---', the fitness (or MIC) increases. Thus, mutation *c* is a beneficial mutation in this context. However, when the same mutation *c* occurs in the background '---*de*', it decreases fitness. Thus, in this genomic context, *c* is a deleterious mutation. This is the definition of sign-epistasis. We learned in the chapter on fitness landscapes that sign epistasis makes the landscape more rugged.

Sign epistasis is rampant when we are talking of mutations *within* a gene. The resulting intramolecular epistasis creates local peaks in the landscapes. Thus, most adaptive walks of populations on a landscape are going to get 'stuck' in a local peak.

The β-lactamase results show us this property of movement on landscapes.

We will now consider another example of movement on fitness landscapes, where a population acquired five mutations in a laboratory condition.

15.3 CASE II: LONG-TERM EVOLUTION EXPERIMENT (LTEE)

The result we will discuss here is from the LTEE with *E. coli* that we discussed in Chapters 13 and 14. As we discussed, in this experiment, *E. coli* is propagated via 1:100 dilutions in glucose-limiting minimal media. As the populations adapt to their evolution environment, mutations fix.

In this work, the researchers analyzed the first five mutations to fix in one of the 12 lines of the experiment. Let us again depict the ancestral strain as '-----' (indicating absence of each of the five mutations) and the evolved strain with the five mutations as '*abcde*' (each alphabet indicating one precise mutation to have occurred). In this case, the five mutations occurred in five distinct genes in the *E. coli* genome.

The order in which these mutations occur in the experiment is (----- ➔ *a*---- ➔ *ab*--- ➔ *abc*-- ➔ *abcd*- ➔ *abcde*). When the fitness trajectory of this path was drawn, it was found that the fitness curve was strictly increasing, as mutations took place along this path. Hence, this path is permissible in a Darwinian sense.

However, we know that for five mutations, the total number of paths is 120. How many of these paths are accessible or permissible in a Darwinian sense?

Note that in this experiment, growth rate of a strain is a proxy for fitness.

Before moving ahead,

- ➔ What does your intuition say about the number of paths which are strictly Darwinian? How much has it been influenced by the previous example we discussed in this chapter.

Somewhat surprisingly, 86 out of 120 paths in this case were accessible in a Darwinian sense. Thus, from a scenario where 15% trajectories were Darwinian, in this case, the number increases to greater than 70%.

How do we make sense of these two results?

Since the publication of these results, we now have data from several other fitness landscapes and trajectories. They all point at the same trend,

a. When we are analyzing mutations *in* a single gene (like β-*lactamase*), sign epistasis is a very strong factor influencing evolutionary trajectories. In such a scenario, the landscape has a large number of fitness peaks, implying that evolving populations are likely to get stuck in local maxima on a landscape.
b. Alternatively, we now know that when mutations are in *different* genes (like in the case of LTEE), sign epistasis is not that prevalent. Instead, the effect of mutations is best represented as negative epistasis. As a result, to a large extent, these landscapes do not have local maxima, and populations evolve with strictly increasing fitness.

The above two statements are, of course, statistical statements. That is, not all trajectories in an intragenic fitness landscape get trapped in a local maxima, and not all trajectories in an inter-genic landscape reach the fitness maxima. However, statistically speaking, protein evolution is largely dictated by sign epistasis and organismal evolution (multiple genes) is largely dictated by negative epistasis.

Thus, protein fitness landscapes are highly rugged, and organismal fitness landscapes are smoother.

15.4 CASE III: *folA* LANDSCAPE IN *E. COLI*

Remember that the main challenge of empirical fitness landscapes is the scale. Remember that if we are talking of a DNA sequence of length k, the total number of sequences is 4^k. In the previous two cases we studied in this chapter, we studied mutations at five sites. In the first case, these five mutations were in one gene, and in the second, they were in five distinct genes. Thus, the total number of sequences considering all possible variations at five sites is 4^7. This corresponds to computing the fitness of ~1000 DNA sequences.

The previous two studies, however, only analyzed fitness of 32 sequences. This was because at each site where the mutation took place, they only analyzed sequences with the original nucleotide and the sequence with the mutated nucleotide. For example, if at a particular site nucleotide `A` changed to `G`, these were the only nucleotides considered at that particular position. Nucleotides `T` and `C` were not considered at that position. The same was true for all five positions, in each of the two cases.

As a result, the total number of sequences analyzed reduces from 4^5 (1024) to 2^5 (32). This smaller number is experimentally much more tractable compared to a thousand. However, how correct is the picture of fitness landscapes that such small-scale experiments tell us?

In our next case, we wish to study what happens to landscapes when they are generated of a much larger scale.

The gene *folA* in *E. coli* encodes for the enzyme folate dehydrogenase. The gene catalyzes a reaction which is an important intermediate for amino acid and nucleic acid biosynthesis. *folA* is an essential gene for *E. coli*. That is, strains lacking *folA* would not survive. Critical to function are three amino acid residues in the protein sequence. These three amino acids, obviously, correspond to nine nucleotides in the DNA sequence of the gene.

An antibiotic, Trimethoprim, targets bacteria by stopping FolA protein from functioning, and thus stopping synthesis of critical metabolic intermediates. However, mutations in the nine-nucleotide region we refer to in the previous paragraph have been known to confer resistance to *E. coli* against Trimethoprim.

Given this property of *folA*, it gave the authors an opportunity to get information for an empirical landscape for the entire *9* base region in the gene. Note that to construct a *9*-base fitness landscape, we need to construct all 4^9 (~262000) sequences. This is exactly what the authors did.

After that, all 4^9 variants were added to a flask, which contained Trimethoprim in nutrient media. Thus, the fitness landscape was constructed in an environment containing the antibiotic Trimethoprim. Equal numbers of each of the 4^9 variants were allowed to grow in this environment for a specific amount of time, after which, the relative frequency of each variant was determined by deep sequencing.

Sequence variants which conferred high resistance to Trimethoprim increased in frequency, while those which were sensitive to the antibiotic would not increase in the environment in which fitness was measured. Thus, by quantifying the relative frequency of each variant, we get fitness of each of the 4^9 variants. This allowed the researchers to construct a fitness landscape of all 4^9 sequences.

What did the folA landscape tell us?

a. *folA landscape is rugged.* So, what did we learn from a high-dimensional landscape of an *E. coli* gene? Remember that if epistasis were not acting in the 9-base region, the landscape would have a single peak. However, it was found that the landscape had more than 500 peaks in it! The landscape is rugged with a large number of peaks. Thus, in an intra-genic landscape, sign-epistasis seems to be extremely relevant.
b. *Most sequences are non-functional.* Remember that in this experiment, >250,000 sequence variants were added to a flask, which contained Trimethoprim. The *folA* sequences, which were either (a) non-functional because the mutations that they carried made *folA* non-functional, or (b) non-resistant to Trimethoprim, did not grow in numbers in the flask. It turned out that >90% of all sequences were non-functional *folA* sequences. Thus, a protein is functional in terms of carrying out the reaction it catalyzes with a very specific sequence only. Even a small deviation from that sequence completely abolishes function. Thus, peaks on fitness landscape are very sharp and narrow.
c. *Most sequences had access to a high fitness peak.* The *folA* fitness landscape had >500 peaks, with most of them with low fitness value. However, a few peaks in the landscape were high fitness. Which peak does a random sequence end up at? There are two possibilities.

One, a random sequence is likely to end up at a low fitness peak because these low fitness peaks are few in number.

Or, alternatively, a random sequence is more likely to end up at a high peak because the 'basin of attraction' of a high peak is significantly greater than that of a low peak. By 'basin of attraction' we mean the number of points which, via evolution's analogy with mountain climbing would end up at a fitness peak. Thus, even though high fitness peaks might be fewer in number, they attract a high fraction of points on the sequence space toward them.

When these two ideas were tested, it was found that due to their large basin of attraction, most of the points on the sequence space had an accessible path to a high peak. By accessible, we mean a Darwinian permissible path, where, from a starting point, a path with strictly increasing fitness can be found to a high fitness peak.

15.5 CONCLUSION

Fitness landscapes are a somewhat enigmatic structure. They have their fans, but also critics.

Some argue that they are useful only in a context where they allow us to imagine an evolutionary process.

Others analyze more than 250,000 sequences to define it for a narrow region of one gene in *E. coli*. Similarly, such landscapes have been attempted for a single gene where protein functionality (e.g., fluorescence for the gene *green fluorescent protein*; or binding ability of a *tRNA*) has been used as a proxy of fitness to understand the structure of a landscape. See references for this chapter for details of these works.

Others yet say that fitness landscapes only make sense if done for a large region of the DNA. If done for a small region of a gene (like *folA*), or for a handful of sites on the genome (like in Cases I and II we studied in this chapter, we miss important detail).

Remember that when a population evolves in a niche, it interacts with the environment. This interaction is bound to change the environment, also. For example, if a member of an *E. coli* population utilizes a molecule of glucose from the environment and releases a molecule of acetate in return, the environment in which it is growing has changed. The environment now has one fewer glucose molecule and one additional acetate molecule in it. But fitness landscapes are drawn for specific environments only. How do fitness landscapes change as the environment itself changes? We can visualize this as a structure which has peaks and valleys, but as the environment is changing, the peaks and valleys are moving in space and size. This link between fitness landscapes and environment is deep, and poorly understood. More importantly, this makes the determination of ecologically realistic fitness landscapes even more challenging.

EXERCISES

1. What is the mechanism of action of β-lactams in gram-negative bacteria?
2. How do β-lactamases protect bacteria against β-lactam antibiotics?
3. In example 15.1, we note that there are 120 possible transitions from '-----' to '*abcde*'. List all 32 transitions.
4. Imagine a fitness landscape for a small part of a gene in *E. coli*. Let us imagine that this landscape looks very similar in its statistical properties to the *folA* landscape. Now, imagine that we change the environment *E* by an infinitesimally

small amount δE. This small change in the environment will bring about a change in the landscape structure. Let us say that the change in the landscape is represented by ΔL. Do you think an infinitesimal change in the environment will always bring an infinitesimal change in the landscape? Or, can you imagine scenarios where an infinitesimal change brings about a qualitative change in the landscape's structure?
5. Can positive or negative epistasis lead to fitness structures with multiple peaks? Why or why not?
6. Find an actual example of sign epistasis where two mutations, when present singly, are each beneficial. However, when present together, they lead to decrease in fitness.
7. Would the results of the fitness landscape in the β-lactamase change if the authors explored all four possible variations at each site (rather than the two they considered between the two alleles they examined). Such a change would mean that instead of exploring 2^5 sequences, the investigation would require analysis of 4^5 sequences. Would you still think that more than 80% of the paths are not accessible in a Darwinian sense?
8. How would your answer change for Case II if all 4^5 sequences were considered?

BIBLIOGRAPHY

Landscapes discussed in this chapter.

β-lactamase

1. Weinreich DM, Delaney NF, Depristo MA, Hartl DL. 2006. Darwinian evolution can follow only very few mutational paths to fitter proteins. *Science* 312:111–4.

LTEE

2. Chou HH, Chiu HC, Delaney NF, Segre D, Marx CJ. 2011. Diminishing returns epistasis among beneficial mutations decelerates adaptation. *Science* 332:1190–2.

folA

3. Papkou A, Garcia-Pastor L, Escudero JA, Wagner A. 2023. A rugged yet easily navigable fitness landscape. *Science* 382:eadh3860.
4. Sarvesh Baheti NR, Supreet Saini. 2025. Variations and predictability of epistasis on an intragenic fitness landscape. *eLife*. doi:https://doi.org/10.7554/eLife.104848.1

Some other papers on experimental determination of fitness landscapes.

5. Sarkisyan KS, Bolotin DA, Meer MV, Usmanova DR, Mishin AS, Sharonov GV, Ivankov DN, Bozhanova NG, Baranov MS, Soylemez O, Bogatyreva NS, Vlasov PK, Egorov ES, Logacheva MD, Kondrashov AS, Chudakov DM, Putintseva EV, Mamedov IZ, Tawfik DS, Lukyanov KA, Kondrashov FA. 2016. Local fitness landscape of the green fluorescent protein. *Nature* 533:397–401.
6. Hietpas RT, Jensen JD, Bolon DN. 2011. Experimental illumination of a fitness landscape. *Proc Natl Acad Sci U S A* 108:7896–901.
7. Li C, Qian W, Maclean CJ, Zhang J. 2016. The fitness landscape of a tRNA gene. *Science* 352:837–40.
8. Acevedo A, Brodsky L, Andino R. 2014. Mutational and fitness landscapes of an RNA virus revealed through population sequencing. *Nature* 505:686–90.

16 What Have We Not Discussed?

16.1 INTRODUCTION

Evolution is a large subject and the variety of mechanisms, manifestations that nature employs to overcome challenges posed by the environment is huge. It is quite impossible for a single book to cover all these aspects. In the preceding chapters, I have covered ideas, examples which I think are exciting and important, as far as evolutionary biology is concerned. However, this list is by no means exhaustive. In this chapter, we will discuss three aspects of evolution that we did not discuss in this book. These are (a) horizontal gene transfer (HGT), (b) speciation, and (c) pleiotropy. Let us start this discussion with the first one.

16.2 HORIZONTAL GENE TRANSFER

In the 1920s, DNA was discovered as the material basis for heredity. In a work published in 1928, Frederick Griffith demonstrated that when a non-virulent pneumococcal strain of bacteria was grown with DNA from virulent strains, the non-virulent strain became virulent. Examination of this experimental result led to the proposal that the DNA from the virulent strain was taken up by the non-virulent strain. This acquisition of DNA from the environment conferred on it the property of virulence.

The paper was also an example of how DNA can be taken up by bacteria from the environment. This fact is very important because it tells us that an individual bacteria can take up DNA and evolve. So far, we have been talking of evolution in the context of progeny acquiring mutations because the DNA was copied incorrectly. Hence, species/populations evolve, not individuals, we said.

Here, though, we note that the DNA of an individual can change via acquisition of foreign DNA. Thus, individuals can evolve, too. This phenomenon is called horizontal gene transfer (HGT).

DNA can be taken up by bacteria from the environment via three main mechanisms.

First, *transformation* – where bacteria uptake DNA from the environment directly,

Second, *conjugation* – where bacteria trade DNA with each other in a contact-dependent manner,

Third, *transduction* – in this, viruses carry genes from one organism/individual to another.

DOI: 10.1201/9781003633662-16

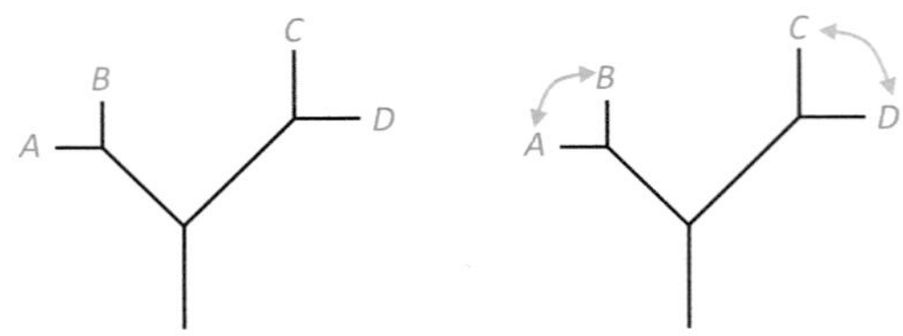

FIGURE 16.1 Horizontal gene transfer allows movement of genes across species, and jumbles up the tree of life. In view of evolution without HGT (left), the four species ***A***, ***B***, ***C***, ***D*** are not permitted to exchange genes with each other. However, in the presence of HGT (right), species can exchange genetic material with each other. In the figure, for simplicity, only the transfer of genes between ***A*** & ***B*** and ***C*** & ***D*** is shown.

HGT radically changes how we think of evolution. In the light of HGT, evolutionary change can take place not only vertically (transmission of change from parents), but also horizontally (an individual bacteria acquiring new genes, and in the process, evolve) (Figure 16.1).

It should be immediately clear why HGT makes the analysis of evolutionary process harder. In the absence of HGT, the only genetic material that can be changed (via mutations) is the genetic material present in an individual. Hence, we know the raw material whose change is going to bring about adaptation. However, in HGT, we do not have this information. A bacterium in soil is surrounded by DNA from plants, other bacteria, insects, and humans. In theory, acquisition of any fragment from this collection could be adaptive, and, hence, increase fitness. Thus, how does one think of a framework which incorporates HGT in a quantitative manner? This remains a challenge.

16.3 SPECIATION

Speciation, or the process by which new species are formed, is a complex area of study. What constitutes a species, itself, is a contentious issue. Imagine a population of *Pseudomonas* diversifying in a stationary test tube, as we saw in Chapter 14. We know that the bacteria become specialists at occupying the three niches via acquisition of mutations. But does that make the three different strains three different species? Or, is it just three different genotypes of the same species? These become subjective calls, and hence, defining species in bacteria is non-trivial.

Think about a sexually reproducing species. In this case, a male and a female mate. Upon mating, their gametes fuse to form a zygote. The zygote then undergoes development to form an offspring, which upon reaching sexual maturity produces gametes – thus completing the cycle. Thus, sexual reproduction in a species is simply the cycling of gametes.

In such a context, defining species becomes easier. In the most widely used definition, two groups are said to be different species if members from them cannot mate and complete the cycle of sexual reproduction we discussed in the previous paragraph.

Hence, while a horse and a donkey can mate to produce an offspring, a mule. But since the mule is sterile and cannot produce gametes, the cycle of sexual reproduction comes to an end with the mule. And hence, horses and donkeys are different species. In such a case, we say that the two species are reproductively isolated from each other. This definition of species is referred to as the biological species concept (BSC).

From our context, we should note that sexual reproduction offers the chance to define species in this fashion. Such a definition is not available for asexually reproducing organisms. Thus, how do we define species and speciation from the context of bacteria? In the chapter on LTEE, we noted that acquisition of mutations allowed *E. coli* to utilize citrate in oxic conditions. The inability of *E. coli* to utilize citrate in the presence of oxygen has been a diagnostic feature of the species. By this yardstick, was a new species born in LTEE? The subjectivity of bacterial species and speciation makes it a fascinating area of study.

16.4 PLEIOTROPY

Our discussion of evolutionary change has been quite limited in one sense. In our discussion, we have focused on constant environments. However, consider a bacterium in soil, and imagine the environmental challenges it faces. During the day, the temperature increases. At night, it's colder. It may face harsh dry weather, but also has sporadic flooding. It is surrounded by chemical agents and predators, which pose a challenge to survival. All these factors are dynamic in nature.

How does adaptation to this dynamic environment differ from the adaptation in constant environments that we studied in the book?

In a constant environment, a mutation that confers benefit is always beneficial. Thus, the qualitative nature of change in fitness it confers does not change with time.

However, in a changing environment, a mutation that confers advantage in the cold temperature of the night might be deleterious in the higher day temperature. Thus, the nature of the mutation changes from beneficial to deleterious in another environmental context.

The fitness effect of a mutation in environments other than the one in which it was acquired is a pleiotropic effect of a mutation. And the phenomenon that a beneficial mutation in one environment confers another effect in another environment is pleiotropy. The root cause of pleiotropy is that one gene often affects multiple traits in an organism. Thus, while a beneficial mutation in a gene will change trait 1. But this mutation also changes trait 2. The fitness effect of the change in trait 2 will show up later, when the environment changes. And depending on the change in the environment, the fitness effect might be beneficial or deleterious.

We know little about how pleiotropy operates. And in the absence of its workings, how mutations manifest in an ecologically relevant context is difficult to predict.

16.5 CONCLUSION

With this, we conclude our discussion of evolution. At least as far as this book is concerned! I started studying evolution 11 years ago, and in some sense, I feel that I am just beginning to learn the subject. For many readers, too, this will be the first foray into studying evolutionary biology formally. The book should be the start and not the end of this learning experience.

BIBLIOGRAPHY

Horizontal Gene Transfer

1. Nguyen ANT, Gorrell R, Kwok T, Connallon T, McDonald MJ. 2024. Horizontal gene transfer facilitates the molecular reverse-evolution of antibiotic sensitivity in experimental populations of H. pylori. *Nat Ecol Evol* 8:315–24.
2. Kosterlitz O, Grassi N, Werner B, McGee RS, Top EM, Kerr B. 2023. Evolutionary 'Crowdsourcing': Alignment of fitness landscapes allows for cross-species adaptation of a horizontally transferred gene. *Mol Biol and Evol* 40:msad237.
3. Arnold BJ, Huang I-T, Hanage WP. 2022. Horizontal gene transfer and adaptive evolution in bacteria. *Nat Rev Microbiol* 20:206–18.

Speciation

4. Retchless AC, Lawrence JG. 2007. Temporal fragmentation of speciation in bacteria. *Science* 317:1093–6.
5. Fraser C, Hanage WP, Spratt BG. 2007. Recombination and the nature of bacterial speciation. *Science* 315:476–80.

Pleiotropy

6. Stearns FW. 2010. One hundred years of pleiotropy: a retrospective. *Genetics* 186:767–73.
7. Pleiotropy Is Not Polygenic Inheritance | Learn Science at Scitable.(n.d.) https://www.nature.com/scitable/topicpage/pleiotropy-one-gene-can-affect-multiple-traits-569/. Retrieved 4 March 2025.

Index

For Product Safety Concerns and Information please contact our EU representative GPSR@taylorandfrancis.com Taylor & Francis Verlag GmbH, Kaufingerstraße 24, 80331 München, Germany